CURING
THE
INCURABLE:
BEYOND
THE
LIMITS
OF
MEDICINE

When you have exhausted all possibilities,
remember this – you haven't.

Thomas Edison (1847–1931)

This book is dedicated to all those facing a life-changing
illness and who are searching for answers, to survivors who
have been a source of inspiration, to my patients
for spurring me on to learn more, and to Judi, my wife,
for her endless patience whilst I was researching and
writing this book.

CURING THE INCURABLE:
BEYOND THE LIMITS OF MEDICINE

What survivors
of major illnesses
can teach us

Dr Jerry Thompson

Hammersmith Health Books
London, UK

First published in 2020 by Hammersmith Health Books
– an imprint of Hammersmith Books Limited
4/4A Bloomsbury Square, London WC1A 2RP, UK
www.hammersmithbooks.co.uk

Reprinted 2021

The information contained in this book is for educational purposes only. It is the result of the study and the experience of the author. Whilst the information and advice offered are believed to be true and accurate at the time of going to press, neither the authors nor the publisher can accept any legal responsibility or liability for any errors or omissions that may have been made or for any adverse effects which may occur as a result of following the recommendations given herein. Always consult a qualified medical practitioner if you have any concerns regarding your health.

British Library Cataloguing in Publication Data: A CIP record of this book is available from the British Library.

Print ISBN 978-1-78161-176-0
Ebook ISBN 978-1-78161-177-7

Commissioning editor: Georgina Bentliff
Designed and typeset by: Julie Bennett, Bespoke Publishing Ltd
Cover design by: Madeline Meckiffe
Index: Dr Laurence Errington
Production: Helen Whitehorn, Path Projects Ltd
Printed and bound by: TJ Books Limited, Cornwall, UK

Contents

About the Author

Dr Jerry Thompson has been working as a doctor for over four decades, mostly in general practice. He now works part-time in general practice at the Welby Practice, Bottesford, in the East Midlands. He has been a long-standing member of the British Society for Ecological Medicine (BSEM). In the last two decades he has been fascinated by people who have recovered from major illnesses, against the odds, often using methods poorly understood by conventional medicine but applying basic principles of good health. At the same time, he became more and more aware of the fact that modern medicine is failing to provide answers for most chronic diseases and for many cancers and yet these diseases have increased at alarming rates. These understandings have led him to believe that a lot more can be done and it is his hope that this book will help people find new solutions for their illnesses based on the best medicine available.

This knowledge exists, but both doctors and patients are often unfamiliar with it or unaware of it. These insights have led him to study nutrition (under BSEM) and the influence of the mind (he has also studied and practised hypnotherapy, neurolinguistic programming (NLP) and the emotional freedom technique (EFT)). He has a special interest in toxicity and was the co-author of *The Health Effects of Waste Incinerators*, published by BSEM. This was well received and has been translated into two additional languages. He has also written many patient leaflets

on common conditions, which are available on his website www.
drjerrythompson.co.uk.

Jerry's knowledge of both conventional medicine (he has
postgraduate qualifications in both general medicine and general
practice) and alternative medicine, and his familiarity with the
experiences of exceptional patients and holistic doctors, have
given him a unique insight into what is possible. His hope is to
make this knowledge more widely known.

Introduction

I am looking for a lot of men who have an infinite capacity
to do what can't be done.

Henry Ford, 1863–1947

This is a book about healing against the odds. It looks at those
people who have inexplicably got better from a potentially fatal
illness and how they achieved it. It's an exploration of some of
the most exciting methods of healing that exist today. It also
looks at the science and logic behind what they did.

For a long time I have been fascinated by these people. We
are seeing more and more of them. I have called these people
'survivors' though they could equally be called 'trailblazers' or
'exceptional patients'. There was a time when I could scarcely
believe these healings were possible. Nothing in my medical
training prepared me for them. Now they no longer surprise me.
They are no longer a rarity. Dozens of books have been written
by these patients. Magazines like *Healing Our World* and *What
Doctors Don't Tell You* (now re-named *Get Well*) regularly give
accounts of healing against the odds. More can be found on the
internet. What was once a trickle has become a flood.

These survivors have described their experiences and they
want us to understand what they did. Just as importantly, they
want the medical community to know. Their discoveries are of
great importance and they know it; something very special has
taken place.

1

By far the commonest experiences are recoveries from cancer. These have typically been against their doctors' expectations. And what is fascinating about this trend is that this has all been occurring outside the radar of conventional medicine. I have long wondered if there was a common thread to these cases. I sensed that we could all benefit from this unique knowledge. I believe these discoveries can shed light on how our body heals. Recent discoveries, as we shall see, have confirmed that many of the methods used by survivors are grounded in science.

I believe they have an important and timely message for all of us, especially for those with a serious illness. I have long wanted to know why one person heals but another does not. I have wanted to understand what works best and most reliably. Success leaves clues. I have wondered what makes the biggest differences. What have been the underlying methods? What have their thought processes been? Are these methods reproducible? How much untapped healing potential exists within the human body? How can we use this knowledge to help treat and prevent cancer and other serious illnesses? And why have these patients succeeded at a time when mainstream medicine has so often failed? Is medicine missing something fundamental?

My approach has been purely empirical – to look at whatever works, however unusual. There is an inevitable emphasis on cancer. Accounts of recovery from cancer far exceed those from other conditions, but this book is not just about cancer. Cases of recovery from multiple sclerosis, motor neurone disease, chronic fatigue syndrome and even Alzheimer's disease have been included.

After reading this book, I hope you will never again believe there is nothing you can do about an illness. I hope you will see that the limits of what modern medicine can do are not the limits of what is possible and that there are ways to reverse even the most serious of diseases.

Anyone unfortunate enough to develop a serious illness needs to be smart when it comes to health. They need to know all the options available. Ultimately, this is empowering, and this is the purpose of this book.

Where have all the cures gone?

The quote from Henry Ford at the start of this chapter was not about health. But what if it had been? This book is also about doing what can't be done; it is about discovering new methods to reverse major illnesses. Could this knowledge perhaps help in the crisis that medicine is undergoing today? For make no mistake, there is a crisis.

Let's imagine travelling into the future and looking back, as a medical historian might do, taking an overview of the medicine of today and noting the patterns. Almost certainly what would stand out would be the lack of success in treating chronic illnesses and also the lack of success in treating cancer. A medical historian would be quick to note that this was happening at a time when health costs were spiralling out of control and when medical systems in many countries were at breaking point, both in terms of workloads and costs. The historian would naturally ask why so much money was being spent and why so little progress was being made. They would wonder why we were losing the battle against those illnesses plaguing the world at this time and would ask if the money had been wisely spent.

As a medical doctor I have become increasingly aware that there has been little real progress in medicine over the last few decades, with a lack of ideas and a feeling of stagnation. Yet I believe it doesn't need to be like this. There are more answers out there than most people are aware of. I am convinced that we already have the knowledge to drastically reduce the burden of chronic illness and cancer. I would like to share this knowledge. Some of it, as mentioned, has come from an unusual source: the increasing number of individuals who have found ways to reverse the serious illnesses that were threatening their existence. I would like to look at not just these spectacular cures but at the latest medical research, at long-forgotten solutions lying unused in medical libraries and at original and successful ideas used by great doctors and great therapists.

Against the odds

What survivors have demonstrated is tremendous versatility; they have used a great variety of methods. But one thing struck me early on about these methods. The strategies they used had parallels with the lifestyles of healthy populations – populations that suffer few, if any, of the diseases that plague modern civilisation.

Let's look at the ground-breaking study by the late HD Foster, Professor of Medical Geography at the University of Victoria, British Columbia, on spontaneous remission in 200 cancer patients.[1] Now make no mistake, these were serious cancers; the majority (53.5%) were metastatic, where spread from the primary site had already taken place. These are cancers that do not normally get better. In reality, the remissions were far from spontaneous but were directly linked to changes patients made to their lifestyles. In this study, 87.5% had made major dietary changes and 56% had used some sort of detoxification. This study strongly implied that their recoveries were directly related to the dietary and lifestyle changes they had made. They typically used a largely plant-based diet, eliminating tobacco, sugar and meat (79.5%), alcohol (75%), chocolate, white flour, milk, tea and coffee (50%).

This was only a single study but its findings are backed up by many similar accounts amongst cancer survivors: a switch to a diet of natural, unadulterated food and efforts to remove exposure to toxic substances. There is other evidence to support the logic of this approach. Populations that naturally eat this type of food suffer little cancer. Hundreds of studies confirm that certain natural foods, notably fruit and vegetables, have anti-cancer properties. In addition, over 150 studies have found that good diet increases cancer survival. Yet further evidence comes from studies showing less cancer in people with higher levels of protective nutrients. These I discuss in Chapters 1, 2 and 3.

Put simply, evidence from a multiplicity of sources has demonstrated the same phenomenon: the powerful healing effect of certain foods on cancer. So, no one should be surprised by the success of Foster's subjects. However, as we shall see, there is a caveat – the more serious the disease, the more radically the diet needs to change.

However, not all survivors have used diet; we will explore recoveries where mental, energetic and spiritual methods were used. Again, as we shall see, research backs up the wisdom of these approaches. So these accounts should not surprise us either.

Good health and where to find it

This brings us back to the basic principles of health. What is good health and how have we strayed so far from it in the modern world? The ground-breaking studies of Weston Price,[2] described in Chapter 2, make it very clear that disease is not our natural companion and that there have always been communities in the world that suffer little disease, lead long healthy lives and have little need for doctors. These communities have typically lived in harmony with nature and their environment. The contrast between their excellent health and negligible healthcare costs and our own poor health and unsustainable health costs could hardly be starker. Most methods of healing in this book have similarities with the lifestyles of these populations and could be described as natural or holistic. Good health, it seems, depends on surprisingly simple elements, like clean air, clean water, natural unadulterated food and an unpolluted environment.

These bring us back into harmony with a world that our bodies evolved to live and thrive in. Even the mental techniques used by survivors have similarities. They are often a way of bringing us back into harmony with ourselves.

Empowering ourselves

When people develop a major disease, they can quickly become anxious, depressed and disempowered. There is a famous, if cruel, experiment in which rats were implanted with cancer cells and then subjected to electric shocks[3]. Some received no shocks, some were subjected to shocks from which they couldn't escape and some were subjected to shocks from which they could escape and learned to avoid. This psychological experience had a profound effect on the rats. In the group who received no shocks, 50% rejected the tumours; in the inescapable shock group only 27% survived; but in those receiving escapable shocks, 70% rejected the tumours.

The result was unexpected. How could the group that could escape shocks do better than those not shocked at all? Not surprisingly, those in the inescapable group did the worst and also had lower levels of immune markers, such as natural killer (NK) cells. I think this research illustrates an important point – having some degree of control over a situation, however unpleasant it might be, is crucial. It stimulates the immune system and aids recovery. Conversely, having no control and feeling helpless depresses the immune system.

To my way of thinking, this means that having knowledge about what you can do about a situation is critically important. In itself it boosts immunity and much else. As this book shows, there is always something you can do. This is both empowering and healing.

However, those who do get better against the odds are still invisible to mainstream medicine. They are statistical outliers and hence get overlooked. In addition, their ideas about diet, mind-body methods, energy-enhancing techniques and reducing toxicity are largely outside the mindset of the medical profession, although this is slowly changing. But success can never be ignored, even if it comes from an unusual source. Many of the discoveries of survivors, notably on the healing properties of diet, are now being verified by science. Despite their huge significance, doctors are typically unaware of these patients.

A different way of thinking

The first step in dealing with any major illness is, of course, to visit a doctor. Most people trust their doctors and this is natural and good, but there are valid reasons to be cautious. I say that as a doctor myself, knowing that the vast majority of doctors will always do their best to help patients.

The reason to be cautious is straightforward: over the last century doctors' track record in treating cancers and chronic diseases has been disappointing. The treatments available have been limited: for cancer this usually involves surgery, radiotherapy and chemotherapy. Fortunately, some useful new methods are appearing. And certainly, some cancers respond well to conventional treatment. However, treatment for many cancers remains poor and can have an adverse effect on quality of life. Similarly, treatments for chronic diseases have major limitations. This suggests the medical profession is missing something fundamental.

You might reasonably argue, how could an ordinary person possibly succeed when the entire medical profession has failed? The answer is that some have succeeded, even when perhaps they had no right to do so. Their hard-won knowledge is now available to us all.

Doctors' knowledge tends to be fairly specific and mainly centred on drug treatments. It has blind spots, the most notable being nutrition. However, nutrition just happens to be highly relevant; for example, there are over 4000 nutrients known to make a difference in cancer[4].

Today it is getting easier and easier for a lay person to learn as much as any doctor about their specific condition, and sometimes more. I know this as I have met such patients and learned from them. I believe it may not be long before the informed layperson knows more about healing with nutrition than the average doctor.

An example of this is our ability to glean life-saving information from social media. People concerned about dementia, especially those with a family history of it, sometimes use genetic tests to assess their risk of developing it, but the results can be scary. People unlucky enough to find they have two copies of the ApoE4 gene (homozygous for the gene) have 10 times the risk of dementia (over 50% risk). But where does this knowledge leave them? Any neurologist will tell them that there is no cure for Alzheimer's disease. The situation is surely hopeless?

One woman found herself in exactly this situation, with this high-risk genetic pattern and already developing frightening symptoms before the age of 50. Fortunately, she heard about the newly developed Bredesen protocol (also known as ReCODE)[5] and had successful treatment. Although it is the only treatment that has successfully reversed Alzheimer's disease, it remains largely unknown. She set up a website called ApoE4.info. The website spread the word and now almost all 600 members are using some variation of ReCODE. The result is that many people with this gene, facing a potentially terrifying future, are now meeting up and swapping encouraging stories and making good progress. The protocol can also be effective for Alzheimer's sufferers without the ApoE4 gene. I believe this trend of finding crucial information through the internet and social media will have an increasing impact on how we practise medicine.

Nevertheless, I think taking medical advice is a crucial and essential first step. This should include a careful evaluation of the diagnosis and how likely any treatment is to succeed and what else can be done. If there is an effective treatment the benefits of which outweigh potential side effects, then go ahead and use it. If it is just a way of reducing symptoms but unlikely to improve life expectancy or quality, then consider other options. These nearly always exist.

Our amazing capacity to heal

Until I started looking into stories of survivors, I had no real concept of the extraordinary capacity of the body to heal. Take the following story of Elaine Nussbaum who developed a sarcoma of her uterus when she was in her 40s.[6] After two years she had nearly reached the end, in pain, bedridden, with a tumour that had metastasised to her bones and lungs. She had been treated with surgery, radiotherapy and chemotherapy, but had deteriorated in spite of all of this. No one had recovered from a metastatic sarcoma of this type before. She was an invalid, in a wheelchair, wearing a brace, sick and depressed, popping 39 pills a day and waiting for death to claim her. I have seen many patients like this and I would have previously regarded this situation as utterly hopeless, with death an inevitable outcome.

 But she did not die. She heard about a Dr Sattilaro who had recovered from prostate cancer using a macrobiotic diet and knew that he had become pain-free after six weeks. She decided to try the diet herself. She also saw a therapist, Shizuko Yamamoto, who had expertise in macrobiotics and shiatsu. And she began to heal.

After six months she was walking, happy, optimistic, free of pain and not taking any pills. Two years later, x-rays confirmed that the tumours in her bones and lungs had gone. Twenty-two years later she was alive and well and went on to write the book *Recovery from Cancer*. She said she felt healthier after the cancer than she did before, a comment not uncommon amongst survivors.

How did she recover when her prognosis was so appalling? Was it the macrobiotic diet? As her therapist told her, 'You healed the cancer, the macrobiotic diet was your tool'. To me, this story was a revelation: it told me that the body's capacity to heal, even from the most devastating illness, is truly awesome. Heal it can, but only if it is given the right conditions.

It is likely that there needed to be an ideal combination of factors in place for Elaine to recover. She kept rigidly to the diet, she had the help of a macrobiotic chef and a therapist whom she trusted, someone who had expertise in macrobiotics and who told her she would get better. She was given shiatsu. She said to herself, over and over, that it was going to work. All these factors may have been important and most likely each one added incrementally to the healing.

Ultimately, any healing depends on the immune system and I now believe the immune system has an almost unlimited capacity to heal under ideal conditions (and, I would stress, *ideal*). Sadly, conditions are rarely ideal. Nevertheless, there have certainly been many dramatic recoveries of this type. There have been hundreds of cancer cures with macrobiotics alone, and although macrobiotics was the method used here, there are similar stories using other methods.

Take the case of Margaret, a 55-year-old retired nurse. By the time she was diagnosed, her breast cancer had already metastasised to her brain, spine and ribs.[7] No surgery was done for she was considered terminal; she was given palliative radiotherapy instead. Soon after diagnosis she had two strange experiences. During one of these she found she was looking down on her own body. She heard a voice state that her experience would help others. On waking the next morning after this event, she experienced a feeling of peace, love and happiness which remained with her. Later, whilst lying in bed, she felt an electric shock which caused her whole body to shake and this was accompanied by a sense of well-being and a feeling that healing had taken place. This was followed by the deepest sleep she had experienced in many years. The experience left her with the conviction she was going to get better, but she knew there was much she needed to do.

She contacted a naturopath who she remembered from a talk she had previously attended. He recommended the Gerson diet (see Chapter 1, page 33). As she later discovered, even he thought she had little chance of surviving. However, she kept to the recommended strict schedule of juicing and enemas. Later she visualised the tumours getting smaller and started meditation. After five months she started to improve. This was followed by a series of healing crises (strange rashes, abscesses and abdominal pains). Her attitude to these was typical of a survivor. With each episode she thought, 'Good, more toxins being released'. Scans and x-rays were later to show that her brain and bones were free of cancer and examination showed that her breast lumps and enlarged glands had cleared. Like Elaine Nussbaum she said she was in better health than before her illness. She remained free of cancer eight years later. She too illustrates the body's incredible healing power, even from the most advanced cancer.

It is difficult to put her healing down to any one therapy. Was it the Gerson diet, some sort of spiritual healing, her positive attitude or her visualisations and meditation? Probably it was a combination of all of these.

It must be said that cases like this are rare, but what is far more important is that they can happen at all. What is so fascinating is this astonishing ability the body has to recover from almost anything. I have been amazed again and again by stories like this.

Sometimes healing defies explanation. Napoleon Hill tells the story of how his son Blair was born deaf, without ears, and without even a bony canal to support hearing. You would think recovery would be impossible in this situation. Unsurprisingly, his doctor told Hill just that. He told him that his son would be a deaf-mute. Hill countered immediately by saying his son would develop 100% hearing. His doctor went on to say, not unreasonably, 'There are some things in the world that neither you, nor I, nor anyone else, can change and this is one of them'. Napoleon Hill maintained his stubborn, irrationally positive position, saying, 'There is nothing in the world I can do nothing about'. He decided then and there that his son would be able to hear and to speak. Amazingly this would later come to pass.[8]

He didn't know how, but knew there must be a way. He worked with his son four hours a day, filling his son's mind with a burning desire to hear, and with prayer. He also took Blair for some chiropractic treatment. Every day he renewed the pledge not to accept his son as a deaf mute. When Blair was 18 months old his father sensed he could pick up a few sounds, but Blair still made no attempt to speak. At three years Hill had some confirmation that his son could hear something, observing Blair turning his head after he snapped his fingers. After playing music on a phonograph, Hill noticed Blair responding to the music. He would put his teeth around the casing of the phonograph. So, Hill played it over and over: this presumably allowed hearing to take place through the bones. Soon after, Blair responded to his father's voice after he placed his lips against his son's mastoid bone, which would again allow the transmission of sound through bone. Later Blair attempted to say words, although these were minimal.

Encouraged by this, Hill started reading Blair bedtime stories designed to make him believe the affliction was an asset, not a liability, and telling him he had an advantage over his older brother. He told him that people would treat him with extraordinary kindness because of his problems. At four years of age he had 65% normal hearing. Gradually, he developed the resourcefulness that Hill had implanted so deeply into his brain. Even Hill himself admitted he could not see how his deafness could be an asset and yet this too came to be.

Blair could still only hear his teachers when they shouted, but Hill refused to send him to a deaf school. What followed was one of those uncanny coincidences that seem to occur so often in the lives of survivors. Whilst he was in college, a company that had heard about his story sent him a hearing device to try (he had had no success with an earlier one). His hearing was transformed. For the first time in his life he could hear normally and now he had 100% hearing just as his father had originally foretold.

Blair wrote back enthusiastically to the company that had sent him the hearing device and was invited to New York to meet them. He then decided to devote his life to helping the deaf and was given a job with the company. He went on to help thousands of deaf people. He also became a successful salesman and businessman. His deafness did indeed become an asset, just as his father had predicted.

This story is by no means unique. Cynthia Ouellette's astonishing account of how she helped her daughter recover from a life-threatening illness and reverse her cerebral palsy (described later – see Chapter 3, page 104), using love, faith and positive suggestions, has many similarities.

These cases and ones like them changed me as a doctor and it has become harder and harder to say that there's nothing more that we can do.

The principles of healing

These are a few examples of extraordinary healing and extraordinary individuals. Several important points strike me about these cases. The first is that the body has the ability to heal from even the most serious conditions under ideal conditions. Cases like these have left me with little doubt that this is so. What follows logically is that if we want healing to take place, then we should aim to create an environment that is as ideal as possible.

This might be high quality food, minimal toxicity and healing thoughts. This is a basic strategy of survivors.

Another key principle is a belief in the ability to recover. This is fundamental to success. The late Louise Hay, author and cancer survivor, recommends putting yourself in the mindset where you know you can be healed, even if you don't know how. Then the right help will come along. As long as you do the work, she says, healing will occur. Napoleon Hill demonstrates this mindset perfectly.

Unfortunately people's ability to heal can be limited by what they believe is possible and not surprisingly this is influenced by what their doctors believe is possible. Sometimes people intuitively sense what they need to do but fail to do it because their doctors, their family or their friends persuade them otherwise. Survivors, however, see it differently and do what they think is right for them, ignoring if necessary the nay-sayers.

Another principle is that the immune system is critically important. It is the sleeping giant that needs to wake up if recovery is going to take place. If the body is going to heal, then ultimately the immune system must do the job. It follows naturally from this that anything that boosts the immune system will help the body heal and anything that damages it must be viewed with suspicion.

Another useful principle is to remove the triggers for an illness. Often the cause of the illness is more important than its name and finding the cause (though not always possible) can make a major difference. An example serves to illustrate this. Dr Patrick Kingsley described in a BSEM lecture once seeing a patient with multiple sclerosis who always became worse in the spring and summer but recovered in the winter. She worked in a flower shop and would take flowers home in the evening. It turned out that she was allergic to the flowers and it was the flowers that were triggering her multiple sclerosis. Once the trigger was removed she rapidly recovered. The cause (flower allergy) proved to be much more important than the diagnostic label (multiple sclerosis). This is an unusual example as the causes of illnesses are rarely this simple, but it illustrates a point. Remove the triggers and healing will take place.

Finding a doctor with the skills to do this, however, is not always easy. Doctors are typically not trained in this way. Another difficulty is that the majority of diseases have multiple causes and multiple triggers. But some can be avoided. To give a simple example, 24 studies have investigated the link between milk and prostate cancer, with 20 finding a positive association. It therefore would make complete sense, after having treatment for prostate cancer, to avoid using milk products. However, this is advice that is rarely given. We will examine this connection and others in more detail in Chapter 3.

Pros and cons of treatment

Many patients with cancer and other serious diseases face a dilemma. They are well aware of the limitations and the adverse effects of conventional medicine. However, they are also understandably reluctant to trust unfamiliar and unfunded complementary treatments. Mainstream medicine typically denigrates complementary therapies, claiming they are unproven, and this is often true. However, it is only half the story.

Some of the alternative treatments can be highly effective, as we shall see, but, at the moment, lack absolute proof. This is a huge problem because it is obviously important to test a remedy fully before it can be recommended. However, it is often impossible to fund studies on natural remedies, partly because only pharmaceutical companies can afford to undertake large trials and partly because, even if the trial should prove positive, natural remedies cannot be patented, so the company funding the trial has little to gain. This conundrum has distorted the search for cures for medical illness more than any other single factor. However, let's just note that highly promising remedies do exist.

What can be said is that for almost every disease there is something you can do. There is more out there than most doctors and most patients are aware of. I hope to make some sense out of this complex area and show which therapies are likely to help and which have good data behind them.

A new approach to disease

But survivors have not only found new ways to treat major illnesses. They have done something else and this is, for me, why they are so important. They have pointed towards a more logical and rational approach to treating disease. To understand this, we first need to look at how modern medicine works.

Conventional medicine has sometimes been described as using the 'magic bullet' approach. After the success of antibiotics it was hoped we would find drugs to treat all major diseases. At first the search for magic bullets seemed to be working. Indeed, drugs can be very useful. Early in my career I witnessed how acid-blocking drugs, such as cimetidine, revolutionised the treatment of peptic ulcers. They were so successful that the commonly used surgical treatment for ulcers became a relic from the past, almost overnight. It was a major advance. At that time, there was an expectancy that further major discoveries would follow. Sadly, this didn't happen. After the 1970s, the supply of new drugs started to dry up. An analysis of new drugs after this time found that only a third gave even a moderate therapeutic advantage.[9] Drugs were proving to be a poor solution to modern diseases.

There was another problem. Drugs initially hailed as wonder drugs turned out to cause more problems than they solved. Typically the problems emerged after a drug had been in widespread use for decades. Examples of this include Valium (diazepam) and hormone replacement therapy (HRT), though they were far from the only ones. Diclofenac, a routinely-used anti-inflammatory drug, prescribed in huge quantities, was found to increase the incidence of heart attacks. What was surprising was that it took three decades to make this discovery. Similarly it took three decades before anyone realised that statins could trigger diabetes.[10]

My excitement about new advances gradually turned to disillusionment as I witnessed how little impact medicine was having on the vast numbers of people being affected by chronic diseases. I also noticed that, although these drugs often relieved symptoms, they rarely made people healthier. I began to wonder if we were on the wrong track.

Perhaps I should have realised that this course of events was inevitable and predictable. Most drugs block enzymes or obstruct specific metabolic pathways. It was never realistic to expect this simplistic strategy was going to solve the complex problems involved in chronic degenerative diseases. Most of these diseases are linked to changes in our modern lifestyle and diet. Sadly, drugs have proved to be a very blunt tool. Many doctors are only too aware of the limitations of drugs and their potential to cause side-effects, but drugs are what they understand and, as they genuinely want to help patients, this is what they give.

However, this approach to medicine should not and must not be confused with looking for cures. Specifically, it cannot be regarded as a logical approach to dealing with serious chronic diseases.

A more rational methodology

Keep this in mind because what survivors have been doing is entirely different. They have been searching for cures. To cure cancer or a degenerative disease, you need a multi-faceted approach. No one drug and no one nutrient will ever cure a major chronic illness. A different approach is needed.

Remember the body has incredible powers of healing once conditions are optimal. We have already witnessed this. But how can we help this happen?

I believe the first key principle is to supply everything essential for health. This is a strategy familiar to survivors. It might be high quality food, vitamins, essential fats, or sometimes an overwhelming reason to live and get better.

The second key principle is to remove anything that is harmful. This may involve identifying toxic substances and/or finding ways to eliminate them or reduce their intake. To give a simple example, if you live under a mobile phone mast you are far less likely to recover from cancer even using the best treatment available, unless you move. You must remove the triggers and anything that hinders the body's ability to recover.

These principles have an inherent logic to them, because, as shown in many studies in this book, it is the absence of essential nutrients and the presence of toxic substances that so often induce chronic diseases, including cancer, in the first place. And correcting these imbalances helps to reverse them.

To illustrate why this approach is important, research studies have found that breast cancer patients typically have lower levels of certain nutrients (these include omega-3 fats,[11] betacarotene[12] and vitamin D,[13] and they are more at risk if they are below a threshold level of vitamin B12[14]) in their bodies. They also have higher levels of certain chemicals (such DDT, the organochloride insecticide dieldren, PCBs and parabens). Those with the highest level of organochlorines in their blood and fat have been found to have between four and 10 times the risk of developing breast cancer. Those who had the highest use of cleaning products and air fresheners had twice the risk of breast cancer[15] and this doubling of risk was also found in those with higher levels of phthalates in their body.[16] Those exposed to high levels of traffic emissions have a higher risk.[17] Various studies[18] have linked breast cancer with hormone replacement therapy (HRT) and drinking milk (see Chapter 2).

It makes logical sense that supplying the missing nutrients and removing the harmful influences will increase the likelihood of treatment being successful. However, these are not aspects of treatment normally considered by doctors. That is why we shall be looking at them in this book.

You could regard these two principles as firstly increasing the power of the body to heal and secondly reducing or eliminating factors that weaken the body. The underlying assumption here is that once conditions are optimal, the body will heal. The aim is to bring it to a tipping point where the immune system can operate optimally and clear the illness. Essentially this is what survivors have done. These are basic principles of healing.

Survivors have used many different methods, but for the purposes of this book I have divided them into those who have used nutrition, those who have used mind-body approaches, those who have used detoxification (ridding the body of harmful substances), and those who have used energy. Most survivors have used a combination of these and there is good evidence, which I will discuss later, that more is better. The classification into these groups is based on what has been the major strategy the survivor has taken.

The first section is about food. I believe much of the information here will be new to the majority of doctors, yet it is fundamental to healing. It illustrates the first principle, supplying the highest quality nutrients, the ones the body requires to function optimally. Chapter 1, on Using food to cure, looks at survivors who were able to cure their illnesses using food as their main therapy. It discusses the diets that have proven effective in treating cancer, multiple sclerosis and other major illnesses. Finally, it discusses the research on specific foods and their disease-modifying properties. For example, many plant-based foods have a range of anti-cancer properties such as protecting DNA, boosting immunity, killing cancer cells, stopping metastases, reducing inflammation and blocking harmful hormones. It also looks at long-lived and other healthy populations and how their diet differs from ours. Chapter 2, on Food and health, discusses individual foods, simplifying it into those foods to avoid, those that have become less healthy and those that promote health.

The second section of this book is on the power of the mind and, some would say, the spirit. Many survivors have used a variety of mind techniques to recover and some have used these methods exclusively. In the last few decades, a body of research has been growing that demonstrates how the mind influences both the body and the immune system, and that changes in our thoughts and emotions will cause changes in our biochemistry on a moment-by-moment basis. This is the science of psychoneuroimmunology (PNI). We also know thoughts and emotions can change gene expression.

Many survivors have been ahead of their time in understanding the significance of these findings. There are many ways to influence a disease by using the mind creatively. Some techniques are well-known, such as visualisation, but some methods have been developed by survivors themselves. Some of the accounts are truly extraordinary and give insight into the incredible powers of the mind.

The third section is about toxicity. This section is unusual within the context of this book in that it contains few stories from survivors. The reason is that, although removing toxicity has been an important strategy for survivors, it has rarely been the only method.

A vast amount of research exists on toxicity, but I believe few doctors will be are aware of it. The data are both fascinating and disturbing. Chapter 6 discusses the hundreds of toxic chemicals to which we are routinely exposed and that can be found in the bodies of every person on the planet. It examines the critical impact this has had, not only on cancer, but on neurological and endocrine disease. Unfortunately, no amount of doctors, drugs or hospitals can produce a healthy population on a polluted planet. Chapters 7 and 8 discuss how to deal with toxicity both by avoidance and by reducing toxicity within us.

The fourth section is about energy. I have included sunlight and exercise in this category. There is a substantial body of research on both. However, other forms of energy also influence health.

Some people have always had the ability to see people's energy fields and to detect disease. By the early 1920s we knew that different species, different organs and even individual cells were surrounded by specific electromagnetic fields. Harold Burr, Professor at Yale School of Medicine in 1929, discovered that in mice an electromagnetic field of cancer occurred before cancer cells became detectable. He later found the same was true of women who developed uterine cancer.[19] He had discovered that changes in energy precede and create disease rather than being caused by disease. It naturally follows that manipulating energy fields has the potential to cure disease.

Scientific research, though still in its infancy, is beginning to unravel the energy pathways of the body and make sense of this intriguing data. Many gifted practitioners have found ways to influence energy and health directly, healing themselves and others in the process. A fascinating and exciting discovery is that groups of people who have a combined intention to heal can have a profound and sometimes curative effect on illness.

If energy changes precede disease, as has been demonstrated by Burr and others, then it naturally follows that energy changes must precede recovery. Anything that allows this to happen must be beneficial. Many simple techniques exist which can increase positive energy. There are exciting new energy therapies and some ancient but highly effective ones. Chapter 10 gives an insight into this emerging field and on how this information can be used practically.

The last chapter, Putting it all together, pulls these divergent fields together. Many survivors have used methods derived from all of these areas. It discusses the evidence that using several strategies is typically more powerful than using just one. In some circumstances, combining them is essential.

Survivors have given us a guide-book on how to tackle illnesses. Often they needed great patience and mental strength to deal with the inevitable setbacks. It was often three steps forward and two steps backwards. Not all have succeeded and some have told us why. Even this has been beneficial, showing us potential roadblocks. Having a good understanding of what works and how to combine methods, is a good place to start when faced with serious illness.

Part I

Change your diet

Chapter 1

Using food to cure

Let food be thy medicine and medicine be thy food.
Hippocrates (460–370 BC)

After Dr Terry Wahls developed multiple sclerosis (MS), she received the very best treatment that modern medicine could offer. Despite this she deteriorated over a seven-year period, eventually having to use a wheelchair. She kept working as a doctor but wondered how long she could continue.

She had read about the benefits of the Palaeolithic diet – that is, eating like a hunter-gatherer. Intrigued and hopeful she started this diet and added supplements such as co-enzyme Q10 and carnitine which supported brain and mitochondrial function. These changes, although helpful, were not enough to stem her decline.

Something else was required and soon. She removed foods that released sugar quickly and added healthy fats (especially coconut oil) knowing these supported nerve and brain function. She also ate nine portions of fruit and vegetables daily (three brightly coloured, three high in sulphur, three leafy green).

In addition she removed gluten and milk, being aware of research showing that these could trigger inflammation. Bone broth, with its high content of beneficial fats and proteins, became an integral part of her diet. She also used exercise where possible, meditation and an electrical therapy called e-stim.

It was a radical change, but it worked. After three months she could walk between consulting rooms with just one cane; after six months she could walk round the hospital without a cane and she could cycle around the garden. After 18 months she could cycle 18 miles. It was an astonishing turn-around.

In her ground-breaking book, *The Wahl's Protocol*[1], she described not only her own story but also those of other people with MS who had made impressive recoveries using the same approach. Initially, what nearly all patients noticed was an increase in vitality and in their clarity of thinking.

By a combination of research, experimentation and intuition she had found that a diet could reverse MS. And she found this diet could also be effective in other autoimmune diseases. It was an immense breakthrough. However, perhaps it should not have surprised us. The clues had been around for a long time.

So was Hippocrates correct? Can we cure diseases simply by eating the right foods? More importantly, can we reverse some of the most serious diseases of our time using diet? To many doctors this idea seems preposterous. But the answer is unequivocal: it can be done and it has been done, time and time again. In fact, this is the most common strategy used by survivors. Food really can act like a medicine and sometimes it can make the difference between life and death.

The best place to start looking for answers is with cancer, for this is where most research has been done. We know that in Foster's group of 200 patients with spontaneous remission (the majority with metastatic cancer), 87.7% had changed their diet.[2] We have seen that Elaine Nussbaum recovered from terminal cancer using a macrobiotic diet.[3] They are far from the only ones. Below are several accounts of people who have reversed their cancers by changing their diet. This is further evidence that food can act like a medicine. However, to put this in perspective, the changes in diet typically have needed to be radical.

One thing that struck me most as I read through these inspiring stories was that some survivors not only recovered from their cancers but also had an unexpected bonus: they ended up feeling better than they had ever felt before. Bernadette Bohan, who recovered from two different cancers over two decades after she radically changed her diet, described how she felt years younger.[4] Good food can do more than cure diseases; it can raise vitality and it can alleviate pain. All this tells us that Hippocrates was on the right track.

Clearly food is far more fundamental to health than most doctors have previously thought.

Is it possible to take this concept a step further: could we live in a world without cancer, heart disease, arthritis and other degenerative diseases? Do we already have the information necessary to do achieve this? The answer to both questions is yes. What's more, this critically important information has been around, though largely ignored, for a very long time. The story must begin with two of the greatest medical pioneers of all time, Weston Price and Robert McCarrison. Few have understood the immense importance of their work.

The food pioneers

Weston A Price

Weston Price has already been mentioned; he was a dentist and one of the most innovative medical researchers of all time. He locked the door of his dental surgery in the 1930s and set off with his wife, travelling around five continents, researching 14 isolated communities over 30 years, looking primarily for the cause of dental decay. Most of these isolated communities were relatively primitive groups (Eskimos, Aborigines, Maoris, African tribes) but some were isolated western communities (in the Outer Hebrides and the Loetschental valley in Switzerland). All these groups had quite different diets but they had one thing in common: they ate foods that were completely natural.

He soon found that none of these communities suffered from dental decay. But he discovered something far more fundamental. The degenerative diseases, so common in the world today, were absent in these communities. There were no cancers, heart disease or arthritis. Gallstones, appendicitis and ulcers were largely unknown, their eyesight was exceptional and childbirth was simple and rapid. Their babies were born in vigorous health and, remarkably, they rarely cried. They lived in harmonious communities with no doctors, dentists or policeman.[5]

The health of these races was exceptional – for instance, he recalled a North American Indian who, after their truck had broken down, walked back 65 miles through difficult terrain, without stopping for food or sleep for 18 hours. He noted Peruvian Indians who would carry loads of 90 kilos (200 lb) on their back through mountainous territory all day and every day. Reading through his accounts, I couldn't help wondering just how healthy we might all be if we all lived this way. Their health was at another level to ours.

These isolated groups had a deep understanding of the relationship between health and food. Before, during and after pregnancy, and during the early childhood years, they were given special foods to boost health, usually fish, eggs and other seafood, but also milk and butter produced from cows fed on rapidly growing grass. They knew this special grass was packed with nutrients. Today we know why: it is especially rich in omega-3 fats and fat-soluble vitamins. Sometimes pregnancy was postponed to coincide with the availability of these high-quality foods. They made sure there was enough time between births to build up nutrition in the mother; usually this was between two-and–a-half and four years. Many groups had access to the sea, but those who did not made great efforts to keep their land fertile; they were aware that this increased the nutritional value of their foods.

However, Weston Price also discovered something else and something more disturbing. Whenever these communities changed their diet to modern food, their health deteriorated rapidly: they developed dental caries; they became susceptible to tuberculosis (TB) and other infectious diseases; their births became longer and more painful. And once the parents changed to a western diet, their children suffered too. Birth defects were more frequent as were dental decay, crowding of the teeth and changes to the shape of their faces. The youngest of the family suffered most, suggesting that their mothers were becoming progressively depleted of something vital for health. Weston Price was not content to speculate that these changes were due to the modern diet. He successfully demonstrated that many of these diseases, including dental decay, could be put into reverse simply by reverting to their original, natural diet.

Here is an example. Price had looked for arthritis in the Native American Indians but failed to find it. The only exceptions were those who ate the 'foods of civilisation'. One was a five-year-old boy crippled with arthritis which developed after rheumatic fever. The boy had been told that he would never recover. Price disagreed. He recommended a diet that removed all white flour products. He added milk and butter from cows fed on rapidly growing grass plus cod liver oil. This was successful and the boy's pain rapidly diminished, his appetite improved and he started to gain weight.

We can sum up Weston Price's ground-breaking work. Populations living on natural foods enjoyed exceptional health with none of the degenerative changes so typical of western societies. He also showed that changing to a western diet initiated chronic diseases and returning to a natural diet reversed the changes.

Robert McCarrison

At about the same time, another great researcher, Sir Robert McCarrison, looked at food from a different angle.[6] He had been struck by the huge differences in health between populations in India. For instance, several of the races in Northern India had exceptionally good health, whereas many in the South suffered poor health with higher rates of TB, cancer and heart disease. He wondered if diet was responsible.

He decided to test this theory in a novel way. He fed these different diets to groups of rats. When the rats were given the diets of the healthiest races (the Hunzas and Sikhs) the rats had no detectable diseases, a very low mortality (1%) and no infant mortality. The rats were cheerful, alert, easily handled and lived together harmoniously. When a similar group of rats was given the diet from Southern India (Madrassi and Bengali), or the typical British diet of the time, the rats developed problems. Their mortality was much higher (30%) and their births were more difficult, with stillbirths and miscarriages. They were stunted, with poor coats, and they developed pneumonia and intestinal disease. They were irritable, would bite their attendants without provocation and eventually began to kill and eat weaker members of their own group.

The Sikh diet consisted of whole wheat, milk, dhal, fruit and vegetables, with meat used sparingly. The diet of the Madrassis and Bengalis consisted mainly of white rice that had been boiled, milled or polished, with little fruit or vegetables. The British diet he used was that of white bread, sugar, boiled vegetables, tinned food, meat and potatoes.

To me it was no surprise that a devitalised diet caused ill-health but what did surprise me was how the diet dramatically changed the rats' personalities and behaviour. It is not hard to see similarities with some of the behaviour we see in western societies today and I suspect that if this experiment were repeated today, with the modern British diet, the rats would become even more unpleasant.

Robert McCarrison came to a simple and profound conclusion: 'I know of nothing so potent in producing ill health as improperly constituted food'. Weston Price put it another way: 'It should not only be a matter of deep concern but of deep alarm that human beings can degenerate so rapidly on using a certain type of food'. He used the analogy of putting petrol in a car; comparing modern food with using ordinary petrol – it gave the energy to get from A to B but did nothing to stop the car slowly deteriorating. Natural food was like special petrol that not only got you from A to B but repaired the car at the same time.

These researchers had demonstrated in separate ways that there was something about natural and unadulterated food which was profoundly different from the refined, devitalised produce that we call food today, and the difference was the impact it had on health and vitality.

Once I became aware of these studies it became impossible for me to practise medicine in the same way again. I knew that, without incorporating diet into my practice, it would be difficult, if not impossible, to heal many of the diseases I saw on a day-to-day basis.

Long-lived communities

Price and McCarrison were not the only ones to come to this startling conclusion. A series of studies, this time on long-lived races, uncovered many of the same findings. These long-lived races commonly live to over 100 years old and typically retain their vigour well into old age. They include the Okinawans and Hunzas, together with the peoples of Barbagia in Sardinia, the Nicoya peninsula in Costa Rica and the Greek island of Ikaria. Other areas known for their longevity, but where the records are somewhat less dependable, include Bama, Georgia and

Abkhasia (an autonomous republic of Georgia), Symi (a Greek island), Vilcabamba (Ecuador) and Campodimele (central Italy).

The studies found that typically these populations ate large amounts of locally grown organic fruit and vegetables (at least 10 portions daily) including many raw foods. And they ate them fresh. They ate wholegrains (as opposed to refined carbohydrates), consumed plenty of essential fats (from fish and/or nuts) and took lots of exercise. They ate slowly, stopping before they were full and typically gave thanks for their food. Another important factor was their highly fertile soils which they treated with great respect. Many (but not all) lived in unpolluted mountainous areas.

Just as relevant was what they didn't do: they didn't eat sugar or processed foods, didn't smoke, didn't drink excess alcohol, didn't overeat and had little meat and dairy produce. They lived in areas where there were no supermarkets.

Like the populations studied by Price, their health was astonishing. For example, the Hunzas are renowned for walking 40 miles a day, up and down mountains, without any sign of fatigue.

These people are living reminders that 'we are what we eat'. Perhaps less obviously, they are also reminders that 'what we eat is only as good as the soil it comes from', a point we shall return to later.

In summary, long-lived populations eat high-quality food which is low in calories and high in nutrients.

In contrast, populations in the Marshall Islands and Mexico have developed some of the highest rates of obesity, diabetes and poor health in the world. This happened after they changed from their traditional diets to a diet high in imported junk food and sugar-laden drinks.

We now have very convincing evidence that high-quality food can effectively prevent degenerative disease. However, it is time to look at whether we can truly use food to *reverse* diseases.

Doctors using food as medicine

In the early 20th century it was found that the Inuit and Native American populations developed a marked susceptibility to TB once they adopted a Western diet. This disease tended to be progressive and fatal. However, Weston Price tells the story of a Dr Romig who had 36 years of experience working with these communities.[5] Dr Romig knew he could not cure TB (there were no drugs for it at the time), but he did have a simple and effective answer. He would send these Indians and Inuit back to their traditional homes, away from contact with westerners, to live on their native diet. Once back on their native diet, he noted that the great majority of them recovered.

He was not the only doctor to discover that serious diseases could be cured by nothing more than a return to healthy food.

Perhaps the best known of these doctors was Max Gerson. As a young man, he suffered from severe migraines and had been unable to obtain relief with medication. He changed his diet to fruit and vegetables and noticed that his migraines went away. He began experimenting, treating people with this diet, free of charge. Many migraine patients did equally well. However, to his surprise, a friend of a patient, using his methods, cured himself of lupus vulgaris. This is TB of the skin and was considered incurable at the time. He later successfully treated the wife of the writer and philosopher Albert Schweitzer, who had severe TB, and Albert Schweitzer himself, who suffered from diabetes.

In spite of his successes he was wary of taking on a woman who asked for help with cancer. She had cancer of the bile duct which was already too advanced for surgery. He told her he did not want to treat her because other doctors were already opposed to him and his unorthodox methods. However, this lady was not one for giving up and wrote a disclaimer stating he was not responsible for the results of his treatment. After six months on Gerson's treatment she recovered.

Gerson went on to treat many other cancer cases with a success rate of about 50%. He was a shrewd observer and made many important observations; some of which have far-reaching implications for medicine.

He noted that whenever one woman with cancer started to lose weight, other members of her family, some of whom were doctors, would feed her with foods not allowed on his diet. He observed that whenever she ate eggs, meat or oil, her cancer re-grew. Once put back on his diet, the cancer regressed. He was learning, empirically, what worked and what didn't.

Sadly Gerson found the medical profession was not open to his methods and failed to comprehend the significance of his discoveries. However, some other doctors followed his lead. The Danish doctor Kristina Nolfi cured her own breast cancer with a 100%-organic fruit-and-vegetable diet.[7] She lived in a tent on an island and when possible tried to get four to five hours of sunlight each day. She went on to cure many other patients using the same regime at the Humlegaarden sanatorium in Denmark, which treated 1000 patients a year, achieving remarkable recoveries in diabetes, heart disease, asthma, epilepsy and cancer. Like Gerson, she fell foul of the medical profession; losing her medical licence for using 'dangerous and unproven' methods.

In New Zealand, Drs Eva Hill and Maude Fere cured themselves of skin and bowel cancers respectively with fruit-and-vegetable diets, and Dr Hill went on to help many other patients using the same methods. In the 1950s, a Hungarian doctor, Dr Ferenczi, had considerable success treating terminal cancer patients with his beetroot diet. The evidence that food could cure cancer and many other diseases of modern civilisation, though still limited, was accumulating. It was becoming hard to ignore.

No-one familiar with the work of Weston Price and Robert McCarrison would have been surprised. Even so, the fact that a natural diet could, in many cases, cure the most serious of diseases, was an astonishing discovery. It had the potential to change medicine for ever. However, doctors of the time were not open to these discoveries. Then, as now, they had trouble assimilating these ideas despite the growing evidence.

Half a century later, a scientist, Professor Colin Campbell, would shed further light on Gerson's careful observations. He was researching the links between diet and liver cancer in children from the Philippines. At the time it was thought that protein malnutrition might be a contributory factor to this deadly disease. However, his research was to turn this theory on its head.

Campbell set out to investigate this link between protein and cancer. Firstly he fed rats with alfatoxin, a potent carcinogen that caused liver cancer. He then divided the rats into two groups: those on a high animal protein diet (20%) and those on a low animal protein diet (5%). The results were unequivocal. All those on the high protein diet developed cancer; none of those on the low protein diet did. He repeated the experiment and found that however much carcinogen he gave, the rats on the low protein diet remained resistant to cancer.

The fact that a low animal protein diet continued to protect, even as carcinogens were increased, surprised me, and I think it is an observation of immense importance. The animal protein he used was casein, found in milk. This promoted all stages of cancer. Significantly, vegetable protein didn't promote cancer. Gerson's clinical observations had been confirmed.

The animal protein-cancer link

This protein-cancer and specifically casein-cancer link was to show up again and this time in a far more dramatic way. Jane Plant, a professor of geochemistry, developed breast cancer in 1987 and by 1993, after five recurrences, it had become terminal and she had with metastatic nodules in her neck. She had tried conventional treatment – surgery, radiotherapy and chemotherapy – but this had failed to halt the progression of her disease.

For some time she had been puzzling over why she had developed breast cancer whilst living a healthy lifestyle with none of the traditional risk factors. At some point she had a light-bulb moment, reasoning that, as breast cancer was very rare in China, perhaps milk products, which were hardly eaten there at that time, were the underlying cause. She removed all milk products from her diet. Because she had cancer nodules, she found herself in a unique position to be able to observe her cancer in a very direct manner. As she changed her diet the tumours melted away and the cancer went into remission.[8] Although this wasn't her last relapse, she lived until 2016, when she died from a blood clot.

Here we have two exceptional observations and a superb piece of scientific investigation, all pointing in the same direction – namely, that milk protein promotes cancer. I have no doubt that this conclusion is basically correct and it is a conclusion that could and should change medical practice.

However there are one or two loose ends to tidy up. Are some animal proteins worse than others? Jane Plant found milk products were especially dangerous; she reasoned that they were high in hormones, especially insulin growth factor 1 (IGF-1), known to promote tumour growth. In fact, the higher the level of IGF-1 in the bloodstream, the higher the risk of cancer, notably prostate cancer.[9] Colin Campbell used a milk protein, casein, for his experiments but noted that similar results had been achieved with other animal proteins. The facts fit with Gerson's observations.

However, before we conclude that animal protein is universally harmful we need to look at another remarkable case history. One man had good reason to believe he had found the perfect diet to cure cancer. His name was William Donald Kelley.

The work of William Kelley

Most great medical discoveries are based on astute observations combined with an ability to understand the significance of these. An example is Alexander Fleming's observation of a mould that unexpectedly stopped the growth of bacteria on the glass dishes he had plated with staphylococcus. He could have regarded this as an annoying contaminant, but Fleming realised that this could be a useful anti-bacterial agent. This, of course, led to the discovery of penicillin.

Kelley was a successful dentist; he had already developed a patent for an orthodontic appliance that didn't require the use of braces. He was unlucky enough to develop pancreatic cancer in his 30s, a cancer which kills over 90% of victims within a year. His cancer had already spread. His situation was dire but he had one small point in his favour. He was able to feel his tumours. He started to note what made them grow and what made them shrink.[10] This was the same method used by Jane Plant several decades later.

Kelley was a methodical observer. He found that his tumours grew when he ate sugar, white flour, red meat and chicken, but shrank when he ate fruit, vegetables and nuts. Carrot juice was especially helpful. He also noted that certain vitamins and minerals helped and some made his tumours worse. Here we have a wonderful combination of astute observation and inspired deduction.

What Kelley, Gerson and Plant had independently discovered was that cancer grows or recedes each time we eat, and this in turn depends on which foods we choose. There is something vaguely comforting about this. Rather than thinking of cancer as an uncontrollable illness, it can be thought of as a disease that we influence, positively or negatively, with every mouthful of food we eat. As we eat food many times a day, this choice has a profound influence on the outcome and to some extent gives us a measure of control. Recent work on the anti-carcinogenic properties of certain foods has made the reasons why this happens much clearer.

Kelley's observations produced dramatic results. To the amazement of his medical colleagues, he started to get better. Here was a great scientist working at breakneck speed, using his own body as a laboratory, and making discovery after discovery.

He was an avid reader and rediscovered the work of John Beard, published in *The Lancet* at the turn of the 20th century (1905). Beard, from his studies of the human embryo, deduced that some stem cells did not differentiate into normal cells and became cancer cells. (A similar theory was later outlined by Professor Wang of Columbia University 100 years later.) Beard noted that in the embryo, stem cells stayed in the 'trophoblastic' state, and in this state, unlike other cells (apart from cancer cells), they did not die. However, the embryo produces pancreatic enzymes at around two months and just at the same time the trophoblastic cells differentiate into normal cells. He proposed that enzymes (enzymes are substances that act as catalysts and speed up biochemical reactions in the body) could be used to successfully treat cancer in humans and animals by reversing this process. It didn't take Kelley long to test this out. He was in for a surprise. When he took the enzymes, the tumours broke down so rapidly he developed a severe toxic reaction. Consulting the standard pharmaceutical manual of the time, the *Merck Manual*, he found that coffee enemas were the mainstay of treatment for toxic crises and he verified that these were effective. They had been used since the time of Florence Nightingale. Recent work has shown that they increase levels of glutathione-S-transferase, a critically important enzyme in detoxification. He continued with his diet, enzymes and coffee enemas and went on to live for another 40 years.

His doctor friends, amazed by his success, sent him other cancer patients to treat. He found the regime worked equally well for these patients and for many other diseases. Over a period of 20 years he went on to treat 455 cancer patients with an overall success rate of 50%. By the standards of the time, these results were exceptional as many of these cancers had been unresponsive to the medical treatment of the time.

Dr Gonzales started using Kelley's methods with great success and had many long-term survivors with pancreatic cancer and various metastatic cancers who have vouched for his methods.[11] Drs Gonzales and Good later did a pilot study using Kelley's treatment. This study was supervised by the National Cancer Institute (NCI). They found patients with pancreatic cancer lived for an average of 17.5 months, which is three times longer than those on standard treatment. This led to a 'phase 3' clinical trial. There were many problems with this trial: the patients having the Gonzales treatment were more seriously ill than controls and the protocol was violated in numerous ways. Not surprisingly, the results showed no benefits and Gonzales felt strongly that his work had been sabotaged.

You might have expected that someone in the cancer industry would have been curious about Kelley's success, especially as pancreatic cancer is generally regarded as untreatable. Unfortunately, as Kelley was to find like many before and after him, the medical profession did not appreciate his discoveries. Instead, they took him to court and banned a book he had written about his findings (*One Answer to Cancer*). They were then, as now, unfamiliar with, and unsympathetic to, the nutritional principles that underpin good health.

As it turned out, the banning of his book proved to be for the best, and this is part of the reason for the detour. Kelley had underestimated the complexity of cancers. Not every cancer sufferer recovered on his regime; as I have mentioned, he had a 50% success rate. Some types of cancer, notably some leukaemias and lymphomas, did not respond to his regime and he failed with some other diseases. Here Kelley, ever the great scientist, set aside his own prejudices and continued to experiment, looking for answers. He went on to find dietary regimes which were effective for those cancers that didn't respond. He found different conditions needed different dietary regimes and worked out that there were 12 metabolic types.

Kelley had found not only that food could cure cancer but that no one diet was satisfactory for everyone. Yet, whilst it was true that no one diet worked for everyone, there was one diet which, far and away, stood out as being the best. This was his original diet, the one he had used to cure himself; this was almost the same diet that had been independently discovered by Gerson. It was highly beneficial in most cases of cancer, especially if combined with enzymes and detoxification.

Different types of meat

This brings us back to the thorny problem of animal protein and cancer. I cannot help thinking back to Weston Price's observations; he pointed out that none of his healthy populations were pure vegetarians. The Native Americans in Alaska were almost pure meat eaters for most of the year and they remained in excellent health with no known cases of cancer. How can we tally this with the first-class observations that meat and dairy promote cancer growth? How did his native Indian population remain in such vigorous health on an almost exclusively meat diet?

I believe the explanation must lie largely in the type of meat they were eating, which was very different from the meat we eat today. In the case of the native Americans, it was wild meat, mainly from moose. They were also careful about which parts they ate, preferring the organ meat. They recognised that certain parts of the animal, such as the adrenal glands, were especially nutritious (we now know, the adrenal glands are very rich in vitamin C) and they made sure they ate those. As for the muscle meat, the part we normally eat today, they had little regard for it. This they gave to their dogs. Like many native populations, they had extensive knowledge of what they needed to do to stay healthy. We will return to the issue of quality of meat and cancer later.

The optimum diet

So what is the optimum diet? The clues are everywhere: in survivors, in healthy populations and in long–lived races. It is a completely natural diet very high in vegetables and, to a lesser extent, fruit. It contains little meat and dairy (except the highest quality meat, such as organic, grass-fed meat and organ meat), good quality fish, little or no sugar, little or no refined carbohydrates and little or no processed food. I suspect the pure plant diets may be the most effective in cancer and the modified Paleolithic diet preferable in autoimmune diseases.

Patients using food as medicine

An ever-increasing number of books have been published by people describing how they cured themselves from major illnesses. Bernadette Bohan has described[4] how she was diagnosed with a lymphoma at the age of 37 and then 12 years later developed breast cancer. She began to wonder why this should have happened to her, not once but twice, and at such a young age. Like many survivors, she decided to learn all she could about health. Once she started to look, she found a wealth of information on the healing properties of a natural diet. She found this information was not particularly complicated or incomprehensible.

She drastically changed her diet, juicing with organic fruit and vegetables, using high-nutrient foods such as sprouting seeds, and making the bulk of her diet fruit, vegetables and whole grains, cutting out foods like meat, milk and sugar. People would remark on how well she looked for someone who had suffered from cancer twice and also undergone chemotherapy and radiotherapy. She observed that as she had changed her diet, her energy level rose, old arthritic symptoms in her arms disappeared and her eyesight became sharper.

So many clues to the cure of cancer lie in the stories of survivors. In Foster's study of 200 people with cancer mentioned above,[2] 87.5% had made major changes in their diet. Nearly 80% of those that had made dietary changes had excluded meat and sugar, and also tobacco. More than 50% had cut out eggs, fish, milk, white flour, tea, coffee, chocolate and oils. Over 80% ate vegetables, notably broccoli, leeks, cauliflower, onions, legumes, carrots and Brussels sprouts, and a high proportion (over 70%) ate certain fruits (grapes, apples, pears, apricots). Also popular were fruit and vegetable juices (carrot juice was used by 53%), wholegrains, alfalfa sprouts, cantaloupes, tomatoes and lentils. Basically, it is impossible not to conclude that these patients successfully reversed their cancers by changing their diet.

We now have a fairly solid body of data on what constitutes the best healing diet for cancer and in addition have strong pointers to the diet most likely to heal an auto-immune disease. However, acceptance by the medical profession is slow. Why should this be? I think, for most doctors, the whole idea of treating disease with food still seems outlandish. So the accumulating evidence supporting this mode of healing continues to be ignored.

On the other hand, science is catching up with these pioneers. There are now more and more research studies verifying the powerful healing effects, including anti-cancer properties, of many foods. This has not been lost on pharmaceutical companies who have been busily trying to develop patented drugs based on these substances. Let's now look at this evidence.

Cancer: the protective effect of fruit and vegetables

There are over 200 epidemiological studies on the link between fruit and vegetables and cancer. The majority (70%) show that the more fruit and vegetables eaten, the less cancer of virtually every type. These studies include 20 'cohort studies', which are generally the more reliable. These show that the higher the fruit and vegetable consumption, the lower the risk of cancer. I will give a flavour of the research.

A case-control study found those who had 28 or more servings of vegetables per week reduced their risk of prostate cancer by 65% (compared with those having fewer than 14 helpings per week).[12]

The Nurse's Health Study, following 88,410 women for 14 years, found that those who ate over six servings of fruit and vegetables daily had a lower risk of non-Hodgkin's lymphoma compared with those who ate fewer than three.[13] A study by Giovannucci et al found those women with the lowest intake of fruit and vegetables had the highest risk of colorectal cancer.[14]

Let's look at breast cancer specifically, for here we find a range of fruit and vegetables reduced risk. These have included:

- mushrooms – Chinese women, half of whom had previously suffered from breast cancer, who ate 10 grams of button mushrooms daily, were 64% less likely to develop breast cancer[15]
- carotenoids, such as are found in carrots, sweet potatoes, tomatoes, leafy greens – those with highest levels had an 18-28% reduced risk compared with those who ate the lowest levels[16]
- high total consumption of fruit and vegetables – those consuming more than 5.5 servings compared had an 11% reduced risk compared with those consuming 2.5 servings or less, with those eating more yellow/orange and cruciferous vegetables having the greatest benefit[17]
- garlic and onion – Puerto Rican women eating high to moderate amounts of garlic and onion reduced their risk by nearly half compared with those with low consumption[18]
- flaxseed – those who had flaxseed at least weekly reduced their risk of breast cancer by 18%.[19]

These foods all made a difference and we might add that fish oils are associated with a 32% reduced risk of breast cancer.[20] I suspect these foods combined make an even greater difference.

However, not all studies found benefits, including a study of cancer and fruit and vegetable intake in Sweden.[21] Unfortunately, the fruit and vegetables we eat most often may not be the most effective in combating cancer. Our most popular choices include potatoes, tomatoes, carrots and lettuce. As we shall see, having a range of fruit and vegetables, eating them in sufficient quantity and having those which have the most powerful properties are all strategies that count.

A remarkable study by Boivin et al tested extracts of a variety of vegetables against different cancer cell cultures.[22] Although different cancer cultures responded differently to different vegetables, a definite pattern emerged. Two families of vegetables had the most powerful anti-cancer effects. The first was the cruciferous vegetables. These include (and I will put these in a rough order starting with those with the strongest anti-cancer effects): Brussels sprouts, broccoli, cabbage, kale, cauliflower and collard greens. The second group with powerful anti-cancer properties was the allium family. This includes (again in rough order of anti-cancer potency) garlic, leeks, spring onions, onions, chives and scallions. Other vegetables not in these two groups but with strong anticancer properties, are celery and beetroot.

However, this study looked only at vegetables. Probably the foods with the most powerful anti-cancer properties of all are mushrooms, which were not tested and are not, strictly speaking, vegetables. Another strong contender is flaxseed, as mentioned in the study above. Many fruits, nuts, herbs and spices (notably turmeric) also have strong anti-cancer effects. Most of these foods work synergistically, acting against cancer at multiple points along the cancer pathway, blocking its development.

Why do fruits and vegetables protect against cancer? It is probably because of the nutrients within them. These often have strange sounding names, such as isothiocyanates, indoles, phenols, carotenoids and limonene. We will look at these later (see pages 47, 76).

Cancer: the protective effect of cruciferous vegetables

Cruciferous vegetables (cabbage, broccoli, Brussels sprouts, kale and cauliflower) have powerful anti-cancer effects as noted. Over 50 studies have been done on these vegetables and the vast majority of them have found a reduced risk of a variety of cancers, including those of breast, bladder, stomach, colorectal and prostate.

For instance, a Chinese study found that women who ate the most cruciferous vegetables had half the rate of breast cancer compared with those who ate the least.[23] A multi-ethnic study found an inverse relationship between the intake of cruciferous vegetables, legumes and yellow-orange vegetables and prostate cancer risk.[24] Another study found that those who had three or more servings per week of cruciferous vegetables compared to those who had less than one serving a week reduced their risk of prostate cancer by 59%.[12] A study comparing myeloma patients with controls found those who ate cruciferous vegetables most frequently reduced their risk of myeloma by 30%.[25]

Eating cruciferous vegetables releases powerful compounds, including sulphoraphones. These cause cancer-cell death and aid the removal of carcinogens from the body. Other important compounds in these vegetables include indole-3-carbinol and phenethyl isothiocyanate (PEITC). These protect laboratory animals from cancer. Glucosinolates present in cruciferous vegetables switch on genes that reduce toxicity. There may well be other cancer-fighting compounds yet to be discovered within this small group of vegetables.

Cancer: the protective effect of nutrients

Again and again research has confirmed that fruit and vegetables and other natural foods and nutrients protect against cancer. Examples include the inverse relationship with vitamin D and cancers of the lung, thyroid, breast, brain, oesophagus and stomach, and with melanoma. A Japanese study found those with the lowest vitamin D levels had a 22% increased risk of cancers compared with those with the highest levels.[26] Similarly, a 10-year study found elderly people with higher levels of carotenoids had a lower risk of cancer and a lower overall mortality.[27]

For those with cancer, the same is true: nutrients protect. Mice with mammary tumours were found to survive longer and have fewer metastases after being given fish oils, and the tumours were 50% smaller.[28] Vitamin C has been known to be toxic to tumour cells in vitro (that is, in lab settings) from 1969,[29] and high-dose vitamin C produces hydrogen peroxide which is selectively toxic to cancer cells apart from those with high levels of catalyse.[30] Dr Lilian Thompson at the University of Toronto has demonstrated that 25 grams of flaxseeds daily reduced the growth of breast tumours. Breast cancer patients with high or moderate concentrations of carotenoids in their plasma have been found to have 23% less risk of recurrence of their breast cancer compared with those with low concentrations.[31]

So what is the message of all these studies? There is an unmistakable pattern to be found: the more nutrients you have on board, the less likely you are to get cancer, and the higher the levels the greater the protection. And the way to achieve this is mainly through eating fruit and vegetables. This is something many survivors have understood intuitively. But there is more. Science is showing us exactly why these nutrients in fruit and vegetables protect us.

There are an astonishing 5000-10,000 phytochemicals within

food, including 4000 'polyphenols'. Many of these have disease-fighting properties, but it is safe to assume that many of the benefits have yet to be discovered by science.

Here are some of the known benefits and how foods and nutrients affect different stages of cancer:

- **Cause cancer-cell death (apoptosis):** vitamin D, dandelion root extract, fucoidan from brown seaweed, bee propolis, phytolexins from many plants, anthocyanins in purple plants such as beetroot, piceatannol (breakdown product of resveratrol), most spices, cruciferous vegetables, garlic, onions, berries, grapes, citrus fruit.
- **Protect DNA:** Resveratrol (in red wine and grape juice and many other plant sources), olecanthol from olive oil, L cysteine (in garlic, kelp and eggs), bee propolis, polyphenols.
- **Inhibit cancer-cell growth:** Carotenoids, indole-3 carbinol from cruciferous vegetables, beta-carotene, ellagic acid (in raspberries, strawberries, walnuts and hazelnuts), green tea, turmeric, garlic, berries, citrus fruits, tomatoes, omega-3 fats, dark chocolate.
- **Reduce pre-cancerous lesions:** Procyanadins in apples
- **Block metastasis:** Pomegranate juice, blueberries, curcumin (in turmeric), sulphorophanes (in cruciferous vegetables and sprouting seeds).
- **Protect the p53 DNA repair gene:** Resveratrol, ellagic acid in nuts and berries.
- **Lower inflammation:** Resveratrol, curcumin, piperine from black pepper, olecanthol from olive oil, epigallocatechin gallate (EGCG) in green tea, tocotrienols (a component of vitamin E), sulphorophanes.
- **Reduce blood vessel formation by tumours (angiogenesis):** Curcumin, piperine, indole-3-carbinol, fucoidan (found in many species of brown seaweed), green tea, turmeric, grapes and berries, omega-3 fats.

- **Improve cellular communication:** Carotenoids, in many fruit and vegetables.
- **Reduce the effect of oestrogen and neutralise the breakdown products of oestrogen:** Indole-3-carbinol (in cruciferous vegetables).
- **Increase natural killer (NK) cells:** Beta-carotene (in many fruit and vegetables, especially those with orange pigment).
- **Restrict IGF-1:** EGCG (in green tea).
- **Block key enzymes in cancer cells:** Capsaicin from chillies, tocotrienols (compounds within vitamin E).

Note these foods come in a variety of colours, sometimes called the 'rainbow diet', and they all act at different stages of the cancer pathway. What strikes me about this research is the wide range of actions plant compounds have against cancer. None of this was known 10 to 20 years ago and we can be sure there will be many more discoveries in this field in coming decades.

There are some key points which are worth understanding. Most of these compounds are unstable and break down rapidly. This means they are difficult to produce as supplements or medicines but work perfectly within food. Ideally, we need to eat some of them with each meal.

Crucially, the effects are reversible: if we stop eating them then we lose the protection. We also know that they work synergistically, so the more the better. For instance, neither EGCG (in green tea) nor curcumin (in turmeric), on its own can kill cancer cells in cultures but when combined they do so. Similarly, curcumin is poorly absorbed but once piperine (from black pepper) is added, absorption is increased 1000-fold. (Note spices have some of the highest concentrations of antioxidants of any foods).

There is another thing we need to know. Which foods have the strongest effect against cancer:

Foods that prevent cancer roughly in order of importance

Mushrooms

Garlic, onion, leeks

Cruciferous vegetables

Turmeric

Flaxseeds

Green tea

Beetroot

Berries

Most nuts

Most spices

Citrus fruit

Seaweed

Ginger

Range of coloured fruit and vegetables

Pomegranate juice

Tomatoes

Omega-3 fats

Foods that promote cancer roughly in order of importance

Milk (breast, prostate, ovarian)

Sugar (all cancers?)

Refined grains[32] (oral cavity, oesophagus, stomach, colorectal, thyroid, larynx)

Meat containing nitrites, such as hot dogs, pepperoni, ham, bacon (colon cancer, leukaemia)

Trans fats (see page 94)[33] (breast, prostate, colon & pancreatic cancer)

Pickled meat and pickled fish (stomach cancer)

Lactose (milk sugar)[34] (ovarian cancer)

Barbecued meat/burnt meat

Alcohol (excess)

Monosodium glutamate[35, 36]

There are some undoubted stars in the plant world. Perhaps the most powerful are mushrooms (notably oyster mushrooms). These can stop cancer in animals and shrink tumours. Medicinal mushrooms are widely used in cancer treatments in Japan and Asia. Dr Kunno from the New York Medical Center found maitake mushrooms combined with vitamin C were highly effective in killing cancer cells and could reduce cancer cell growth by 90% in cancer cell cultures, while a study using a maitake extract in patients with advanced cancer showed a significant improvement in 74% with breast cancer, 67% with lung cancer and 47% with liver cancer.[37] Numerous other bioactive compounds from a variety of mushrooms have been shown to kill cancer cells in cultures.[38] Other research has found that lentinon extracts from shiitake mushrooms can increase survival, enhance cancer cell death and reduce recurrences in hepatocellular carcinoma.[39] The compound active hexose correlated compound (AHCC) is a mushroom-based product used in over 700 hospitals in Japan, has been subjected to multiple clinical studies and shown dramatic increases in survival in many cancer patients, doubling survival time in advanced liver cancer.

A similar mushroom-based product called Biobran has remarkable properties. It is known to increase natural killer (NK) cells, and there are dozens of anecdotal accounts of recovery from cancer, including metastatic cancer, after using this product.[40]

However, mushrooms are far from being the only foods with powerful anti-cancer effects, as the list shows. Others include turmeric, garlic, cruciferous vegetables, green tea, brightly coloured fruit and vegetables, seaweed, omega-3 fats and citrus fruits. The data are strong on all of these. I would anticipate that these will be beneficial in many other chronic illnesses also. However, variety is important. With cancer, what is needed is protection at multiple stages of the cancer pathway and compounds that act synergistically.

Conclusion

To sum up, we know for certain that fruit and vegetables prevent cancer, we have identified many of the nutrients within them which have activity against cancer and we understand how they block various stages of the cancer pathway. All this powerfully validates those cancer therapies, such as the Gerson regime, which have advocated using these foods as medicine, and attests to the inherent logic behind their methodology. All this reinforces the old saying, 'garbage in, garbage out'. In other words, you can't produce the highest level of healing without the highest quality of building blocks. Survivors, as ever, have been ahead of their time on understanding this.

It is surely time to look again at the potential of food, both to prevent and to cure disease. The methods used by Gerson and Kelley are inexpensive compared with today's cancer treatments and would not be hard to put into practice. It would be interesting to speculate about how much more progress could have been made in the fight against cancer if the medical profession had been open to these methods from the beginning.

Chapter 2

Food and health

There is no way you can heal your body if you don't feed it useful healing foods.

Dr Patrick Kingsley

Food and disease

Whether we look at Weston Price's isolated populations (page 27), McCarrison's rats (page 30), exceptionally long-lived peoples (page 31) or those patients who have successfully used food to treat cancer, the same conclusions stare us in the face. Food has a profound impact on health.

The massive Global Burden of Disease, Injuries and Risk Factors project emphasises this. It investigated the causes of disease and premature death between 1990 and 2013 in 188 countries and found that poor diet was the single biggest factor shortening life, on average by 9.7 years. Smoking was in fourth place, shortening life, on average by 5.8 years.[1]

At a time when we have been searching, largely unsuccessfully, for more than half a century for treatments for chronic diseases and have spent over a trillion dollars in a largely fruitless search for a cure for cancer, this is information of immense importance. As we have seen, diet underpins health more than any other single factor. So, if you are seriously ill, food is one of the first places to look for an answer.

Health problems start in the kitchen

People often say to me that you can't win with food. They tell me there is so much conflicting information you might as well give up. However, food is not really that complicated. It is true there is much misinformation, but a good consensus does exist on which foods are healthy and which are not.

This chapter is divided into three main sections:
1. Foods to avoid, due to their health-damaging properties
2. Foods that have become hazardous, mainly due to modern farming practices
3. Healthy foods.

This classification simplifies healthy eating. Anyone with a major disease should aim to eat 75-80% of their foods from the last category. Even for the rest of us, the majority of our food should come from this group.

Foods to avoid

It is astonishing that, for most of us, 55% of our calories come from just three food sources: sugar, refined carbohydrates and processed vegetable oils. Equally astonishing is the fact that these same foods have absolutely no nutritional value, containing only 'empty calories'. We are talking about over half the foods we eat. Not only are they largely devoid of vitamins, minerals and essential fats, but, as we shall see, they can positively damage our health.

For anyone with a serious illness, these are the foods that it would make sense to avoid. As for the rest of us, we should keep the quantities low.

Sugar

Weston Price's 'healthy communities' had no added sugar and

long-lived communities eat very little.

William Kelley (page 37) observed his tumours grew after eating sugar, and white sugar was deliberately avoided by 79.5% of Foster's cancer survivors (page 42). They believed this would help cure their cancers. But does research back them up?

Firstly, sugar has been shown to depress immunity. It does so rapidly and dramatically.

Two studies of young adults looked at their ability to deal with bacteria after ingesting sugar, one after 100 grams of sugar,[2] and the other after 24 ounces of soda (66 grams sugar).[3] There was rapid suppression to 50% of normal in both cases, with a peak at two hours in the first case and 45 minutes in the second. The effect lasted five hours.

Studies on rats have again shown a 50% drop in the ability to produce antibodies on a diet containing as little as 10% sugar, with greater amounts of sugar causing a proportionally greater drop in immune function.[4]

However, of even more interest is the link between sugar and cancer. In 1931, Otto Warburg won the Nobel Prize in Physiology for discovering that cancer cells feed off sugar using a mechanism called 'anaerobic glycolysis'. Cancer cells require three to five times more sugar than normal cells.[5]

Could sugar make us more prone to cancer? A prospective study in Sweden found people with higher glucose levels were more prone to later developing melanoma and cancers of the pancreas, endometrium (womb lining) and urinary tract, and this effect was independent of obesity.[6] A review of 21 western countries found higher sugar intake was linked to higher rates of breast cancer.[7]

Other correlations make the case stronger. Insulin and IGF-1 are growth hormones which stimulate cancer growth and can switch off the mechanism for cancer cell death (apoptosis). These hormones rise as sugar increases in the diet.

If sugar is important in cancer, we might expect to see an

increased cancer risk with higher levels of insulin and IGF-1. This is exactly what we do find. There is both an increased risk of cancer[8,9,10] and a worse prognosis.[11, 12]

However, the 'acid test' is what happens to cancer on reducing sugar intake. In a landmark study, mice were inoculated with cancer cells and given diets with varying amounts of sugar. The results were unequivocal. Those on a low-sugar diet were 16 times more likely to survive than those on a high-sugar diet. In mice on a high-sugar diet, 16 out of 24 died; of those on a medium-sugar diet, eight died; but of those on a low-sugar diet, only one died.[13] These results have huge relevance to cancer treatment.

Does this happen in humans? Clearly the same experiment would be unethical. One way around this is to look at cancer patients on treatments which artificially increase glucose levels. These include treatments using steroids (typically dexamethasone) and these are indeed associated with a poorer prognosis.[14, 15] We also know that depriving cancer cell cultures of sugar triggers apoptosis.[16, 17] The implication is crystal clear: whether you have cancer or you just want to prevent it, sugar is something to avoid. Foster's survivors were ahead of the game.

Sugar plays a part in other major diseases, most obviously diabetes but also cardiovascular disease. In one study, those who consumed more than 21% of their calories in the form of sugar were found to have twice the cardiovascular mortality of those who obtained only 7% or less of their calories that way.[18] (The National Diet and Nutrition Survey (see page 380) found the average consumption for UK adults was 12.1%.) Most of the diets used by survivors from diseases other than cancer have been very low in sugar.

It stands to reason that one of the most basic steps in improving health is reducing sugar. However, when I talk to people about sugar, they tell me that they don't eat it. 'I don't eat cakes and biscuits, and I don't even put sugar in my tea,' they say. And this is the crux of the problem. Over half of the sugar we eat is hidden sugar; over 80% of foods in a supermarket have added sugar.

In fact, in the last 20 years the amount of sugar we buy as sugar has gone down, but the amount we consume has risen sharply, due to hidden sugar. Some foods we eat, such as soups and breads, have double the amount of sugar they once had. The average sugar intake in the UK is nearly 22 teaspoonfuls a day.

Many people are surprised by how much sugar is found in everyday foods. A single cola drink can contain 10 teaspoonfuls of sugar, an energy drink 15 to 19 teaspoonfuls, a fruit juice up to 14 teaspoonfuls, a portion of pizza 8 teaspoonfuls, a packet of couscous 6 to 10 teaspoonfuls, a serving of sauce 1 to 3 teaspoonfuls, baked beans 6 teaspoonfuls, bran flakes 3 teaspoonfuls and a typical 150-gram tub of yoghurt can have 3 to 7 teaspoonfuls.

Most breakfast cereals, including mueslis and those advertised as being 'healthy', are laced with sugar. Foods labelled as 'low-fat' (see page 93) are major culprits. Sugar is contained in almost anything that comes in a packet or tin. The average ready-meal may contain eight different types of sugar and be up to 15% sugar in total. Sugar can be found in savoury foods such as sauces, canned fish and canned vegetables. It's also added to meat. Fruit concentrates are added to baby foods, giving babies a taste for sugar.

The first step in dealing with sugar is recognising it. Table sugar is called sucrose, but sugar has many forms and names, including: glucose, maltose (in beer), lactose (in milk), dextrose (glucose in corn), fructose (fruit sugar), molasses, rice syrup and polydextrose.

Though our bodies have hardly had time to adjust to so many sugars, we are now being exposed to novel sugars, such as sugar alcohols, developed from the breaking down of starches; these include sorbitol, maltitol and mannitol. These can be converted by enzymes to maltodextrins, which are added to soft drinks and baby foods. Anything that ends in 'ose' or 'ol' is likely to be a sugar.

Read labels: any food in a packet or tin will give the sugar content per 100 grams. If you remember that one level teaspoonful is 4 grams you can soon work out if it is high in sugar or not.

Table sugar is 50% glucose and 50% fructose. High-fructose corn syrup (found in many soft drinks and most processed foods) may be the most dangerous sugar of all, because of its higher fructose content (55%). Unlike other sugars, fructose is largely broken down by the liver but once the liver becomes overloaded it starts to malfunction. (Fructose from fruit is less harmful because the fibre slows absorption and it contains other beneficial nutrients).

In summary, sugar is the first food to cut out of your diet if you want your health to improve. Start enjoying the taste of food without sugar. And enjoy the extra vitality.

Refined carbohydrates

Refined grains are not eaten by healthy and long-lived communities but are some of the foods that tragically destroyed the health of Weston Price's isolated communities once they were introduced to the western diet (page 29). Previously these groups had used freshly-ground grains for their bread and in their food.

Kelley noticed his tumours grew after eating white flour and 65.6% of Foster's survivors removed white flour from their diets. Does science back them up?

Levi found that the third of the population who ate the most refined grains had nearly double the rate of cancers of the oral cavity and pharynx, nearly four times the risk of oesophageal cancer and a four-fold risk of cancer of the larynx (compared with the third eating the least). In contrast, whole grains reduced the overall risk of these cancers by 50%.[19] An Italian study looked at refined grain in the form of cereal, pasta and rice. They compared the third of the group who ate the most refined cereals with the third who took the least. Again they found a higher incidence of cancers of the pharynx, oesophagus and larynx (50% increase) but also an increase in cancers of the stomach (50% increase), colon (30% increase) and thyroid (100% increase).[20] The authors reviewed the literature and noted wholegrains were protective against a variety of cancers whereas refined cereals increased the risk of other cancers (breast, endometrium and lung).

It seems the instinct of Foster's survivors was right. And it's not just cancer. A meta-analysis of 21 studies found whole grains reduced the incidence of cancer, type 2 diabetes, cardiovascular disease and obesity.[21] But again, what we need to know is whether reducing or stopping refined grains helps recovery from cancer. The following studies shed some light on this.

'NOP mice' have a genetic mutation which gives them a very high probability of developing breast cancer. Researchers looked at what happened when they were given either a low-carbohydrate diet or a diet similar to the typical Western diet (with a similar mix of carbohydrates). The odds of these mice getting cancer turned out to be dramatically different. On the diet equivalent to the standard Western diet, about half of the mice developed cancer within a year, but only 15% of those on the low-carbohydrate diet developed cancer. Their chances of developing cancer were reduced to less than a third of expected. However, perhaps more importantly, even when they did develop cancer, they were far less likely to die from it. Of the low-carbohydrate group, the death rate was 27% compared with 70% in the group on a standard diet (the mortality was again a third of that expected).[22]

There is more. Another study on mice inoculated with prostate tumour found those given a diet high in refined carbohydrates had nearly twice the tumour growth.[23]

What, however, do we mean by 'refined carbohydrates'? This category includes white or bleached flour products, such as bread, pasta and cereals, white rice and crisps.

Why should consuming these foods make a difference and why should wholegrains be better for our health? The reason is that wholegrain and wholemeal products still contain the germ layer of the wheat, where nearly all the vitamins, minerals and essential fats are stored. Another benefit is that it contains health-protective fibre.

Refining grains has been very popular with the food industry as it gives them a long shelf-life, which allows easy transport and storage. However, once the grains become devitalised, even insects won't touch them.

Consumption of refined carbohydrates, because of the speed with which they break down into sugar, leads to insulin release, higher levels of circulating insulin and ultimately insulin resistance. This leads to the secretion of insulin-like growth factors (IGF-1). These can promote cancer growth as we noted with sugar.

How much do we eat? In the US, the National Health and Nutritional Examination Survey determined that the amount of calories which come from low-quality carbohydrates went down from 45.1% to 41.8% between 1999 and 2016,[24] but they remain a major part of our diet.

There are other problems. Over 98% of bread produced today is made by the Chorleywood process; this includes most wholegrain bread. The process uses a lot of poor-quality ingredients: hydrogenated fats, additives, sugar and higher amounts of yeast.

Most breakfast cereals consist of refined carbohydrates. Nearly all contain large amounts of sugar and they are typically high in salt. Even without the added sugar, the industrial processing necessary to produce cereals from grain also produces yet another hazard, acrylamide, a carcinogen linked with cancer of the ovary and uterus. Any process where grains are subjected to high temperatures, such as in the making of crisps or cereals, will produce this carcinogen. It is even present in many baby foods and there is no safe limit. The US Environmental Protection Agency has labelled acrylamide as an extremely hazardous substance and the European Commission was set to limit its level in food but backed down after strong lobbying by the food industry.

Gluten

For anyone with a serious disease there is another important reason why wheat could be an issue. Originally, wheat contained 10% gluten; now, following a switch to mutated forms of dwarf wheat in the last 50 years, the gluten content has risen to 80%. During this time, the incidence of coeliac disease in the UK has shown a steep rise (from one in 8000 in 1950 to one in 100 today); this is likely due to changes in wheat and in bread-making. This is no small matter. For instance, 54% of neurological patients have antibodies to gluten compared with 12% of healthy people, and 16% of these previously undiagnosed neurological patients[25] have been found to have coeliac disease after gut biopsies. For many patients with neurological or autoimmune diseases, removing gluten can be an essential step in their recovery.

Refined carbohydrates – summary

In summary, refined carbohydrates are bad for health. Read the labels, look for wholegrain (this means at least 30% of the wheat must be wholegrain and it must have more wholegrain than refined grain within it) for your bread and pasta. With rice, use long grain rather than short grain. Avoid most breakfast cereals. The colour of the bread is a poor guide: brown bread, granary and multi-grain bread are not wholegrain breads; they contain refined flour, often with colourings such as E150 added. Grains like barley, millet, spelt and rye tend to be less refined.

Hydrogenated fats

These fats were absent in Price's healthy communities and are largely absent in long-lived cultures. Foster's survivor's lived on natural foods so their intake would have been close to zero.

Hydrogenated fats are formed whenever fats are heated to high temperatures, such as in the processing of cooking oils and margarines. It is theoretically possible to produce them by prolonged frying at high temperatures, either by stir-frying or deep-fat frying. Frying produces acrylamide and has been found to increase the risk of cancer in some (but not all) studies.[26]

Professor Willett estimated these fats were responsible for 30,000 premature deaths annually in the USA.[27] The Harvard School of Public Health found hydrogenated fats doubled the rate of heart attacks. A further study suggested they were responsible for 6-19% of cardiovascular deaths in USA and 2700 deaths annually in the UK.[28] Animal studies show they cause a variety of problems, including reduced sperm counts, lowered immunity and increased complications in pregnancy.[29, 30] They are thought to be a cause of macular degeneration.

They are banned in some countries, and from baby foods in the UK. Some stores, including Waitrose and Marks & Spencer, have banned them from their own brands.

Key sources of hydrogenated fats are, as I have said, cooking oils and margarines, but they can also be found in a wide range of processed foods, such as biscuits, mayonnaise, pastries, pies, crisps and cakes. Any food sitting on a supermarket shelf with a long shelf-life is likely to contain hydrogenated fats. These fats are not always easy to spot. Look for the following on labels: 'trans fats', 'partially hydrogenated vegetable oils', 'shortenings' or 'vegetable fats' – these are all hydrogenated fats.

Emulsifiers (substances used to combine oil-based and water-base foods) typically contain mono- and diglycerides, which are forms of trans fats, but products containing these can be labelled as being free of trans fats. The clue would be 'partially' or 'fully hydrogenated oils' on the list of ingredients, the higher up on the list the greater the amount.

When cooking, butter, lard, animal fats, coconut and nut oils are a good choice. Unrefined oils have lower smoke points and are not suitable. Hydrogenation can occur at around 176°C (350°F). Frying can reach this temperature and can produce hydrogenation if prolonged. Olive oil has a smoking point of 160°C (320°F) depending on the type (light olive oil has a higher smoke point then extra virgin olive oil), so hydrogenation can occur. Refined vegetable oils have higher smoke points but have been preheated to high temperatures in their manufacture so already contain hydrogenated fats. Always avoid re-using cooking oils.

Today many manufacturers have recognised the public concern about hydrogenated fats and are taking them out of some foods. However, this is not quite such good news as it seems. Hydrogenated fats are being replaced by 'fractionated fats', created by a process which also involves heating and altering oils and fats. It may be safer than hydrogenation but could turn out to be just as bad. Only time will tell. So, I think the answer is to be wary of all processed fats.

And here it makes sense to include a word about saturated fats. Over the last few decades, saturated fats have had a bad press and were thought to be a factor in heart disease. Two major meta-analyses have concluded that they do not cause heart disease[31, 32] and, in contrast, one of these studies found that hydrogenated fats increased both cardiovascular and all-cause mortality.[32]

In summary, the real danger comes from processed or hydrogenated fats, not from saturated fats, and the lesson here is the more unnatural and processed the food, the more our health suffers.

An added problem is that sugar, refined carbohydrates and hydrogenated fats are commonly combined in processed foods.

Processed and ultra-processed fats, oils and starches

Few people are aware that these highly processed ingredients exist in food. Even fewer are aware of the huge increase of these substances in the modern diet. These materials have never been present in the diet of healthy populations and have been avoided by survivors.

Where do they come from? About one-third of wheat, 50% of corn and about 80-90% of soya is grown to feed livestock. Altogether 80% of the soya and most of the corn is genetically modified. These plants are broken down by industrial processes using high temperatures and chemicals producing protein, such as soya meal, for animal feed and by-products which are added to processed foods. These include processed starches (especially from corn) and processed fats and oils (especially from soya and rapeseed). These by-products can be labelled as hydrolysed vegetable protein, vegetable oil, soya flour, soya protein isolates, emulsifiers and plant sterols. They find their way into processed foods (60% of processed foods contain soya), sausages, soups and pet food.

What is staggering is the increase of these substances in the food supply. Soya oil was responsible for 0.02% of calories in the US in 1909, but by 2000 this figure had sky-rocketed to 20% of all calories consumed.[33] In the UK, soya, corn and sunflower oils increased from 1% in the 1960s to 5% by 2000.[33]

Their dangers are largely unknown but research in mice is worrying. Soya oil caused 25% more weight gain than coconut oil and 9% more than fructose (fructose is already under intense scrutiny as it is thought to be a major contributor to the obesity epidemic). Soya oil also caused fatty liver, metabolic syndrome and diabetes in the mice.[34]

These foods, with their low nutritional value and long shelf-life, are a new and worrying addition to our diet. My own opinion is that they should not be there. The long-term effect on our health is unknown, but we can be virtually certain it will be negative or at the very least rob us of our vitality.

Processed foods and ready meals

Unfortunately, with food, what you don't understand can harm you. Few people look through labels on packaged foods or ready-meals. If they did, they would see many ingredients with strange-sounding or incomprehensible names. Most of these foods contain a combination of different sugars, processed fats, salt, starches and additives such as thickeners, stabilisers, separators, sweeteners, artificial flavourings, artificial colourings and preservatives. Virtually all of these are health-damaging, and who knows what effect they have in combination. Recent studies have found those who had eaten the most processed food had higher rates of cancer.[35]

Anyone with a serious disease should avoid processed foods with their unwholesome combinations of sugars, chemicals and processed fats, starches and oils. If you see foods with a list of ingredients that include chemical names or names you've never heard of, then leave them on the shelf.

Preservatives, additives and chemicals in food

Long-lived communities simply don't use preservatives and additives. Now the average person eating a western diet consumes nearly 5.5 kg (12 lb) of additives each year. There has been considerable debate about the safety of these chemicals. The food industry considers them safe, but none has been tested for chronic health effects or for synergistic effects (the additive effect of a cocktail of chemicals), so this bland reassurance is not worth the paper it is written on.

Numerous studies have indicated that combinations of chemicals amplify toxicity. Worse still, toxic effects occur for mixtures of chemicals even when all the individual compounds are kept at safe levels. In one study, rats were given three commonly used additives. When only one was used there was no effect. When two were combined the rats stopped growing, lost their hair and developed diarrhoea. When all three were used, the rats developed rapid weight loss and all died within two weeks.[36] To me, this sort of experiment tells us two things: firstly, we know next to nothing about the safety of these chemicals, especially in combination; secondly, we should not be using them in the first place.

Recent studies have shown that additives can cause hyperactivity, something long-suspected by parents but denied by the food industry.[37]

Pesticides

Pesticides are designed to kill insects by interfering with an enzyme essential for nerve function. However, these substances are unable to discriminate between the nervous systems of insects and humans. During the time they have been in use, diseases of the nervous system have shown some of the steepest rises of all illnesses. In the last few decades, Parkinson's disease and Alzheimer's disease have shown major increases (by several hundred per cent).[38] In children, there have been similar sharp rises in hyperactivity (ADHD), autism and learning disabilities. Over 100 published studies have found pesticides to be a causative factor in Parkinson's disease. As a recent meta-analysis found, they increased the risk by 46%.[39]

Pesticides accumulate in the body over time. Their effect is long-term, insidious and unpredictable. The problem with these substances is that no one has tested them for long-term safety, no one has looked at their potential to produce chronic disease and no one has tested their safety in combination. As with additives, we know virtually nothing about their safety.

Fifty pesticides are known to be carcinogenic and 60 are known to cause birth defects. Most people associate pesticide exposure with fruit and vegetables, but in reality residues are greater in milk, meat and fish, with the highest residues in farmed salmon (see Chapter 8).

Levels of pesticides are greater in raw than in cooked products.[40]

We ingest an average of 22 grams of pesticides a year; these poison our nervous systems and some of them will never leave our bodies. To my way of thinking, adding known poisons to our food and soil, when we have no knowledge of their long-term dangers, can only be described as madness. The best way to avoid this problem is to buy organic wherever possible.

It is true that the positive effect we get from all the phytonutrients and vitamins found in fruit and vegetables outweighs the negative effect from the pesticides. However, this in no way alters the fact that it makes no sense to deliberately poison our food.

Foods to avoid – conclusion

To sum up, sugar, refined carbohydrates, processed fats, processed starches, chemical food additives and pesticides are all substances that are both toxic and without virtually any nutritional value. They are bad news, especially to those who already have a serious disease.

Out of this hazardous group, two stand out as being especially problematical, mainly because they are so widely used in our foods but also because of their dangers. These are hydrogenated fats and high-fructose corn syrup. They are best avoided wherever and whenever possible and should have no place in anyone's diet.

Foods that have become less healthy

The danger in this group of foods that have become less healthy is less obvious. These foods, once regarded as healthy, have undergone a great change in how they are produced. This group includes meat and dairy products.

William Kelley (page 37), Max Gerson (page 33) and Jane Plant (page 35) all independently made the same astute observation: cancers increase in size after eating meat and milk. Professor Colin Campbell provided more evidence on the link between animal protein and cancer.

Red meat

Meat was deliberately avoided by 79.5% of Foster's cancer survivors (page 42). Both Gerson and Kelley noted eating meat increased the size of tumours. Most long-lived and healthy populations love meat but eat it only occasionally. In addition, the type of meat they eat is very different from the meat we eat. It comes from wild animals or from lean, free-roaming domestic animals that haven't been artificially fattened. Weston Price's communities ate a diverse range of natural foods. Most ate little meat but some, as mentioned in the last chapter, hunted and ate natural game. They often ate organ meat (liver, heart, entrails, brain), which is higher in omega-3 fats and other nutrients.

There is, however, a problem with meat. The Nurses' Health Study and the Health Professional's Follow-up Study,[41] and the much larger NIH-AARP Study[42] have all noted an association between meat consumption and increased mortality from cancer and heart disease and lower life expectancy. Some of the risk appears to come from charred meat or meat heated to high temperatures. Processed meats, including bacon, ham and salami, have the strongest association, thought to be due to the nitrosamines in these meats.

Vegetarians have an 11% lower risk of cancer and this is even lower in vegans (by 19%).[43]

Meat production has changed dramatically in the past few decades. Nowadays, two-thirds of the meat is factory-farmed and produced from animals bred to put on weight as fast as possible. Selective breeding has produced this rapid weight gain, but this has not been the only change. Drastic modifications in animal feeds mean cows, once fed on healthy grass, are now fed on protein concentrate from soya and corn. The soya and corn are mostly genetically modified (90% in the case of soya, as noted above).

The result of this change has been predictable and inevitable. There has been progressive nutritional depletion of the meat we can buy. Studies have shown a 30-80% decline in key minerals in meat, such as iron and calcium, since the 1940s.[44]

The changes can be large: studies of beef from pasture-raised cattle, compared with intensively-reared cattle, have found 300-400 fold higher levels of omega-3 fatty acids,[45, 46] and 300 to 700-fold higher levels of beta-carotene.[47, 48] In addition, grass-fed cattle have been found to have three times as much a-tocopherol (a form of vitamin E)[49] and higher levels of glutathione (an important antioxidant) and superoxide dismutase (a key enzyme in the detoxification process). These just happen to be nutrients that are essential for immunity and that help to protect us from cancer.

Compounding the problem of nutrient depletion is the issue of toxicity. Altogether, 143 residues of drugs and pesticides have been found in meat; 42 of these have been found to cause cancer, 20 to cause birth defects and six to cause mutations. This problem of toxicity and nutritional depletion is sadly one we will see over and over again with modern food production, though not just in meat production. It is the combination of these twin perils that many consider to be a major predisposing factor for cancer.

There are other issues. Antibiotic resistance, squandering

of the world's precious resources of grain (one third of the total), exhaustion of water supplies, depletion of fish stocks, pandemics of major disease, cruelty on an unimaginable scale, environmental degradation (the cost of the clean-up of this is estimated at $4.1 billion in the USA) – these can all be laid at the door of factory farming.

Just as seriously, food producers are putting us all in danger. We are now at risk from both increasing antibiotic resistance and the unknown hazards of GM crops unscrupulously fed to factory-farmed animals (and not declared on the label). This is far from a minor consideration: research has shown that rodents fed GM soya lost their ability to reproduce within three generations.

Sadly, meat has been changed beyond recognition. We have travelled a long way from the meat eaten by our ancestors and are continuing in very much the wrong direction, if health is our primary objective. The changes that have been made have been reckless, unethical, and ultimately self-destructive.

However, the problems of factory-farmed meat should not blind us to the fact that animal products can be healthy. Organ meat has always been prized, and ideally should come from organic or grass-fed animals. Another excellent food is bone broth. Here bones are boiled for four to 24 hours, producing a particularly rich source of nutrients which are hard to obtain from other sources. Both organ meat and bone-broth were extensively used by Terry Wahls in her recovery from MS (page 25). She was originally vegetarian but during this time her health declined. However, when it comes to cancer, the observations of Gerson and Kelley suggest meat is a food it would be wise to avoid (pages 34, 37).

In summary, keep meat consumption low and look for 'organic', 'pasture-fed', 'grass-fed' or 'outdoor-reared' on the label.

Chicken

Kelley also observed that chicken specifically increased growth of his own tumours. Chicken was once rightly regarded as a healthy, lean meat with relatively high levels of omega-3 fats. Not any more. The change in these birds has been nothing short of dramatic. Now, according to the UN, 80% of chickens are factory-farmed.[50] Taking half the time to grow, compared with 50 years ago, they also grow twice as large. Their bones and organs cannot cope with the colossal growth rate and large numbers of these young birds are crippled and suffer from heart failure before they reach slaughter weight at seven weeks.

Data from the Food Standards Agency and the Institute of Brain Chemistry and Human Nutrition have found a chicken in 1896 had 1.8 grams of fat per 100 grams of body weight whereas it now has 22.8 grams per 100 grams, with a higher saturated fat content than red meat,[51] making its reputation as a lean meat undeserved. Whilst the fat has gone up, the protein has gone down.[52] Today's fast-grown chickens have significantly fewer long-chain omega-3 fats (half as much in chicken breast) compared with slow-grown chickens.[53] This means today you would need to eat at least two to four standard chickens to get the same nutritional benefit as eating one chicken in the past, or one of a slow-growing variety. Sadly, intensive mass production has destroyed the very benefits that chicken once promised.

Ultimately, the quality of the chicken depends on the quality of the food the birds are given to eat, and on their ability to exercise (as the quality of the muscle meat depends on how active it is). Both of these have undergone a steep decline.

There is another concern with chicken. Chicken consumption has a stronger association with cancer of the pancreas,[54] leukaemias and lymphomas[55] than does red meat and fish. The likely cause is transmission of oncogenic poultry viruses. A number of these avian viruses (such as avian leukosis virus, reticuloendotheliosis virus and Marek's disease virus) can cause visceral tumours and sarcomas in poultry. They are known to cause cancers in vitro (in lab experiments) in human cells. In addition, poultry workers have a three to nine times greater risk of developing cancer of the tonsils and/or nasal cavity and myelofibrosis.[56]

In summary, most chicken has sadly become a poor-quality food. Eat organic where possible or avoid it altogether.

Milk and butter

We learned in the last chapter how Jane Plant's metastatic tumours melted away once she stopping consuming milk products (page 35). We also saw how Professor Campbell found that milk protein stimulated tumour growth in rodents (page 35). In addition, we know 62% of Foster's survivors avoided milk. However, milk has not always been a problem food. The story of milk and butter is a perfect illustration of what not to do with food.

The Swiss in the Loetschental Valley and the Maasai in the Great Rift Valley of East Africa both knew the best milk and butter came from animals fed on rapidly growing grass. Animals intuitively understand this themselves and great herds of wildebeest migrate across Africa in search of the richest pasture. Caribou travel 3000 miles annually, searching for the new growth of cotton grass before giving birth, so they can suckle their young on the richest milk.

Cows and goats thrive on this fast-growing grass and produce milk of exceptionally high quality. This milk was considered indispensable for pregnant women and young children in the Loetschental Valley. The fatty part of the milk, with its very high levels of fat-soluble vitamins and essential fats, was especially valued. (Note, these vitamins are partially removed when milk is skimmed.) However, today milk has changed beyond recognition; it is positively associated with some types of cancer and with heart disease. What has happened? And why has it changed so much?

There are several reasons. Firstly, cows are selectively bred to produce far greater quantities of milk. They naturally produce about 1000 litres of milk a year, but 30 years ago were managing 5000 litres a year. Today, the average dairy cow produces 7000 litres a year, and some high-yielding cows produce 10,000 litres a year.[57] Secondly, cows are fed on poor-quality grains as opposed to grass.

The outcome of both of these changes is predictable: progressive nutrient depletion. Between 1940 and 2002, the following minerals had all declined in milk: iron, copper, sodium, potassium, magnesium, phosphorus, calcium and copper. Milk from pasture-fed cows contains far higher levels (50-184% higher) of omega-3 fats and of carotenoids (60-436% higher)[58] than does milk from cows fed on grains.

However, nutrient depletion is far from the only or even the most serious concern. Today, more milk originates from pregnant cows than in the past due to artificial impregnation of cows after birth. This has an unfortunate and sinister consequence: milk now contains high levels of unhealthy hormones. One of these, insulin-like growth factor 1 (IGF-1), is raising alarm bells as it promotes both tumour growth and tumour metastasis, and inhibits apoptosis (cell death). Levels of this have been steadily rising in milk and small increases raise the risk of several common cancers.

Research studies have noted this link between milk and cancer. Altogether, 24 studies have investigated the link between milk and prostate cancer, with 20 showing a positive association. On average, these have shown a doubling of prostate cancer risk,[59] but also a higher risk of cancer recurrence.[60] Recurrence in breast cancer was also increased by 49% in another study.[61] Other studies have found links with breast and ovarian cancer.[62] Milk consumption is linked to Parkinson's disease, and each daily cup of milk is estimated to increase the risk by 17%.[63]

Milk consumption has also been linked with heart disease. Seely found the food with the strongest correlation with heart disease mortality in 24 countries was milk (both milk sugar and milk protein).[64] Grant investigated coronary heart disease and diet in 32 countries and found much the same: the strongest correlation was with non-fat milk in males and milk carbohydrates and sugar in females.[65]

However, the problems with milk don't end there. Homogenising and pasteurising milk mean exposing it to very high temperatures and pressures that alter its quality. (While pasteurisation only requires 60°C, much pasteurisation uses 'high temperature short time' (HTST) processes, which go up to double this temperature.) These methods are similar to the process involved in hydrogenating fats.

Sadly, the dairy industry has set its sights on quantity not quality, pushing dairy cows to their limit. This has been bad for cows and bad for our health. Sadly, one of the most prized of all foods has been changed beyond recognition to a food that almost everyone should avoid. It is a terrible indictment of modern farming methods. So, in summary, if at all possible, avoid milk. Organic milk is possibly an option, but with cancer, total avoidance of milk is best.

Foods that have become less healthy - conclusion

Whether we look at milk, red meat or chicken, we find the same pattern emerging. We have cheaper products on the shelves, but behind this seeming benefit lie a multiplicity of problems: nutrient depletion, increased toxicity, environmental degradation and animal cruelty.

From the perspective of health, these changes have been a calamity; these foods are nutritionally inferior to those of the past and are putting us all at risk of a range of serious diseases.

However, these products still have the potential to be healthy if produced in the right way. Butter and milk from animals fed on fast-growing grass, organ meat from animals free to roam and bone-broth are examples of this.

Foods that can heal

It is some relief to find that there are foods that can boost our health. In this category are many fruits and vegetables, seeds and nuts, and wholegrains. With some reservations (see below) we can add fish and eggs.

Fruit and vegetables

Foster's survivors (page 42) consumed fruit and vegetables in large quantities and Kelley witnessed that his tumours regressed after eating fruit and vegetables (page 37).

Fruit and vegetables are known to reduce the risk of the big three killer diseases: cancer, heart disease and stroke. More than 200 studies have been done on the link between fruit and vegetables in the diet and cancer, including 20 cohort studies.[66] Over 70% have demonstrated a protective effect against cancer. Those who eat the least fruit and vegetables have about double the risk of cancer.[67]

What is fascinating to me is that there seems no upper limit to this benefit. It doesn't stop at five-a-day: there appears to be no threshold. The large Health Survey of England found each serving of fruit and vegetables made a difference, with seven servings daily being inversely related to total mortally (drop of 33%), cardiovascular mortality (31%) and cancer mortality (25%).[68] Overall, vegetables had a greater benefit on mortality,[69] with raw vegetables having a stronger health benefit than cooked vegetables. Frozen and canned fruit and vegetables showed a negative effect in this study, possibly because of the added sugar in the case of canned produce.

The Health Survey of England found only 28% of adults and 18% of children today eat the recommended five-a-day. In the UK, we eat half as much as do people in France, Italy and Spain. One-fifth of our children eat no vegetables.[70]

Long-lived races eat large quantities, usually over 10 portions daily. These are typically organic and eaten fresh, as soon as ripe. In contrast, we typically buy our fruit and vegetables from supermarkets and they may have been stored for up to one year. This is important as fruit and vegetables lose 50% of their vitamins in four to five days.

We are beginning to understand just why fruit and vegetables protect against cancer. The Nutrinome Project, developed by Professor Beliveau at the University of Montreal, has investigated how extracts of various fruit and vegetables inhibit the growth of different cancers in the laboratory.[70] Garlic slows cancer growth at concentrations as low as one part per thousand. Garlic, leeks, spring onions, broccoli, Brussels sprouts, cabbage, kale, cauliflower and beetroot (in roughly that order) are the vegetables with the strongest ability to inhibit cancer growth. Mushrooms and various fruit and spices also have powerful anti-cancer properties, as discussed in the last chapter.

These anti-cancer effects of fruit and vegetables are thought to come from substances called 'phytonutrients' ('phyto' is Greek for 'plant'). Eating a good selection of fruit and vegetables should provide an intake of 5000 or more phytonutrients, including polyphenols and terpenoids (carotene and lycopene).

What has come to light is the importance of synergy: the beneficial effects multiply when different foods are eaten together, as noted in Chapter 1 (page 48).

Knowledge about the benefits of plant-based nutrients is rapidly expanding, including the way they help intracellular communication and up-regulate useful genes (for instance, activating antioxidant genes). Here again, different strands of evidence point in the same direction:

- Higher consumption of fruit and vegetables in long-lived races
- The statistical association of lower cancer rates with higher fruit and vegetable intake
- Evidence that extracts of fruit and vegetables inhibit cancer growth in the laboratory
- The discovery of compounds within fruit and vegetables with specific anti-cancer properties
- The ability of these substances to switch on beneficial genes.

Collectively, this is powerful evidence, vindicating the clinical observations of pioneers such as Gerson and Kelley.

Vegetables usually have higher levels of minerals than do fruits. However, fruits do contain greater levels of antioxidants. Vegetables mix better with other foods, whereas fruit eaten with other foods can cause fermentation. They are often best eaten separately. Fruit and vegetables with multiple colours have the widest range of antioxidants.

There is another thing to consider about fruit and vegetables. The quality depends completely on the quality of the soil. In the rush to produce more, with intensive farming, the inevitable has happened. The quality of the soil (see below) has deteriorated as has, in turn, the mineral content of fruit and vegetables – this has declined significantly.[71]

This problem of vitamin and mineral depletion has been exacerbated by long storage times and the practice of growing fruit under plastic; this reduces levels of antioxidants, such as flavonoids.

Despite their many benefits, fruit and vegetables sometimes cause problems for some people. Plants contain chemicals that protect them from being eaten. Some individuals with irritable bowel syndrome (IBS) react to substances called fermentable oligosaccharides, disaccharides and monosaccharides (FODMAPS). These are found in a wide range of fruit and vegetable and cause gut fermentation, triggering IBS. Other patients with osteoarthritis are made worse by the nightshade family of vegetables (potato, aubergine, peppers, paprika, curry and nicotine). Others are susceptible to oxalates found in many fruit and vegetables, which form tiny crystals, giving rise to kidney stones, chronic muscular pains, brain fog, urinary irritation and vulvodynia (chronic pain in the vulva).

However, the recommendation for most people is to eat as many different fruits and vegetables as you can, with as many different colours, and eat them when as fresh as possible. Eat organic whenever possible. Few things are more beneficial.

Fruit and vegetable juices

Many of Foster's survivors (page 42) drank freshly-made fruit and vegetable juices daily. A wide variety of juices were used, with over 50% having one of the following juices daily: grapefruit, apple, carrot, grape, orange, tomato and green-leaf juice.

The Gerson diet is basically a diet of fruit and vegetable juices. Kelley (see page 37) also used juices extensively, observing that carrot juice reduced the size of his tumours more than any other single food.

Maximilian Bircher-Benner, a Swiss doctor, developed health problems as a young man, suffering from jaundice. He recovered after changing to a natural diet. Encouraged by this, he began to treat his patients with what he called 'living foods'. These included raw foods and juices. The treatment proved highly effective for a wide range of diseases, including arthritis, diabetes, heart disease, kidney disease, eye diseases and other disorders. He went on to found a clinic in Zurich in 1897 which continues to practise to this day, treating patients with raw food and combining this with exercise. Fresh juices were one of the cornerstones of his dietary treatment.[72]

Jason Vale, author of the *Super Juice Me* DVD and book, is

a modern-day equivalent and has devised the 28-juice plan. He uses this system in juicing retreats but also recommends it for home use. He has found this regime is deeply healing and has reversed many chronic diseases, including diabetes, psoriasis, depression, eczema, Crohn's disease, ulcerative colitis and fibro-myalgia. He has noticed that most people make profound changes in their health when they go on his juice diet. He says it accomplishes two things, both crucial for healing: it removes all the toxicity going into their bodies, and it replenishes them with high-quality nutrients. These changes allow the body to heal.

Juices allow the nutrients they contain to be easily assimilated. A particular benefit may be their high enzyme content as these are deficient in the average diet. Using juices is like flooding the body with high-quality nutrients and enzymes. A 500 ml glass of juice is equivalent to 10 portions of fruit and vegetables.

Another benefit of juices is their ability to make the body more alkaline, known to enhance the healing process and believed to accelerate the removal of toxic materials.

Fruit juices (and, to a lesser extent, dried fruit and very sweet fruits) can release sugar rapidly. For this reason, care needs to be taken, especially in diabetes, neurological diseases (which are often made worse by sugar hits) and obesity. Smoothies may be the better option for fruit whereas vegetable juices are usually fine. However, Jason Vale, who has much experience with treating diabetics with juicing, has found this is not a problem with fresh juices. However, there is a trap for the unwary: freshly-made juices are entirely different from commercial juices. Commercially-made juices can be 90% water, often with large amounts of added sugar, and have been noted to increase mortality.[73]

Juices have their highest concentrations of nutrients just after they have been made, and enzymes will only be present in fresh juices. Use organic ingredients where possible because juices concentrate pesticides as well as nutrients. Freshly-made juices are one of the great secrets of health and have been an important component of many anti-cancer regimes. The fact that they taste so delicious is an added bonus.

Raw foods

Raw foods and juices have a deserved reputation for healing. They have helped reverse many serious diseases. In fact, we are the only species on the planet that does not live entirely on raw food, apart from domesticated animals.

A dramatic example took place, many years ago at the Royal Free Hospital in London. At the suggestion of one of the doctors, a patient bedridden with severe rheumatoid arthritis was sent to the Bircher-Benner clinic in Zurich. The treatment there proved to be a complete success and the patient recovered fully.

Amazed by what had happened, the staff at the Royal Free Hospital decided to do a trial. They selected 12 patients with severe arthritis who were considered to be incurable. The treatment involved two weeks on a strict raw-food plant-based diet. This consisted of uncooked fruit, vegetables, nuts, cereals, herbs, honey, egg yolk, seeds and cold-pressed oils. After this, some cooked foods were introduced but meals always started with raw food. No painkillers were used during the time. The trial was filmed. By the time it was completed seven of these patients had made a full recovery, three had made a partial recovery and two had not been helped.[72]

A fascinating feature of the treatment was that some patients developed 'healing crises' after six to seven weeks. During these episodes they had severe pain and fever. Healing crises occur with many natural methods of healing and are important to recognise. There is a real danger that the treatment could be stopped just when success is imminent (see later example in Appendix III). After going through these crises, the patients rapidly recovered.

These results were astonishing and I know of no orthodox

treatment even moderately comparable with these results. Sadly, I think this sort of trial, which involved long stays in hospital, will never be repeated.

However, many health clinics in Europe do use similar treatments and reputedly get excellent results in a variety of diseases. Dr Joseph Evers treated 600 people with multiple sclerosis with a raw diet and these were monitored at sanatoriums and hospitals in 1947.[74] Of those treated, 42% showed improvement or complete recovery. Most of those who did not recover had already developed irreversible changes before the treatment had been started. He went on to treat over 10,000 people by 1970, with similar outcomes, writing two books about his work.

The research of Professor Werner Kollath gives experimental backing for raw food.[75] He gave animals a diet of processed foods virtually devoid of minerals and vitamins. Surprisingly, these animals grew normally and seemed healthy until they reached adulthood. After this, they developed a variety of degenerative diseases of the type commonly seen today. It was interesting that these illnesses could not be reversed by giving nutrients but could be reversed by raw foods, if used early enough.

An even more dramatic demonstration took place in 1950. Dr Masanore Kuratsune was the head of the medical department of Kyushu University in Japan. He put himself and his wife, then pregnant, on a very low-calorie diet (700 to 800 calories) consisting of brown rice, dried fruit and vegetables. It was the same diet given to British prisoners of war. First they ate the raw-food version of the diet. Remarkably they remained in good health. They then switched to the same diet but this time it was cooked. Now they began to develop all the symptoms suffered by POWs.[76] This was a somewhat reckless piece of research, but nothing could better illustrate the healing qualities of raw food. Perhaps the simplest way for anyone with a chronic disease to test this is to eat only raw fruit and vegetables for one month.

Nearly all chronic diseases will benefit.

To sum up, many serious diseases have been reversed with raw foods and we all need some raw food in our diet. Long-lived races know this and typically eat plenty.

Nuts and seeds

The diet of Foster's survivors was not especially high in nuts and seeds, with 32% eating almonds regularly and 19.5% eating sunflower seeds. Kelley noted that his tumours receded after he ate nuts (see page 37).

One of the largest studies, published in the *New England Journal of Medicine* in 2013, following over 100,000 men and women between 1980 and 2010, found that those who ate nuts daily reduced their overall mortality by 20%, their cardiovascular mortality by 29% and their cancer mortality by 11%. The more nuts they ate, the greater the drop in mortality.[77] What is interesting is that the benefits occur with surprisingly small quantities.

Another large study, this time in the Netherlands, of 120,000 men and women, found significant benefits for those who ate 15 grams of peanuts, tree nuts (half a handful daily) or peanut butter.[78] Those who ate the most nuts, compared with those who ate none, reduced their mortality from cancer, diabetes and neurodegenerative diseases. The biggest reduction was for neurodegenerative disease (44%). Peanut butter, however, had no effect on mortality.

There is one downside: nuts contain fats and fats can go rancid. Once rancid, nuts are not a good choice. This means they are best kept in the fridge or at least away from light. Ideally, the best time to eat nuts is when they are first extracted from their shells.

Seeds are rich in essential fats, zinc, manganese and magnesium. Data on their impact on disease are unfortunately sparse.

Flaxseed has powerful anti-cancer properties, as noted in the last chapter (page 49), and is a useful source of omega-3 fats. Nuts are an important source of essential fats and contain zinc and other key minerals. Eat nuts unsalted and unroasted, as heat destroys essential fats. Almonds are also high in vitamin B17 and have a reputation for reducing the risk of cancer. Be aware, however, that many almonds are now produced in California under artificial conditions in areas of very high pesticide use. The atmosphere is so toxic that no birds or insects can survive there. It seems unlikely almonds grown this way could retain their health benefits.

Apricot kernels deserve a special mention. They are a staple food of the Hunza, a race in which cancer is thought to be absent. These are especially high in vitamin B17 and some patients have used apricot kernels to help heal their cancers, typically using 40 kernels per day. Dr Philip Binzel used this as the mainstay of his treatment and his cancer patients had excellent five-year survival rates of over 80% for primary cancers (standard treatment gave a 20% survival) and of over 60% for metastatic cancer (standard treatment gave less than 2% survival).[79]

Sprouting seeds

Sprouting seeds are one of the most nutrient-dense foods on the planet. There are many varieties, including alfalfa, mung beans and wheat grass.

Fruit and vegetables have sometimes been categorised as living foods. Strictly speaking this is not true as they start dying as soon as they are picked. Not so with sprouting seeds; they are still alive and this brings very high nutrient levels. The levels of phytonutrients in sprouting seeds can greatly exceed those in the mature plant. Cruciferous vegetables contain glucosinolates, which convert into sulphorophanes. Both substances inhibit cancer.[80, 81] However, the sprouts of cruciferous vegetables contain about 50 to 100 times as many of these compounds as the parent vegetables, making them even more valuable.

The super-healthy Hunza leave lentils and beans out in the sun until they have started to sprout and only then do they eat them. Sprouting seeds can be regarded as one of nature's superfoods. They also happen to be cheap and easy to grow. Their use has been popular amongst cancer survivors.

Fish, seafood and eggs

Seafood and eggs almost deserve a separate category. This is because they have also been subject to industrial farming, and in the case of fish, toxicity. This has inevitably reduced their benefits. However, in the main they still remain healthy foods, though there are exceptions.

Fish and seafood

Many of Weston Price's healthy communities loved seafood and knew how good it was for their health. Certain items, such as fish eggs and shellfish, were especially prized for critical times such as pregnancy, and for young children. In contrast, 67% of Foster's survivors avoided fish (page 42).

Numerous studies confirm that fish is good for us. It has been shown to reduce the risk of cancer in even small amounts,[82] and eating more than one portion a week reduces the risk of stroke.[83] Studies have found an inverse relationship between fish consumption and mortality from coronary heart disease.[84] The American Academy of Neurology noted at their 70th annual meeting that it reduced the risk of multiple sclerosis by 45%.

It seems fish has many benefits. These benefits have been put down to its high nutrient content and especially its omega-3 fats (see below). However, the situation is not quite as simple as it seems. Fish are not without their problems. They often have a long food chain leading to a build-up of toxic chemicals, such as mercury, PCBs (polychlorinated biphenyls) and dioxins. Almost all fish are contaminated with microplastics, ingested from the eight million metric tonnes of plastic that finds its way into the oceans annually. Researchers at the University of Ghent have estimated that seafood eaters will consume 11,000 pieces of microplastic each year.[85] The medical consequences of this are unknown.

Some studies have shown that oily fish reduce the risk of heart attacks,[86, 87] but others have paradoxically shown the opposite.[88] The reason for this paradox is thought to be mercury. Guallar has noted that the relationship between fish consumption and heart attacks depends on the ratio between beneficial fatty acids to mercury in the fish eaten.[89] Those with the highest intake of mercury had double the risk of myocardial infarct.

This is typical of the dilemmas of life today: by polluting the world we have turned one of the most nutritious foods into a potential health hazard. Generally, the largest fish, such as tuna, swordfish, halibut and marlin, have the highest levels of mercury and other pollutants. Oily fish, such as herring, sardines and mackerel, are good choices, being high in the crucial omega-3 fats.

When it comes to fish, this is not the only or even the most serious problem. Over 50% of fish bought today are farmed. They are fed artificially and, due to the overcrowded conditions, chemicals are used to keep them healthy and give them colour. At least four of these chemicals are known carcinogens and some are endocrine (hormone) disruptors. An added problem is antibiotics, given to fish to prevent disease.

Farmed fish are typically fed on fishmeal. It takes 3 tonnes of wild fish to produce 1 tonne of farmed fish. This has led to an increase, rather than decrease, in fish taken from the wild, putting a further strain on depleted fish stocks. Another problem is environmental degradation, an entirely predictable consequence of this practice.

Fish farming reduces nutrients (omega-3 fats) and increases

toxicity, with higher levels of chemicals such as PCBs, PBDEs (polybrominated diphenylethers), pesticides and antibiotics. Farmed salmon typically contain the hazardous colouring agent astaxanthin and farmed trout may contain steroids. Even more worrying, in one study, four out of seven samples of smoked salmon contained the radioactive waste product technetium-99.[90] Farmed fish cannot be regarded as a healthy choice.

However, the biggest issue regarding fish is the diminishing supply. Great shoals of fish still swim in these oceans, sardines by the billion off the coast of South Africa, North Atlantic herring in such large numbers (up to three billion) that they can be seen for tens of kilometres, and in the Caspian Sea, tens of millions of mullet. But all is not well in these once teeming and fertile oceans. The numbers of all large fish have plummeted by a staggering 90%, and 82% of all fish stocks are under threat. Over one third (27 million tonnes a year) of the vast haul of the fishing industry is regarded as waste or bycatch, thrown out as trash (reaching approximately 80% with shrimp fishing). We are now in a position where we could wipe out all the fish in the sea by 2050. For this reason, the amount of fish we eat and whether it comes from a sustainable source have become increasing concerns.

It is also important to mention that fish stocks are declining rapidly just at the time when we are beginning to appreciate the value of fish for our health.

In summary, eat some oily fish, avoid farmed fish, especially salmon, and use sustainable sources of fish wherever possible. Fish just make it into the healthy category but increasing toxicity and the rise in farmed fish are worrying trends.

Eggs

Eggs of all kinds are eaten regularly by long-lived populations. However, 70% of Foster's survivors deliberately avoided eggs (page 43).

Eggs contain many beneficial nutrients: lutein, xeaxanthan

(useful in macular degeneration) and choline deserve a special mention.

Eggs are generally a healthy food, but this needs qualification Results of studies of those eating eggs have been conflicting. A recent study of 30,000 people eating eggs in the USA showed a 27% increase in heart attacks and strokes and all-cause mortality.[91] In comparison, a study of 500,000 people in different parts of China found an 18% reduction in cardiovascular disease and a 28% reduction in strokes in those eating eggs.[92] A meta-analysis of those eating eggs in 2016 found a non-significant reduction in heart disease and a 12% reduction in strokes.[93] I think these contradictions are because eggs of different quality are being eaten.

Again, the same logic applies here as it does with meat and milk. The quality of the egg depends intimately on the quality of the food given to the hen. Manufacturers acknowledge this. They now offer omega-3-enriched eggs laid by hens fed on a special diet. Perhaps one day the food industry will realise that the same logic applies to us. Just as with hens, the quality of our health depends on the quality of the food we eat. If we eat enriched food, our health will be enriched; if we eat poor quality food, our health will be poor.

However, I would not recommend eggs to cancer patients. Gerson observed that eggs caused tumour growth in his cancer patients. In addition, some studies have shown an increase in hormonal cancers (breast, ovary, prostate[94]) in those who ate more eggs.

I believe eggs just about deserve to be in the healthy category, providing they are free-range or, better still, organic.

Fats: the good and the bad

Essential fats were prized by Weston Price's healthy populations (page 27). They found them in fish, milk and meat, notably the organ meat and milk from animals allowed to roam, and especially those feeding on fast-growing grass. As mentioned, Weston Price's 'isolated societies' (page 27) made special efforts to obtain enough of them, particularly during critical times, like pregnancy.

Deficiency of essential fats is probably the single commonest nutritional deficiency so eating enough of the right fats is vital for health. Removing bad fats from the diet is almost as important.

The fats that are essential in our diet comprise omega-3 and omega-6 fatty acids. We need these for multiple body functions, the most notable being in our cell membranes (20% of these membranes are formed from essential fats). We cannot manufacture them so a food source is crucial to good health.

We know from healthy societies that a healthy ratio of omega-6 to omega-3 fats is about 2.5 or 3.5 to 1. (In the current western diet the ratio is about 19 to 1, though much of the omega-6 is unusable – see below.)

Keeping things simple, we only need two essential fats: alpha linolenic acid (ALA), which is an omega-3 fat, and linoleic acid (LA), which is an omega-6 fat (although some people find it difficult to convert ALA into EPA (eicosapentaenoic acid) and have to consume omega-3 in the EPA form, which comes mainly from oily fish). All other fats that our body needs are secondary and can be made from these. Good sources of ALA are flaxseed and cold-pressed flaxseed oil and good sources of LA are sunflower seeds and cold-pressed safflower or sunflower oil. We should aim to have more omega-6 than omega-3 at the ideal ratio given above (twice to three times as much).

However, essential fats, because they go rancid and have a short shelf-life, have proved inconvenient to food manufactures and are often selectively removed from foods. They have been diminishing in our food for three reasons:

1. There has been a massive increase in processed seed oils, such as sunflower, safflower and rapeseed (canola) oil, and oils derived from corn and soya as noted above.

Here essential fats have been replaced by processed fats.

2. Farm animals are being fed wheat, corn and soya rather than grass. This has led to a major decline in omega-3 fats in meat, as noted above.

3. Mass processing of grains has removed most of the essential fats.

Oily fish remains an important source of omega-3 fats but farmed fish have lower levels of these fats. Other sources are nuts and seeds.

However, there are some traps for the unwary. There has been a tendency amongst many in the health field to extol the virtues of omega-3 fats and demonise omega-6. It is true that deficiencies of omega-3 fats are common, but lab tests now frequently show deficiencies of omega-6 fats as well (but paradoxically an excess of processed omega-6 fats, which the body cannot use). Here is an example of why this happens.

You can buy cold-pressed sunflower oil at a health-food shop. It is an excellent product containing much-needed omega-6 fats. You can also go to your local supermarket and buy a product with exactly the same name on the bottle: sunflower oil. This oil has been heated to a high temperature and the essential fats have become damaged and oxidised, forming harmful hydrogenated fats. Same name, different product; and the two have a totally different impact on health. Finally, when we take in hydrogenated fats, we actually increase our need for essential fats.

In summary, deficiencies of essential fats are common and the best sources of these are nuts, seeds, cold-pressed seed oils and oily fish (sardines, herrings and mackerel).

The health of the soil

However long we talk about healthy foods, we must eventually come back to the health of the soil. Ultimately, how healthy a food is, as in the case of fruit and vegetables, depends on the health of the soil, and in the case of meat, it depends on the quality of the feed given to the animal, which in turn depends on the soil. In other words, the health of the soil and our own health are intimately linked.

Farmers in the past lived by the adage 'Look after the soil and everything else will look after itself'. Long-lived populations understand this perfectly and take great care of their soils. Sometimes they are blessed with fertile soil, but this has not always been the case. The Hunza had to fetch soil from rivers thousands of feet below where they farmed, fertilising their land with carefully-prepared natural compost, which included organic manure from animal and human waste. Nothing was wasted. Soil erosion was kept to virtually zero. Now they have some of the finest soils in the world and it is thought this is largely responsible for their exceptional health.[95]

In a key experiment, Robert McCarrison (page 30) fed large numbers of animals on crops fertilised by stable manure and next with crops where chemical fertilisers had been used. The animals fed on the former flourished; those fed on the latter fared poorly.[96] This was ground-breaking research; it should have changed the way we farm. Sadly, it did not.

Soil is formed as minerals break down from below and work their way up, combining with decaying organic material from plants and animals and also with air (air makes up 50% of the soil).

Today, depletion of the earth's topsoil is one of the biggest problems facing the planet. It takes 500 years to produce 2.5 cm (1 inch) of topsoil. In the last 200 years, the once fertile plains of America have lost 75% of their topsoil, going from 53 cm (21 inches) to 15 cm (6 inches). Every 16 years, another 2.5 cm (1 inch) is lost and this process is accelerating. In addition, the minerals within it are being depleted.

At the Rio Earth Summit the official report noted, 'There is deep concern over the continuing declines in the mineral values in farms throughout the world'.[97] They produced data showing that over the last 100 years, mineral levels had fallen by 72% in Europe, 76% in Asia and 85% in North America. The cost of soil degradation in the UK has been estimated at £1.4 billion per year. A 2015 United Nations report stated that we may have as few as 90 harvests left before our soil is unfit for farming. Then we may starve.

There is only one reason for this massive decline: intensive farming and, in particular, its reliance on artificial fertilisers. Plants require about 70 to 80 minerals from the soil and we require 52 for our health. Artificial fertilisers put back three: nitrogen, phosphorus and potassium. This type of farming is like continually taking money out of the bank and putting none back. Future generations will not thank us for leaving them with nothing in the account.

This ever-worsening problem of decreasing minerals has gone largely unnoticed, but minerals are, as ever, essential for health. For instance, magnesium protects against heart disease, chromium protects against diabetes and zinc is essential for immune function.

The soil has also become toxic due to chemicals accumulating within it. We have noted that cancer has often been regarded as a disease of both nutrient depletion and toxicity and it is perhaps no surprise we are suffering from an epidemic of cancer. What happens to our soil, sooner or later, happens to us. If we seriously want to stay healthy, the starting point has to be the soil.

What can we do to help prevent this impending catastrophe? The obvious answer is to use organic produce wherever possible. We should do it both for ourselves and for future generations.

Organic farming and nutrients

Organic farming raises the levels of protective nutrients: it produces higher levels of vitamins, minerals and other natural substances, such as glutathione. Many of these, such as selenium[98] and beta-carotene,[99] help to protect us against cancer. However, when it comes to cancer, the greatest benefit may be the higher levels of phytonutrients in organic produce. Substances, such as resveratrol, anthocyanins and salvetrols, which have powerful anti-cancer properties, are produced by plants to protect themselves against bacteria and fungi. Levels decline once pesticides and herbicides are used.

A recent study following 1340 people for nearly five years found that those who ate the most organic food had 25% fewer cancers and 73% fewer non-Hodgkin's lymphomas (the latter tallies with the higher incidence of these lymphomas in farmers, thought to be due to pesticides). This protection remained whether the participants had consumed organic food of high or low quality (e.g. ready meals).[100]

Another advantage of organic produce is the absence of toxins, such as pesticides. A study by Newcastle University reviewed 343 papers comparing organic with non-organic produce. They found organic produce had higher levels of antioxidants and phytonutrients (flavanones 69% higher, flavonols 50% higher and anthocyanins 51% higher). Harmful substances were lower (cadmium was 48% lower, nitrates were 30% lower and nitrites 87% lower). Pesticide residues were four times lower (some pesticide lands on organic crops from nearby spraying).[101]

Organic farming is by far the cheaper option if we factor in the health and environmental costs of intensive agriculture. Sadly, at the moment industrial agriculture is heavily subsidised whereas organic farming receives little or no help. Again, if we want good health and lower health costs, this makes little sense.

Food labelling

We all need to know what we are eating. This gives us control over our health. This means labels are important. A key point is that the healthiest foods (such as fruit, vegetables, seeds and nuts) don't need labels with lists of ingredients. Anything with more than five chemical names on the packet is best avoided and the ideal is to have none.

The pictures on food labels are often typically misleading. An example would be pictures of cows grazing freely in idyllic surroundings when the product is from a factory farm. If the truth was made clear, the unacceptable face of food production would start to change.

Perhaps this is why food companies fight tooth and nail to avoid honest labelling. The most notable example of this relates to GM foods. Over 70% of food in the USA now contains GM produce. Most of the meat we eat is from animals fed GM crops and yet this is omitted from the label. In the USA, 80% of animals are factory-farmed (and hormones and antibiotics routinely used). The USA is fighting to remove the country of origin from labels so that we can no longer assess the health risks we are being exposed to.

I believe we deserve better. We should expect and demand honesty and integrity from food producers. As things stand, I believe it is best to have a certain attitude when reading labels on food. This is the same attitude you need when interpreting estate agents' jargon. Almost nothing should be believed. In fact, it is best to deliberately turn most labels around.

Here are some examples:

'Low fat': Removing fat from food makes it taste like cardboard. Expect these foods to be packed with sugar and the more fat removed, the more added sugar. Some low-fat products can have a six-fold increase in sugar compared with standard products.

'Low in saturated fats': Read this as high in sugar but sometimes it can mean that health-destroying hydrogenated fats have been added.

'Sugar free': This means free of table sugar – that is, sucrose (see page 58). Other compounds which break down into sugars, such as sugar alcohols and maltodextrin, can be included. Artificial sweeteners and other chemicals are the rule in sugar-free products.

'Natural flavours': These are anything but natural and can contain up to 100 chemicals, including excitotoxins and GMO-derived products. It has no legal meaning.

'Free of trans fats': It may surprise you to learn that small amounts of trans fats are allowed under this label (less than 0.5 gram per serving in the USA). Emulsifiers, flavourings and colourings can all contain trans fats. Look out for 'monoglycerides' and 'diglycerides', which are types of trans fats that are usually not labelled as such.

'Enriched': This usually means depleted of nearly all nutrients with a few artificial vitamins thrown in.

'Natural': This has no legal meaning; read as, 'We are trying to pull the wool over your eyes'.

Eating healthily

When I first started researching food, I found it hard to believe that over half of the foods we were eating were not only virtually devoid of nutritional value, but had harmful effects as well. Was there any wonder that our health was so poor? These are foods that healthy populations simply don't eat. The first step to eating healthily is to reduce these foods. This means less processed food, less sugar and less refined carbohydrates.

In many ways, what is happening is very simple: the more we process and adulterate our food, the more unhealthy it becomes and the unhealthier we become. However, processed foods are not always easy to avoid; they are tempting, tasty and addictive. But reducing them will pay dividends and those dividends will be increased vitality and better health.

Think carefully about milk and meat. These foods have changed beyond recognition since the advent of factory-farming, as we saw earlier in this chapter.

With milk, the association with cancer and heart disease is too strong to ignore. The link between meat and cancer is weaker, but survivors faced with cancer have typically eliminated meat from their diet. Gerson and Kelley have given us first-hand observations of how cancer grows when meat is eaten, as described in Chapter 1. Buy organic, pasture-fed or grass-fed produce wherever possible. However, there are meat products of value, including organ meats and bone broth.

Fish, if not farmed or deep fried, is usually a good choice, but toxicity is an increasing issue; take care with large and/ or predatory fish, such as tuna, which can have high levels of mercury and other pollutants. Pollutants can also be concentrated in fish oils.

Increase foods known to enhance health, such as fruit, vegetables, seeds and nuts. Certainly aim for at least five portions a day, but remember, healthy populations eat far more than this and there is no known upper limit to the health benefits. If you have a serious illness, aim to make 70-80% of your food come from the healthy groups. (Note this is vastly different from the so-called 'balanced diet' promoted by government agencies and the food industry.)

Keep in mind that throughout most of our history we have evolved to live on a low-carbohydrate diet with the occasional sugar treat in the form of honey and seasonal fruits. In some diseases, such as neurological diseases, diabetes and autoimmune illnesses, reducing spikes in blood sugar levels is necessary for healing, so care needs to be taken with some types of fruit.

If you are suffering from a major illness, then go for the healthiest and most nourishing foods you can find. Drink fresh homemade fruit and vegetable juice on a regular basis. Few things taste better and few foods are more beneficial for your health. Consider adding superfoods such as sprouting seeds and increase the number of raw foods. Try two months eating only plant-based foods.

It is not always easy to make healthy choices. A useful strategy here is to pick the best option available. If organic chicken or eggs are not available, or affordable, then use free-range. If you want to cook with oil, use butter or coconut oil, not sunflower, safflower or other processed oils (which are already partially hydrogenated). If organic fruit and vegetables are not available, buy local and seasonal produce.

I have noticed an interesting trend with healthy eating. Once people have built up a number of good recipes with healthy foods, they start enjoying food more and often say they would not go back to their old ways of eating. But be patient, this takes time.

Summary

There is a theme running through modern food. It is a story of the progressive adulteration of almost everything we eat for the sake of producing higher and higher quantities of food of a poorer and poorer quality. It is a story of food supply flooded with sugar, chemicals and poor-quality ingredients. It is a story of plants grown on increasingly depleted and poisoned soils. It is a story of animals treated as inanimate objects, whose sole purpose is to put on weight as rapidly as possible or to produce unnatural amounts of milk regardless of their welfare. The impact of these changes on our health has been inevitable and disastrous.

Many people are tempted to give up when it comes to trying to eat healthily. There are so many problems, they are so wide-ranging and we have travelled so far from what is good for us. Many people are confused by all the contradictory messages they hear, but eating the right food is really quite simple. The more natural, unadulterated and fresh it is, then the better it is for us. Unprocessed is better than processed, fresh is better than frozen, organic is better than non-organic, raw is generally better than cooked and a short shelf-life is better than a long one.

The healing properties of food can still astound us. The benefits of high-quality food outstrip those of almost any other method of treatment. Survivors have demonstrated that this is so. Many have literally turned their health around, reversing the most serious diseases that face mankind. Furthermore, we are now beginning to understand why food is such a powerful healing agent. High-quality foods contain a host of healing nutrients. These can block all the stages of the cancer pathway, act synergistically, change and up-regulate genes, improve intracellular communication, reduce inflammation, and remove toxins. Little by little, science is catching up with the food pioneers, confirming what they have been telling us for so long and giving us a logical explanation for the extraordinary healings that we have seen.

We have many of the answers, but how do we use this information? For most of us, the best way forward is to gradually introduce a healthier diet. For people with a serious chronic disease, a more radical change is usually needed, consuming only foods that heal and eliminating those that harm.

Part II
Use your mind

Chapter 3

Belief, expectation and purpose

Once you've made a decision, the Universe conspires to make it happen.

Ralph Waldo Emerson

The story of the unfortunate Mr Wright has been told many times but bears repeating. Suffering from a lymphosarcoma (a cancer of white blood cells and lymphoid tissue) that had failed to respond to treatment, Mr Wright knew he was dying. He had heard about and desperately tried to obtain the new drug Krebiozen which some believed to be a miracle cure for cancer. Although he did not meet the criteria for the drug, being too ill, he repeatedly asked for it, and his doctor reluctantly agreed. The drug was duly given. The response was so unexpected and his recovery so rapid that he left the hospital 10 days later in excellent health. Two months later the news broke that Krebiozen was of doubtful value and Mr Wright's cancer returned on cue.

His doctor, Philip West, however didn't give up on him but instead persuaded Mr Wright to try some new highly concentrated Krebiozen. In reality, he simply injected him with water. Again, Mr Wright responded miraculously, staying in excellent health for another two months. When the news finally broke that Krebiozen was useless, Mr Wright relapsed and died within two days.[1]

This is a remarkable story, but think about what happened here: it is surely extraordinary. His body demonstrated that it already possessed the ability to cure his cancer, not once, but twice. The rapidity of his recovery shows how awesome the body's healing powers can be. He also relapsed twice, and just as quickly, once he discovered the drug was worthless, presumably because his mind switched off his immune system.

To me, the most remarkable fact about this story is that it proves he always had the ability to cure himself of cancer, he just needed the right prompt to make it happen. He had to believe it could happen. Was this innate ability unique to Mr Wright?

The power of the mind

Almost nothing, apart from food, has more impact on health than our minds. And sometimes its influence can be extraordinary. There is a well-documented condition called 'multiple personality syndrome' in which a person can switch between two or more personalities. The differences can be dramatic. For instance, in the case of one individual, one personality had epilepsy complete with an abnormal electroencephalogram (EEG) whereas the other had no epilepsy with a normal EEG. In another case, one personality had a severe allergy to oranges whereas the other was completely unaffected by them. In yet another, one personality was blind whilst the other had perfect vision. Over the years, many cases like this have been documented. As different personalities take over, they can literally switch a disease on or off in a moment.[2]

But why is this rare condition relevant to healing? It is relevant because it turns medical thinking on its head. The normal medical understanding is that disease is down to faulty mechanisms within organs, cells or genes. This strange disorder proves that this is not true. It tells us it is our mind rather than our body that really controls health and that disease can only exist if it resonates with and is compatible with a particular personality. We don't understand how this happens, but a mechanism clearly does exist; it can turn an illness on and off and it is controlled by our mind.

What we do understand is that our thought processes powerfully influence our biochemistry, our immune system and even our genetic expression. In fact, a whole new field of medicine, called psychoneuroimmunology (PNI), has documented this evidence. We will look at aspects of this in the next chapter.

Despite these advances, the mind is still regarded with some suspicion by mainstream medicine. However, survivors have not been slow to turn this knowledge to their advantage. And one of the most basic characteristics of survivors is a belief that they can get better.

Belief

Belief matters. In one study, men who rated themselves as being at low risk of heart disease had around a third of the expected deaths from heart attacks and strokes of men of a similar age, even when all other risk factors were equal.[3]

Hirshberg and Barasch[4] interviewed patients who had had spontaneous remissions from cancer and asked them what they thought were the most important factors in their recovery. Topping the list was a belief in a positive outcome. This view was held by 75% of patients.

Not all survivors have had this belief from the beginning. Many initially had had periods of intense doubt. But they had also had a vague feeling somewhere within them that they could recover and this became stronger with time. They accepted the possibility of the illness getting worse but refused to accept its inevitability. However, the first step was making a decision that they would get better. And this decision had to be supported by an underlying belief that it was possible.

In the Introduction we saw three examples where belief was a crucial component in recovery. However, can a single-minded belief do more – can it heal another person?

The story of Jennifer related by her mother, Cynthia Pike Ouellette, in the book *The Miracle of Suggestion* gives us the answer.[5]

Jennifer had been born 11 weeks premature and weighing only 0.9 kg (2 lb); she suffered from hydrocephalus, fits, respiratory distress and jaundice. The doctors gave her no hope of survival. They later changed their minds, stating that she would end up severely handicapped, with brain, lung and eye damage and, even more devastatingly, mental retardation. Her time in the Neonatal Intensive Care Unit was one of daily crisis. During this time, her mother maintained an unshakeable faith that Jennifer would recover. As she (Jennifer's mother, Cynthia) could not touch Jennifer, the only way she could communicate with her baby was by talking. Whether a premature baby can understand the human voice is unknown, but Cynthia remained undaunted. She repeatedly told Jennifer she would be fine and that her body was healing itself.

Jennifer eventually left the hospital at nine weeks. By the seventh month she had developed cerebral palsy just as predicted by the doctors. Regardless of this, her mother was convinced her suggestions had made a difference. She decided to use this strategy more methodically, regularly using words such as, 'You are a perfectly normal creation,' 'You are perfect, whole and healthy'; 'Your spine is perfect, whole and healthy'; 'You have perfect control of your hands'; 'You are capable of doing anything you want to do'. She added tape recordings of these statements.

She coached herself to deliberately think of her daughter as healthy. If a visitor asked 'What's wrong with Jennifer?' she would say 'Nothing is wrong; she is a healthy baby.' And she believed it. And Jennifer eventually became what her mother had always believed – a healthy young girl. The power of Cynthia's belief won through, even when there was nothing in the outside world to support it.

The Bavarian scientist, Max Pettenkofer, demonstrated the power of belief in a different way. He had his own ideas about bacteria and thought that Robert Koch's new theory (that cholera was caused by microrganisms in the water) was utter nonsense. He challenged Koch to give him a concentrated sample of the organisms, cultured from a cholera victim, mixed in water. He and several of his colleagues then drank the solution. Apart from mild diarrhoea, they suffered no ill effects.

History proved Pettenkofer wrong: cholera is indeed caused by bacteria. However, he did remind us of something of equal value: that when the mind believes it cannot develop a disease, it rarely does. This experiment was not a one-off. It was repeated by the Russian pathologist, Eli Metschikoff, who drank a solution of millions of cholera bacteria, this time to prove that it was not the bacteria that mattered most but the host. As with Pettenkofer and colleagues, he had only mild diarrhoea and, as intended, he proved that it was the person with the illness not the illness itself that mattered most.

Hippocrates observed much the same, in ancient Greece, when he said it was more important to know what sort of person had the disease than to know what sort of disease the person had.

Consider this story from Bernie Siegel's book, *Love, Medicine and Miracles*. A mother, with young daughters, was diagnosed with leukaemia and told she would die within a year.[6] However, rather than accepting the diagnosis, she told them she wasn't going to die and was going to stay alive until her daughter's wedding. She proved to be as good as her word and she was there at her youngest daughter's wedding eight years later.

To believe that you will be healthy at a future wedding

presupposes you will be healthy before that time too, a belief which can powerfully affect health. It is interesting that other survivors have used somewhat similar strategies, such as imagining giving a speech telling people how they made a miraculous recovery.

So beliefs are important and they can affect health in a positive or negative way. There have been recorded cases of people dying after being wrongly diagnosed with cancer and given only months to live. They died as predicted, presumably after giving up hope. This is not unlike the scenario of a person dying after a witch doctor points a bone at them telling them they are going to die.

Take the following case. A woman was diagnosed with terminal cancer and given two months to live. In desperation she went to see psychic healers. The healing was performed and she was told by the healers that she had been successfully healed. She didn't believe them and died two months later, as predicted. At postmortem, no cancer could be found. Here was miraculous healing of terminal cancer, but even this wasn't enough: the combination of her doctor's prognosis and her own beliefs did what her cancer had failed to do and tragically proved enough to kill her.

The opposite can happen. The book *Chicken Soup for the Soul* describes the story of Angela. She was struck by a serious disease of the nervous system at the age of 11. It was considered incurable and she was expected to spend the rest of her life in a wheelchair. She was put in a specialised unit where, amongst other treatments, she was taught visualisation. She spent hours visualising that her legs would move again. One day, while imaging the movement coming back into her legs, the impossible happened – her legs moved, the bed moved and she screamed with delight, 'I've moved my legs'.

No one told Angela there had been an earthquake that had shaken her bed, but from that day she began to be able to move her legs. She went on to make a complete recovery.[7] A belief, whether factually based or not, has its own peculiar power.

The Tarahumara Indians in Mexico have a tradition of long-distance running and are known for their endurance, often running the distance of two marathons at a time. They have a belief, most peculiar-seeming to us, that they reach peak condition at 60 years of age. A team from Harvard decided to investigate and performed extensive tests on their physiology and fitness. Much to their surprise they confirmed that the 60-year old runners were indeed the fittest: fitter than the 40-year-olds who, in turn, were fitter than the 20-year olds. I am sure we could all benefit from a belief like this.

Suffice it to say, some force exists within all of us that can influence health and illness. Furthermore, the effect can be so powerful that it can produce anything from a rapid healing of cancer to dying from nothing apart from a mistaken diagnosis. So how do we use this awesome power? Fortunately, data from both research and from survivors have given us clues.

However, let's step back for a moment and imagine a person with, say, terminal cancer believing they can recover. Notice there is something distinctly odd about this belief. It defies medical statistics. It is irrational, even crazy. Yet it is this crazy, irrational, but highly valuable, belief which is so commonly found in survivors.

However, could it be that those who believe they will recover have intuitively sensed something that we don't yet fully understand and the medical profession doesn't understand? Could we, at some level, already know that we have innate healing capabilities far beyond anything that we presently believe?

What are we capable of?

Some people have always been aware of the power of the mind. Tibetan monks have the ability to visualise fires in their abdomen and raise their body temperature; they demonstrate this by going out into the ice-cold Himalayas wearing only loin cloths. In India, some people drive large poles through their skin and then hang from these poles. Others walk across red-hot coals without ill effect. On Good Friday, in the Philippines, some Catholics crucify themselves with two- or three-inch nails. Although the church discourages this practice, the experience is positive enough that some individuals repeat it year after year.

The late Jack Schwarz, a mystic and clairvoyant, had the ability to see inside his body from an early age. He learned how to control pain during his time in a concentration camp (see his book *Voluntary Controls*). He could lie on a bed of three-inch nails with a 180-lb man lying on top of him without ill effects. The doctors measured the changes in his body using EEG recording, cardiovascular monitoring and galvanic skin responses whilst he performed these feats. He was able to run large sailor's needles through his biceps without blood loss and without any change in his physiology.

He explained to investigators how he did it: he imagined the needle was being pushed into his chair whilst it was actually going into his body. By changing his mindset he could switch on the bleeding and bleed profusely, if he so wanted. He could then switch it off again just as easily. He had the same lack of physiological response when subjected to cigarette burns; these then healed rapidly. He could control his pulse rate and his blood pressure, and heal within hours of injury, and was unaffected by toxins injected into his body. This gives us an inkling of the power of the trained mind to influence the body. Yet no one can yet explain how this was done.

Ultimately, however, it is the immune system which must heal us. Have we underestimated its powers? We can also get some idea from a study done on mice. These mice were given injections of S180, a highly virulent mix of sarcoma which normally causes tumours to grow rapidly and kill the mice within two months. One strain of mice mysteriously developed resistance to the S180 cells when injected. The researchers kept injecting more and more S180 but each time the immune system of the mice simply stepped up a gear. Their immune system eventually became so powerful that within a 24-hour period it could reject a cancer weighing 10% of its body weight. This is equivalent to clearing a cancer a hundred times greater than the worst seen in humans, within a day. At least, for some types of mice, curing cancer is easy.[8]

We know that the immune system is an intelligent system with the ability to learn. As the mice studies illustrate, its capacity to heal is vast. For instance, it is known that the immune system is capable of producing 80 million antibodies a second.

But is it only mice that are capable of these remarkable healings? Dr James Hull, a dentist living in Newport, had a strong family history of cancer. True to form he developed cancer at the age of 50. This was a stage 3 bowel cancer which had spread to his lymph nodes. He had extensive surgery but his doctors felt it would be terminal. The next year he developed an aggressive pancreatic cancer. He was told to put his affairs in order. Seven years later he developed a melanoma. Soon after he was found to have tumours in his liver but decided against surgery. Each time he recovered.

He should have died but he didn't. Investigations by Professor Sewell of Cardiff University School of Medicine found his T cells had an astonishing ability to kill cancer cells. Not only did they cure his cancers but his T cells were highly effective in killing cancer cells taken from other patients. It turned out that he was not the only cancer survivor to demonstrate this ability, though none did this to the same degree. He formed the Continuum Life Sciences charity to investigate this extraordinary phenomenon.

I believe it is hugely valuable to understand that the body is far more flexible, creative and durable than we presently give it credit for.

We already know the body can produce chemicals every bit as powerful as any pharmaceutical drug. For instance, in response to pain it can release dynorphin, a morphine-like substance 200 times stronger than morphine. This might explain stories of soldiers at Anzio beach on D-Day, many with horrific wounds, who seemed oddly free from pain. I suspect it can produce hundreds of other chemicals we know much less about.

Let's just note for now that the body has, within itself, untapped healing potential which we are only just beginning to understand. Of course, doctors will rightly say that curing terminal cancer happens rarely. However, far more important is the fact that it can happen at all. Perhaps this is why there has never been an illness that doesn't have some survivors.

We might use the analogy of running the four-minute mile. At one time this was considered an impossible feat so no one attempted it. After Roger Bannister proved it could be done, his record was broken within a few months. Now hundreds of people from the USA alone have run the mile in less than four minutes. Some of this is down to better training, but much is down to the belief that previously didn't exist – that it is possible. Once we know something can be done, and once we understand how to do it, then we can start to replicate it. I consider we are getting close to reaching this tipping point with cancer and other major illnesses.

Attitude

Attitude and expectation (see page 111) are closely linked with belief. The Simontons, who worked with many terminal cancer patients (see www.simontoncenter.com), are best known for their work on visualisation. They made the observation that those cancer patients who had positive attitudes towards their treatment did better. More surprisingly, this attitude proved a more reliable indicator of the success of treatment than the severity of the patients' disease.[9] In contrast to patients with a positive attitude, only two of their patients with a negative attitude did well.

I might add that, for those facing a major illness, not to mention the prospect of receiving many unpleasant treatments, keeping a positive attitude is a tough call, if not almost impossible. Any suggestion to be positive under these circumstances could easily be resented.

A longitudinal study of personality, the Terman study,[10] gives an interesting slant on this: being conscientious and disciplined was strongly associated with good health and longevity. To my mind, rather than being positive, a more realistic goal, in the face of a serious disease, is to be committed, well informed, determined and sometimes perhaps a bit bloody-minded.

Expectation

There is another aspect of the mind that is similar to belief and attitude. This is expectation. Survivors typically have an expectation that they can make a difference and get better; the Simontons' positive patients believed their treatments would help them. And research has confirmed that expectation has an unexpected power.

Rosenthal investigated expectation in a novel way. He falsely selected a group of children as being 'intellectual bloomers' and their teachers were duly informed. Those picked as bloomers did indeed blossom and gained IQ points. Rosenthal performed a similar experiment on rats, randomly labelling some as intelligent. Again he let their handlers know. The outcome was exactly the same: those labelled as intelligent did well, finding their way through mazes better than those labelled as dull.[11]

Why is this worth knowing? The reason is that expectation in serious illnesses can often be very negative, especially when it comes to cancer. This negative expectation can come from doctors, loved ones or the media. The take-home point is that if you want to get better from an illness, it is best to surround yourself with people who believe you can recover and to believe the same yourself.

During my career as a doctor I have frequently been amazed and sometimes appalled at how patients have been told horror stories by well-meaning friends and relatives. This is doing them a disservice. The last thing anyone with a serious illness needs is to be surrounded by people picturing and expecting the worst. Furthermore, this can sometimes stop the patient going along with their own intuition about what they want to do.

Rosenthal's studies on expectation make clear what many have intuitively suspected. Letting others feel sorry for you and expecting the worst is a poor option if survival is your goal.

Medical statistics and expectation

Medical statistics also count as a potentially negative expectation and deserve a special mention. There are two very good reasons for ignoring survival statistics, especially if the prognosis is bad.

The first is that medical statistics are made up from a diverse group of people. The group may include people who develop the disease at different ages, who smoke, who are on a poor diet and who have other major illnesses. Some may be depressed or have widely diverging mental attitudes, and all have different genes. Essentially, all the people within those statistic are dissimilar in many ways. The treatments may also have changed. Each person is unique and their risk will be different. Any person reading this book would not fit into these statistics by virtue of the fact they are looking for innovative ways to recover.

The second reason is that this information takes the mind in the opposite direction from where it needs to go. It moves it towards disease and fear and away from hope and recovery. Survivors often sense this, and decide they are going to ignore the statistics and be the ones to beat the odds.

I also realised, that as a doctor, I needed to be very careful of what I said to patients. It was all too easy to squash hope at a time when it is most needed. And my research kept reminding me that there was always hope.

Changing belief

A belief is just a thought we regard as true that we keep thinking. We get what we focus on, if we give it enough attention. So one way to develop a belief that we will survive is to keep repeating the thought or phrase in a manner that we can accept. This brings us to affirmations.

Affirmations

Few things make as big a difference to our lives as the words we say to ourselves. This is especially true when it comes to illness. These repeated phrases, known as 'affirmations', can enhance health or impair it. Yet how can words make a difference? After all, it is believed that it is the subconscious part of the mind that is responsible for healing, and the subconscious works with imagery rather than words.

Notwithstanding this, affirmations can work, as the Jennifer story illustrates. Affirmations are also convenient and easy to use. Over time they can have real power. The author Robert Collier sums this up neatly with the statement: 'One comes to believe whatever one repeats to oneself sufficiently often, whether the statement is true or false.'

The driving force behind a successful affirmation is positive emotion. It is, therefore, worth taking time to choose affirmations that resonate, that are believable and that generate the most positive emotions. Words on their own, without emotion, have little power. So once you have an affirmation that works for you and feels good, keep repeating it.

Advertisers pay millions to feed us their suggestions. They know how effective they are, especially when repeated enough, even if they seem idiotic to us.

Here are a few examples of affirmations:

- 'I feel whole, healthy and healed'
- 'My immune system is all-powerful, functions perfectly and deals with any disease easily, effortlessly and perfectly'
- 'I am now filled with vitality, strength and energy'
- 'I now draw towards me everything that I need for my complete and total recovery'
- 'I am free of cancer.'

I love Albert Schweitzer's affirmation – 'My body is a very inhospitable place for any disease' – and Catherine Ponder's – 'I do not accept this condition. It is nothing. It has no power over me; it cannot be. My health cannot be limited'. For times when worries are getting the upper hand I like: 'Even though I have concerns, my body is healing me perfectly'. The fomat 'I am' or 'I am now' is a useful one for affirmations. These are best said with meaning. A variation is to imagine shouting them from the rooftops and feel them echoing through your body.

With any chronic and serious disease, you must be prepared for a relapse or an unpleasant surprise at some point in the illness, so 'Whatever happens, I can and will handle it' can be a very useful affirmation.

An interesting and powerful variant is to give thanks in advance for the healing. An appropriate affirmation might be: 'I give thanks for my continuing health and my radiant vitality'. This strategy has been used by a number of survivors. The best-selling book, *The Secret*, tells of a woman diagnosed with breast cancer. She relates how she would say each day, over and over again, 'Thank you for my healing', and she truly believed she was already healed. Her body healed in three months without using chemotherapy or radiotherapy. Although she used other strategies also, this method struck me as simple and elegant.

Affirmations need to be believable. If not they invite mental back-chat which can create counter-productive unconscious imagery. Here's an example. Imagine a person telling themselves 'I am slim' but a voice in their head answering back: 'You're not slim; you look like a lump of blubber'. The chances are that this will bring up negative imagery of blubber rather than the imagery of looking slim and great, and it's likely that the negative imagery will win out.

For some people, positively-framed questions work as well as, if not better than, affirmations. Examples would be: 'What will make me feel healthy and energetic?' and 'What can I do today that will boost my health and immune system?'

Simple, sharp, brief affirmations, with punch, can be some of the most useful as they generate strong positive emotions quickly. Examples include 'Get out', 'Go away' (as if spoken to the disease), 'No, no, no, I do not accept this' and 'I can beat you any time'.

A particularly good time to use an affirmation is before going to sleep when they can sink into the unconscious.

My experience is that affirmations work best and are more believable when you have started some other heath-enhancing activity.

The most marvellous set of affirmations I have ever heard comes from Louis in Bernie Siegal's wonderful book *Love, Medicine and Miracles*.[6] After being diagnosed with an aggressive hormone-responsive breast cancer when she was 13 weeks pregnant, she decided to carry on with the pregnancy. She 'listened to her body' and would do whatever the messages seemed to indicate, such as 'move fast' or 'drink orange juice'. However, she also told her body what to do. She told her immune system to protect her; she told her body to be well and every night she told it to reject cancer; she told her food to make her strong and her vitamins to go to the right places; and she told her other breast to behave. She felt her body and mind had become integrated in a way they had never been before. Despite the aggressive cancer and having a baby who developed heart problems, she went into remission for six years, far beyond her doctor's expectations, before she finally died.

Sense of purpose

A sense of purpose is another factor we know is important for survival. The Health and Retirement Study found that those individuals with the lowest score on life purpose had twice the mortality of those with the highest scores.[12] Having something to live for can extend life.

It might seem obvious that we have no control over the date we die, but we may have more choice than we think. Six times as many people die in the three months after their birthday than do so in the three months before. There are more deaths in January after the Christmas period, and there was an excess of deaths after the millennium. It's as if people decide to survive long enough to enjoy dates which are significant to them.

The astrophysicist Steven Hawking's life-story is well known. At the age of 21 he started to develop strange neurological symptoms. At first he was simply told it was not multiple sclerosis. But it was worse. It was amylotrophic lateral sclerosis, also known as motor neurone disease. This is a disease out of our worst nightmares; one in which the body wastes away in a relentless downhill course. He was told he had two and a half years to live.

Few people have survived for longer than this from this horrible disease so the odds were stacked against him, yet he lived for another 55 years. His achievements as a scientist are outstanding and include his acclaimed work on black holes, being the youngest Fellow of the Royal Society, winner of the prestigious Milner prize and the publication of his best-selling book, *A Brief History of Time*. However, no less of an achievement was his long-term survival from a disease that typically kills within a few years. How did he achieve this? No one knows for sure, but a passion to bring his unique scientific theories to the world may have been instrumental in slowing the course of his disease. Certainly, there may have been other factors, such as falling in love and having the support of his first wife, Jane, especially around the critical time when he was first coming to terms with the diagnosis. He said that listening to Wagner's *Die Walkure* (about the doomed Siegmund) had a deep emotional impact on him and gave him great comfort.

How is this relevant? It is about meaning. It is about the difference between living just to survive, and living because you want to achieve your passion in life. Finding this sense of purpose activates our survival mechanisms.

How can this be achieved? One way is to ask questions, such as: 'What it is that I want to do most with my life?' 'What do I really enjoy?' 'What would make all this worthwhile?' and 'What is the reason I want to get well – what will I do with that extra time?' Once you know the answer to these conundrums, then do it. Imagine doing it, imagine loving doing it.

The meaning of illness

It is obvious from accounts of survivors that many of them were keen to understand the meaning of their illness and some eventually came to see it as a gift, although this was typically only after a period of heartache. Doctors rarely see illness this way. Larry Dossey records his initial surprise when several cancer patients described cancer as one of the best things that ever happened to them.[13] He noted his confusion that what he thought was the arch-enemy, cancer, was something that some patients were actually grateful for.

I might add from my own experience as a doctor that it is unusual for patients to describe cancer this way, but it seems to be more common in survivors. Some of them have viewed their disease as transformational, forcing them to re-evaluate their priorities.

Remission

It is interesting that the word for a period of recovery in an illness is 'remission'. Re-mission literally means renewing a sense of purpose or mission. Many of those who have survived against the odds changed their lifestyle and typically started doing what they enjoyed – they changed their mission, if you like. Take the case of Dermott O'Connor who had been diagnosed with multiple sclerosis. Although he used many approaches to treatment he also changed from working in a banking job that he hated to becoming an alternative therapist.[14]

Denise Linn described her shock after being told she had breast cancer in her book, *The Soul Loves the Truth*. When she later looked at her life she admitted, with some astonishment, that she was quite willing to die (she had previously had a positive near-death experience). So she asked herself a different question: 'Am I ready to really live?' – and realised that she needed to make some big changes in her life. She decided to savour every moment and, instead of putting other people's needs before her own, she decided to take care of herself. She healed after one month without any other treatment.[15]

For Shavani Goodman, the effect of cancer was even more dramatic: she heard a message coming from inside telling her: 'Either live a life of joy or I'm checking out on you'.[16]

Survivors often use the approach of 'following your bliss' or 'singing your own song'. Many wanted to spend their time doing things they felt passionate about, being true to themselves and living out unfulfilled ambitions.

You would think fighting a major illness was a big enough challenge in itself, but oddly enough some survivors have decided to take on extra challenges, and sometimes this has had the effect of stopping the disease in its tracks. Why should this be? It is surely extraordinary. Maybe, for most people, it needs a major illness to push them out of an unsatisfying but safe lifestyle into one that involves major and often scary changes, catapulting them into a more fulfilling life.

Not wanting to live

The opposite situation is not having a reason to live. Dr Norman Shealy noted that 75% of his cancer patients reported that they had wanted to die in the six to 24 months before diagnosis.[17] If someone still has an underlying death wish or feels they don't deserve to live, then this must influence the outcome. Not everyone wants to live, and it may not even be the right outcome for everyone.

However, most people faced with a life-threatening disease do want to live, but the motivation can be far stronger for some than others. The will to live is something very real and plays an important part in survival. It may need exploring.

Can a change of location heal?

A change of location has many parallels with a change in purpose. Dan Buettner, in his book *The Blue Zones*, relates the tale of Stamatis Moraitis, a Greek immigrant to the United States. Stamatis, a smoker, developed lung cancer in his early sixties. His doctors gave him six to nine months to live. Deciding against cancer treatment, he and his wife moved back to his parents' house on the island of Ikaria; returning to die. He adjusted to the relaxed Ikarian lifestyle, tending the garden and vineyard when able, meeting up and drinking wine with old friends in the evenings, and going to church on Sundays. To his surprise, he didn't die but started to feel stronger. Ten years after his diagnosis he returned to America to see if his doctors could explain how he could have lived so long. They couldn't; they were all dead. Thirty-five years later he was still alive and going strong, eventually reaching the ripe old age of 100.[18]

Ikaria is known for its longevity. Some of the factors thought to be important are the high quality food (locally grown, organic fruit and vegetables, olive oil, goat's milk and herbal tea), the mountainous terrain making exercise a necessity, the relaxed lifestyle and the close social connections. All of these probably played a part in his recovery.

Martha Beck tells the story of Katherine, in the book *Finding Your Own North Star*. Diagnosed with metastatic ovarian cancer, she had the terrifying experience of overhearing a doctor tell a colleague, 'She's a dead woman'. As she felt her life was over and, guided by what felt right, she moved from New York to a small town in Northern California, selling or giving away most of her possessions in the process. She moved there because she felt the area was so beautiful. She connected with the people there and eventually began working again. Ten years later she was free of cancer.[19]

Strategies of survivors

Those who have survived major diseases often made major changes in their lives. It is difficult to listen to their stories without feeling profound admiration. In fact some have commented that their colleagues have occasionally had a sneaking envy for what they have accomplished. They have something to tell us all.

What survivors have done has varied hugely. In this chapter we have seen that belief in recovery and a sense of purpose are important. We will explore other strategies in the next chapter. Many may seem obvious at first sight but are still worth including. Here are a few of their ideas:

- Accept the disease but not the prognosis.
- Take control of some aspect of the problem or something else (some have taken up a different challenge – such as climbing a mountain or running a race).
- Allow others to help.
- Join a support group.
- Get the best possible information you can.
- Participate in the decision-making regarding treatment and know your options.
- Slow down and appreciate life; live in the moment.
- Make time for yourself and make self-nurturing a priority, at least for the first three months.
- Keep a positive attitude but allow yourself to have bad days.
- Let go of resentment, anger or any negative emotions and heal any relationships that need healing.
- Listen to your body.
- Take one step forward, knowing that more help often appears further down the line.
- Take one day at a time.
- Act on any dreams and do what you really want to do.
- Give something back.
- See yourself as healthy.
- Go within to heal.

There is probably no one method that works for everyone. Survivors have often used their intuition to sense what would work best for them individually.

Chapter 4

How the mind heals

As man imagines himself to be, so shall he be, and he is that which he imagines.

Paracelsus (1493–1541)

Joe Dispenza describes in his book *Evolve your Brain* how he injured his back when his bicycle was hit by a car at high speed whilst competing in a triathlon. He had multiple compression fractures and was told he had a 50% chance of never walking again. Several different surgeons told him he needed immediate surgery with a laminectomy combined with Harrington rods. As a chiropractor he knew the rods would seriously limit his future mobility and probably cause him chronic pain. Even if he rested on his back for six months he was warned that he was at risk of instant paralysis from just standing up. It was a scary scenario.

However, he was aware of the phrase, popular amongst chiropractors, 'The power that made the body heals the body'. He discharged himself from the hospital against medical advice and put himself on a regime of raw food, meditation and visualisation. He imagined the joy of being healed and his spine responding perfectly. He studied hundreds of pictures of normal spines to imprint these on his mind. He asked friends and relatives to come in and put their hands over his spine to heal him (see later). He then used an incline board (a board where he could rest on an incline – a bit like a chair where you can go from nearly horizontal to upright) which he gradually raised; later he started swimming. Within 10 weeks he was back to work. His spine had healed completely.[1]

Most people assume that when they develop a disease such as cancer that they have a body which is out of their control. As we have seen in Chapter 2, this is only partly true. Pioneers such as Kelley and Plant observed that their cancers changed from hour to hour; varying in a consistent fashion depending on the foods they were eating. The same is true for the mind. Certain states of mind, like certain foods, are naturally healing whereas others have an opposite effect. In other words, we have the power to influence an illness both with our diet and with our mind on a moment-to-moment basis. This gives us another tool when fighting any disease.

Top athletes have known for years how important mental states can be. They have been quick to seize on any advantage that could give them a competitive edge. Often that difference is in the mind, and now most top athletes and sports teams have their own psychologists to help give them this cutting edge. Why should we not do the same when faced with a major illness? After all, it could make the difference between a successful outcome and an unsuccessful one.

Many of the mental strategies that survivors have used are based on two simple ideas. Both are backed by a substantial amount of research:

1. The body goes into healing mode once it becomes relaxed, and conversely healing of the body stops when we are under stress.
2. Thoughts are creative and can modify health.

Stress, relaxation and healing

Let's look at the evidence. We already know that stress increases the incidence and severity of many diseases. A meta-analysis of nearly 300 studies found that stress lowered immunity.[2] Stress increases inflammation, which in turn increases the risk of cancer. It activates the 'fight or flight' response, triggering the sympathetic nervous system, releasing hormones such as adrenaline, noradrenaline and cortisol, and reducing levels of growth hormone. Both adrenaline and noradrenaline block the body's ability to destroy tumours. One study showed tumours grew 225% faster in stressed mice.[3] However, it isn't just that we produce harmful chemicals when under stress. We also produce less of those anabolic hormones essential for healing and repair, as raw materials get diverted to produce more adrenaline and cortisol.

Stress triggers the release of an inflammatory cocktail, including harmful forms of eicosanoids, and cytokines, which in turn increase endothelial growth factor, a cancer promoter. Stress alters the expression of genes linked with inflammation, switching on 70 genes and switching off another 100, reducing DNA repair and regeneration. Natural killer cells (NK) are depressed. Suffice it to say that stress alters our biochemistry in a negative way.

It is obvious that if we want to promote healing, then reducing stress becomes a priority. However, there is more to stress than meets the eye. In the previously-mentioned study on rats subjected to electrical shocks (see Introduction, page 6), those that learned to avoid the shocks rejected their tumours three times as often as those that couldn't. What's more, 20% more of these rats rejected their tumours compared with those rats not subjected to any shocks. Here the stress proved beneficial and adapting to it had a positive survival effect.

A study of Harvard graduates found good copers (those

who had few symptoms when under high levels of stress) had significantly higher NK cell activity than poor copers (many symptoms under high levels of stress), suggesting again that it is not just the stress we are under, but our ability to cope with it that determines immunity.[4] So reducing stress, or adapting to it in a positive way, can enhance our ability to fight a disease.

Let's just note for now that, although stress can be harmful, it is not just the stress but how we deal with it that counts. However, we can take this a step further.

Is relaxation the answer?

Is it possible that we could do the opposite: deliberately switch on healing? The work of Herbert Benson, who developed our understanding of the relaxation response, has given an unequivocal answer. We can. When relaxed, the body releases a very different set of chemicals and hormones to those produced under stress.

During the relaxation response, the parasympathetic system is stimulated, hormones like dopamine and chemicals such as endorphins are released, boosting immunity and well-being. NK cells are increased. Gene expression changes in a way that favours cellular repair and reduces inflammation. All these changes promote healing.

Benson was a cardiologist. He had observed that many people with heart disease became worse under stress. He knew relaxation induced slowing of breathing, heart rate and blood pressure and reduced the need for oxygen. It also produces coherence in the two hemispheres of the brain.

He initially discovered that five things were needed to induce the relaxation response:

1. repetition of a word, phrase or sound
2. a quiet environment
3. progressive muscle relaxation from the feet upwards

4. slowing of the breathing
5. ignoring other thoughts that enter the mind and continuing to return to the word or phrase.

The relaxation response achieved in this way is similar, if not identical, to many types of meditation. Later he found that that just repeating a phrase and disregarding other thoughts worked almost as well.

Benson discovered that the relaxation response created a beneficial response in a variety of illnesses, including asthma, hypertension, ulcers, diabetes, angina, insomnia, rheumatoid arthritis, muscle and joint pain, palpitations and depression. It helped in many types of chronic pain.

It also changed gene expression. A study of 19 long-term practitioners of techniques which induced the relaxation response (meditation, yoga and repetitive prayer) and 19 novices (who received eight weeks of training), found these practices altered over 2000 genes in a beneficial way (both up-regulation and down-regulation) in experienced practitioners and over 1500 in novices. Even one session resulted in changes in gene expression. The gene expressions altered were those associated with oxidative stress, inflammation and energy metabolism. Clearly something remarkable happens when we relax in this way on a consistent basis.[5]

Other healing states

Relaxation is not, however, the only mental state that can heal. Other positive states can do the same, although the data are not as strong. Laughter increases NK cells and reduces cortisone levels.[6]

Valuable as the relaxation response is, I think there is something more fundamental going on here. Throughout our life, we are either, partially or wholly, in stress mode or in relaxation mode.

The difference is important. When in relaxation mode, whether it is the relaxation response or some other calming activity, we are stimulating the parasympathetic nervous system. This initiates healing. When we are under stress, the opposite occurs: the sympathetic nervous system is triggered and healing ceases. If this continues, inflammation develops, and later some kind of disease.

For anyone with a serious disease this is priceless knowledge. We can switch on healing when we need to. This can be achieved by doing activities we find relaxing, whether it be walking, reading, being engrossed in a hobby, having a bath, being in nature, enjoying friends, listening to music or just being in the moment. Slumped in front of the TV will not do it. However, doing the relaxation response may still be the fastest and most effective way to switch on the body's powerful healing mechanisms.

Meditation

Meditation and the relaxation response are similar. Meditation has been found to reduce the incidence of 17 different diseases. A study of a group of 2000 subjects in the USA who used transcendental meditation found that they had 80% less hospital admissions from all categories.[7] Overall, mortality was reduced by 23% and cardiovascular mortality by 30%. Meditation slows the aging process with studies showing that those who had practised meditation for over five years had a 12 year reduction in biological ageing, whereas those who had done so for less than five years were five years younger biologically.[8] Some studies suggest meditation can slow cell aging and even lengthen telomeres (shortening of telomeres occurs with age).[9] Sleep improves, immunity is enhanced and inflammation lowered. Delta waves in the brain, produced by meditation, add to the benefits, flooding the body with frequencies that promote cellular repair. Suffice it to say that there is plenty of evidence that meditation is good for you.

There is another advantage to meditation that gets less publicity but may be just as important in an illness. It allows moments of intuition and insight and, as many survivors have found, these can often be the turning point in an illness, leading them in a new direction.

Sometimes the effects of meditation can be dramatic. Ian Gawler, an Australian vet, developed an osteosarcoma (an aggressive bone cancer) on his leg. He needed to have his leg amputated but unfortunately the tumour had already spread to his lungs, leaving him coughing up blood. He developed bony metastases which were visible over his ribs and sternum. His doctors told him they could do no more. He experimented with various alternative therapies and ultimately went on to make a remarkable recovery. He considered the most important component in his recovery was meditation.[10]

Gawler was introduced to meditation by Ainslie Mears, an Australian doctor. Mears taught cancer patients an intensive form of meditation and found that 10% had a 'remarkable slowing of the growth of their tumours'.

Gawler did a lot of meditation. He started with five hours daily for three months, then reducing it to one hour daily. As he did this he noticed his bony metastases begin to shrink and later he made a full recovery.

There is an important principle here. If you meditate to cure a disease, it may not happen. If you meditate to relax and to be at peace with the illness, then recovery is paradoxically more likely. But how could something as simple as meditation cure a cancer, particularly one as aggressive as an osteosarcoma?

Clearly meditation puts the body into parasympathetic mode and this allows healing to take place. If we could stay in this state, completely calm, without negative thoughts and without thoughts of disease, it has been speculated that healing would occur automatically. Clearly this is a tall order but meditation gets the ball rolling.

The benefits of relaxed states

There is a very simple truth here. Stress produces chemicals which adversely affect health whereas relaxation releases chemicals that aid healing and recovery. So a fundamental strategy in healing is to make time for, and to induce, relaxation.

There is, however, a second and somewhat different strategy: thoughts are creative and modify health.

Thoughts are creative

At first sight, the idea that our thoughts can create changes in our body seems far-fetched, but think again. There are commonplace examples of this; the most obvious is the unmistakable changes that follow sexual imagery. Another is blushing. And science confirms that our thoughts do alter our biochemistry.

In one experiment, students were given information about visualising white blood cells and asked to follow an audiotape giving suggestions on visualisation and relaxation. After six sessions they were able to noticeably alter the number of neutrophils in their blood, either increasing or decreasing them.[11]

Another example comes from the Institute of HeartMath. This Institute was formed to investigate the effect of thought and feelings on the human body. In one study, they showed that it was possible to alter isolated DNA samples by exposing them to strong emotional fields produced by the experimenters' thoughts, without any direct contact with the DNA.

They used a technique in which the experimenters quietened their minds, created a positive and coherent mental state and held the intention of either winding or unwinding molecules of DNA. By doing this they were able to move the DNA in the direction they intended, purely by the power of their minds.

This is intriguing but is it enough to make a difference in a major illness? Can we deliberately make a disease go away with our thoughts? Can we visualise recovery?

Visualisation

Carl Simonton, a radiologist, stumbled upon visualisation by chance, whilst treating a man with throat cancer. The cancer had progressed to the extent that he was unable to swallow and he was now wasting away. He was given only a 5% chance of surviving five years. As conventional treatment was not expected to help, Simonton, in desperation, suggested visualising his immune cells cleaning up the cancer, leaving only healthy tissue. The patient agreed, doing visualisations daily. In two months the cancer had completely gone. He remained free of cancer for a follow-up period of six years and went on to successfully visualise clearing his arthritis from his legs.

Simonton was impressed but puzzled. He went on to use visualisations with other cancer patients, but his success varied. He described his experiences in his classic book *Getting Well Again*.[12]

Garrett Porter developed a malignant brain tumour when he was 10 years old. He was expected to die as radiotherapy had failed to shrink the tumour. At the time, a psychologist, Pat Norris, was researching the effect of visualisation and taught him how to do this. She first showed him some basic visualisations, such as imagining cutting a lemon and putting a piece of it in his mouth. This made him salivate, as should happen if someone can visualise well. It was a good start. Garrett was fascinated by *Star Wars* and he imagined his T cells (immune cells) as spaceships and the tumour as an invading planet, an alien invader. His spaceships would approach their target, fire their laser guns and watch as damage appeared on the planet, which then released its cells. He did this visualisation every night, complete with the sounds of the missiles hitting the target.

One night, about five months after he had started, his T cell cruisers were unable to locate their target. He had nothing to fire his missiles at. A subsequent CAT scan revealed the brain tumour had disappeared. He is not the only person to sense the disappearance of a tumour during visualisations before it was medically confirmed.

Such a dramatic outcome is probably uncommon. It may have helped that Garrett was an excellent visualiser, but the fact that it occurred at all is extraordinary and reminds us of how awesome the power of the mind can be.

Dos and don'ts of visualisation

So why have some patients succeeded whereas other have not? Major reviews of the scientific literature, notably by Drs Achterberg and Lawlis,[13] can help us here. Suffice it to say that these studies have confirmed what some survivors have already told us: that visualisation does work, at least for some. Successful visualisers formed large, clear, bright compelling images and saw things as if they were actually there.[14] Unsuccessful visualisers formed small, fuzzy, distant pictures, often using a questioning tone of voice, imagining the scene as if they were not present. (This is the difference between imagining travelling along a roller-coaster or looking down on yourself in the same rollercoaster). Typically, visualising needs to be repeated for several weeks before any changes occur, so patience is also needed

Examples of visualisation

There are different types of visualisation. The first is imagining the tumour being destroyed. This can be realistic, such as seeing the white cells as bristling with energy and power, relentlessly hunting down cancer cells and smashing them to pieces. Or it can be creative, such as with Garrett Porter's spaceships destroying an enemy planet.

Another type of visualisation is to imagine you are in great health. Running along a beach seems especially popular. Remember a time of great vitality and health, feel the emotions and then amplify them and amplify them again. Send any good feelings through the roof. Being realistic is not the aim. The goal is to maximise the good feelings, pushing vitality up to its limits. It's handy to remember those times when you have felt great and store them for future use.

Other options are breathing in white or beautifully coloured light, seeing the body as pure, healthy and healed. A variation is to see all the cells and organs looking healthy and working in perfect harmony. Another is to imagine you are connected with anyone and everyone exhibiting great health and vitality, or anyone and everyone who has cured themselves from a similar disease.

Another option is to imagine a time after the illness is gone, perhaps telling friends how you got better or the specialist telling you that you are cured (see pages 105, 134).

Music can amplify the effects. For instance, using stirring music whilst imagining an army blasting away at tumour cells until no more are left.

An excellent resource is David Hamilton's book *How your Mind can Heal your Body*. This has an appendix with a large number of medical conditions and suitable visualisations for each of these. He suggests visualising for 10 minutes three times a day.

Shivani Goodman (page 118) used a technique similar to visualisation to reverse her breast cancer. Initially she used visualisations for an hour three times a day, later doing it daily. She believes it takes about three weeks to have an impact on the subconscious mind. This figure of three weeks matches accounts by other survivors.

Assume the feeling of the wish fulfilled

In the 1950s, Neville Goddard, usually known as Neville, was asked to see a young man in hospital with terminal heart disease. The resulting weakness and weight loss had left him looking like a skeleton. He had been told he had only months to live. Neville was well aware of how thought patterns and emotions impact on health. This was decades before people discovered concepts like visualisation or creating your own reality. His most well-known sayings were: 'Assume the feeling of the wish fulfilled' and 'Persist in the assumption that your desire is already fulfilled and your world will inevitably conform to your assumption'.

The way he dealt with this patient was inspired. He simply asked the young man to imagine the face of the hospital consultant once he was cured and imagine seeing him shaking his head and saying over and over again 'I don't believe it'. The young man, perhaps having nothing to lose, took Neville at his word, assumed the feeling of the wish fulfilled and persistently imagined this positive scenario. He duly got better, amazing his doctor in exactly the fashion Neville had predicted. Neville gives several other astonishing examples of the use of these principles in his books.[15]

This is a wonderful example of the mind's ability to heal, even when things look desperate. The difference between this and other techniques, such as visualising an illness healing, is like the difference between the phrase 'I am healing' and 'I am healed' – the latter feels more solid.

An important quality with these methods is persistence – the aim is to have more positive thoughts about the illness than negative. It is no good putting aside half an hour a day to visualise great health and spending the next eight hours worrying about it (which is effectively visualising poor health).

The trick here, as Neville pointed out, is to hold firmly to that imagined reality even when nothing in the present supports it. In his words: 'An assumption, though false, if sustained, will harden into fact'. It is accepting the diagnosis but radically altering the prognosis. It is painting with thought.

I think these are acquired skills and may be much easier for some people than others. What is important though is that they have been used with success.

Notice this is not like using a drug or surgery. It is more akin to a skill that needs to be developed. Notice also that it combines relaxation and creating health: both put the body into healing mode. Although we don't understand how it works, we do know it can work and we know how to maximise its power.

So here we have seen unequivocal cases where patients have used their mind to create another reality, against the expectation of doctors, and have cured major diseases. But can others heal us with the power of their minds?

Extraordinary healing

There is an astonishing sequence in Gregg Braden's DVD, the *Science of Miracles*. This DVD shows a Chinese woman with bladder cancer being treated in what is known as a 'medicine-less' hospital in Beijing. The Chinese usually go to these hospitals when conventional methods have failed. Here they are taught about healthy eating, breathing exercises and movement techniques.

However, they also use a remarkable type of healing and this is what was being filmed on the DVD.[17] In the room shown, there is a photographer recording the procedure and a technician using equipment scanning the bladder. Three *qigong* healers (*qigong* means energy work) then attempt to heal a woman who has bladder cancer. The healers begin to heal the cancer using the power of their minds. They repeat a word and they feel themselves to be in the presence of a woman who is already healed of cancer. They repeat a phrase which roughly translates as 'already healed, already healed'.

On the scan is a split screen showing the tumour as it was, on the left, and as it is, in real time, on the right. The image on the right monitors the 3-inch (7.6 cm) tumour as it begins to change, first beginning to quiver, going in and out of view until it finally disappears. The time from the start to the disappearance of the tumour was 2 minutes, 40 seconds.

German filmmakers later noted another cancer that disappeared in just 11 seconds.[16]

After the tumour has been healed the *qigong* practitioners bow, clap and then simply ask for the next patient to be brought in.

Now this is not a one-off occurrence; the clinic has treated hundreds of people this way and they have a 95% success rate at five year follow-up, providing their patients stick to the recommended diet and exercises.

An important message given by the healers is that this is not something a patient needs to travel to Beijing for. The healers achieved the healing by generating a positive state and holding fast to an image of the woman as already healthy and healed (a point we will come back to later). The suggestion is that this is something that could be achieved by anyone. I must confess to having some reservations about this last statement. However, I will, in Chapter 11 (Energy within and around us) give other examples of group healing, but not using *qigong*. So this form of healing is by no means unique.

Now I am aware that most people would find it hard to accept that a cancer can be cured in this way, never mind in less than three minutes. The danger, however, is this could be dismissed as a miracle. But if a miracle is achieved consistently and achieved hundreds of times, using the exact same technique, can we really regard it as a miracle? There is a methodology at work here, even if we don't fully understand how it works, and one which merits investigation.

Of course, these findings would need to be followed up and tested in other settings and in other countries. I suspect that western patients would find it harder to believe in this type of therapy. For the Chinese, it is a part of their traditional medicine.

However, I do also believe that perception could change quickly. I think it would be fair to say that it wouldn't take too many demonstrations, especially on prime-time TV, showing a rapid, successful treatment of cancer, before a lot of people would want to give it a try. Once it had proven consistently successful, then beliefs could change rapidly.

The quantum world

In fact, as Gregg Braden explains with the *qigong* healings, this method should be regarded as a technology, predictable from today's scientific knowledge. To be specific, it can be predicted from quantum physics.[17] It has been said that quantum physics is not just stranger than you think but stranger than you *could* think and has baffled some of the world's greatest minds. Although it is strange, keep in mind that this is a form of science that underpins most other scientific disciplines.

In experiments scientists have discovered that neither a particle nor a wave really exists until observed. (See *Quantum Healing* by Deepak Chopra for more on this.[18]) If the scientist looked for a wave he found a wave, if he looked for a particle he found a particle. Until the observation was made, there is only a mass of infinite possibilities, and it is observation that determines which of the many possibilities comes into being.

But this quantum world gets even stranger. Another feature of it is non-locality. This means quantum events in one place instantly affect those in another, however far apart (more about this later). Everything is connected and a change in one part causes a change in the whole. Odder still is that fact that quantum events appear to break our normal rules of time. What the scientist decides to observe affects the behaviour of the particle not just at the time of their decision and the time after that decision, but also at the time before that decision was made. The equations of quantum physics allow for this, but it strikes us as spooky and counterintuitive. What this means is that the building blocks of our universe are a lot weirder and reality a lot more fluid than we think. On a positive note, it allows for a much greater range of outcomes than we might previously have considered possible.

Many authors have pointed out that our thoughts, speech and behaviour are quantum events. These are creating, at any one time, one or another reality out of multiple possible realities.

This means that, at any moment, one option we always have is unlimited possibility. What we are talking about here is something very exciting and very profound. The mind can be used for the deliberate creation of an alternative outcome. This is not just a theoretical possibility; the above stories clearly demonstrate that it can be done. Jennifer's mother believed she would get better when reality told her the opposite (page 104). Hers was a total belief in this outcome. As Neville pointed out, reality then had to change to conform to her beliefs.

If we take the above example at the Beijing clinic, multiple possibilities existed for how the woman's bladder cancer would develop. The most likely outcome was that the tumour would get worse. As long as everyone, doctors and patient included, assumed and believed that this must happen, then this outcome would come to pass. And, of course, this is what usually happens.

To change this reality requires an opposite thought of considerable intensity. During the *qigong* healing, powerful thought forms created by the healers, coupled with a belief by the patient that she would be healed, combined to bring into existence an almost miraculous outcome, namely complete healing of the tumour. Once the patient saw the healing take place in front of her own eyes, her own belief was reinforced.

Most people find it is difficult to believe that thought can alter matter so dramatically. This is understandable. And it does take a lot more than positive thinking to heal a major disease; it needs an intensity of focus, combined with a very strong belief, such as happened in Beijing. In my opinion, few people possess this strength of belief. But this isn't the point; the real message is that it is always a possibility. We have a powerful and almost magical tool at our disposal.

Now we are beginning to see a pattern. We have *qigong* healers who imagine their patient to be totally healed and watch as their patient returns to health; we have survivors who disbelieve their doctor's prognosis but choose to believe they will get better and do so; we have seen Mr Wright heal once he was convinced he was taking a curative drug; and we have Cynthia Ouellette seeing her seriously ill child as totally healthy with extraordinary results. This is using the formula: 'Don't tell it as it is – tell it as you want it to be'. This is the pattern of using the mind to successfully create health.

When not to visualise

You may say, 'Are you asking me to imagine I'm in vibrant good health when I'm racked with pain and feeling terrible?' Although the answer has to be yes, it is admittedly a difficult feat to pull off. Times of pain or overwhelming symptoms are not the best time for positive images of health. The best policy at these times is distraction. Do anything you can to keep your mind off the disease. Leave other mind techniques for a time when your energy is higher. Then maybe start with imagining less pain or feeling better than the day before. This should start things moving in the right direction.

Of course, in any major disease, it is inevitable that some worries and fears will be present. Remove your attention from

⹁se before they build up: starve them of energy. Then switch to a positive phrase or visualisation when you can.

Creating health: the snowball effect

Let's go back to the previous examples of imagining great health or that a cure has taken place. Something else is happening. These images are not just creating health at the time of the thought, but are also setting a 'snowball' in motion. They generate positive emotions. They activate the relaxation response. They attract thoughts of a similar nature. They produce optimism and hope. They attract health, healing and useful information. They set a direction.

These thought patterns often attract synchronicity. These are the happy coincidences that help in the fight against disease. As we shall see, synchronicities are common in the life of survivors. We will come back to these later (page 157).

Creating health: A summary

Clearly the mind has powers way beyond what we can fully comprehend. How can we access these and find the best healing strategy to rid ourselves of disease?

Any type of visualisation can help. I particularly like the Neville technique, which may be the most powerful.

I will try to condense the essential elements of his recommendations: First, think of a scenario that implies healing has already taken place. It could be friends congratulating you on your recovery, on how well you look or your doctor exclaiming a miracle has taken place. It could be as simple as giving thanks that you've healed. All these have been used. Secondly, think of a phrase or single event that sums it up. Keep it as simple as possible, one that you can easily visualise. If it is a single sentence, Neville suggests using no more than three words, such as: 'Isn't it wonderful', 'It is done', 'Thank you, thank you'.

Thirdly Use this phrase whenever you can and, as much as you can and experience the wonderful feelings which go with it. You could end with something emphatic like: 'And it is over'. Keep repeating it until you believe it has taken place and it starts to harden into reality. He suggests a relaxed state is necessary and trying too hard and getting tense are counterproductive. The best time to do this is last thing at night before going to sleep. Here, as I have said, it will go straight into the subconscious without resistance.

This method can be combined with other methods such as the relaxation response, meditation, visualising a disease healing or visualising a positive state of health.

Chapter 5

More on the mind

*It seemed to me that, if I wanted to be the one case in
500 to survive, I'd better do something more than be a
passive observer.*

Norman Cousins

Evy McDonald, a nurse and hospital administrator, developed
amyotrophic lateral sclerosis (motor neurone disease) in 1980.
This is a disease regarded as being uniformly fatal. Indeed, Evy
was deteriorating as expected and was given six months to live.
She described her body as 'a bowl of jello in a wheelchair'. She
hated her body and was not looking for a miracle cure. All she
wanted to do was to make peace with herself before her death.
However, she made a series of decisions which led to one of the
most remarkable healings of all time.

She decided to write down all the negative things she felt
about her life and body. It was a long list. Then she wrote down
what she liked about herself. It was a very short list. Then, each
day, she sat down with all her negative feelings, accepted them
and then gave them to God. She would then focus on, praise and
love some part of her body as she looked in the mirror. Initially,
she found this very difficult. Each day she would add to the list
of positives. The whole process would take about 20 minutes.

In addition, she decided to forgive anyone she needed to

forgive. It was also a long list, going way back in time. At the end of the day she would ask herself if she had been of service to anyone and had she done it without expectation of reward. She also tried to live and celebrate each moment.

Over time her positive list grew longer. At some point her negative feelings just disappeared and she felt great love and compassion for herself. About this time, her limbs started to get stronger and soon she was walking again.

She was in new territory. Never before had anyone recovered from ALS. It was a first. She has remained free of the disease ever since that time.

There are many methods of healing using the mind. Some can be thought of as mental strategies and some as strategies to enhance immunity. In addition, some methods could be described as psycho-spiritual. Let's look at the various strategies people have used.

Releasing emotions

It has long been known that negative emotions can impair healing. This approach comes up repeatedly in accounts of survivors. Dr Fawzy gave 40 patients diagnosed with melanomas a six-week course of therapy, teaching stress management and coping skills. He noted they had better immunity (enhanced natural killer cell function) after the therapy. Six years later the rate of recurrence and death in the therapy group was a third of that in a control group.[1]

Researchers from Denmark noted that in two women, breast tumours reduced to half their original size within a few hours of a therapy session when painful memories were identified and processed. The cancers were later removed so the long-term benefits were difficult to assess.[2]

Lawrence LeShan tells the story of a 32-year-old patient with malignant melanoma which had metastasised to his throat, making eating extremely difficult. During therapy he was encouraged to relive an unusually traumatic incident from his childhood where he had witnessed his father shooting an adult, someone who had been warm and kind to him. This memory had been partly repressed. After recalling the incident he had an acute emotional reaction and afterwards the tumour started to regress. Remarkably, the cancer disappeared within four days.[3]

It seems that negative emotions and repressed memories do have the capacity to impair immunity. This could be any strong negative emotion, such as anger, guilt, fear, self-criticism or self-doubt, or it could be an unresolved emotion, an internal conflict or a traumatic memory.

Brendon Bays in her book *The Journey* describes how she developed a large abdominal tumour originating from her uterus. This puzzled her as she ate a good diet, was well aware of the importance of positive thinking and had done plenty of previous therapy on herself. However, she reasoned that if some part of her had created the tumour, then some part could remove it. This, to her, meant she needed to contact the part responsible for creating it.

She was aware of the work of Deepak Chopra (page 137) and the theory that somewhere there could be faulty programming or faulty cell memory, probably from a traumatic emotional event in the past. She let herself be guided to the right therapist. She put herself on a raw-food diet. Significantly, the only people she confided in regarding her illness were those who shared her belief that she would get better.

During therapy she 'surrendered inwardly and allowed herself to expand into the stillness' and an intense childhood memory came up, one which she thought had been cleared in previous therapy. Strong emotions surfaced and she was able to fully experience these and release them; after this, she forgave her parents for what had happened. She felt weak and strange for three days but noticed the abdominal swelling was getting smaller day by day. Within seven weeks, the tumour had gone.[4] She went on to help many others using the same techniques.

Many people have a suspicion about what caused their illness. Sometimes they sense it was a major stressful event – one that has happened or is still happening. If this is the case, then we have evidence that releasing that negative emotion can make a difference.

There are many ways of releasing negative emotions and different methods will suit different people. Often an experienced therapist will be needed. Hypnotherapy has a long history in the field of releasing past emotions. Other methods include the energy psychology methods such as the Emotional Freedom Technique (see Chapter 10). These can be surprisingly rapid.

Brandon Bay's method is another useful technique as is the Sedona method. However, here is another simple method which might get things started. The benefits have been well-documented and it has been shown to boost immunity.

Write down, on a piece of paper, all the negative events that could be upsetting you. First, ask yourself if there is anything you blame anyone for or feel guilty about. Write these things down or write down any other strong negative emotions you have about anything or anybody and describe them in detail, with as much emotion as possible.

After putting the events on paper, read them the next day.

The following day, add any more events you can think of. Use all your emotions to describe these.

Keep going – reading one day, writing the next – until there is nothing left to write down. Once this list is complete, destroy the paper in a symbolic way: – burn it, shred it, bury it. The symbolism is important and helps to release the emotions.

One study found patients with asthma and rheumatoid

arthritis, who used this method for five days, improved for six months following completion of this process.

The body as feedback

The best-selling book, *You can Heal Your Life* by Louise Hay, describes the symbolic meaning of differing illnesses.[5] To give an example, Hay believed cancer can be seen as the body being eaten up because of hatred, long-standing resentment or deep grief. The location of the cancer gives a further clue to the underlying cause. For instance, the breasts represent mothering and nurturing and femininity whereas the lungs represent inability to breathe, being smothered or overprotected. Although I don't believe this approach would be right for everyone, the late Louise Hay was a perfect example of how useful this approach can be.

After writing her book she was shocked to develop vaginal cancer. Having suffered abuse in childhood, including sexual abuse, she believed that the resulting deep resentment and lack of self-worth had led to this particular type of cancer. She could simply have blamed the men in her life who had abused her, but she knew she had to change at a more fundamental level.

Before she developed cancer she had taught the principles outlined in her book and had observed that changing the underlying mindset often led to healing. It was therefore an unpleasant and unexpected surprise when she developed cancer herself. However, she at least had an idea of what to do, even if time was not on her side. First, she made a decision that she was going to get better. This decision led on to a series of synchronistic events (more on synchronistic events later). For instance, certain therapists were in her view attracted into her life. She also used colonics and a healing diet.

However, she considered the most important element of her healing to be releasing the pattern that created the illness in the first place. She reasoned that letting go of the resentment and boosting her self-esteem would ultimately change the underlying pattern which she thought had created the disease. As she believed that lack of self-love had created her cancer, she used repeated affirmations that she loved and approved of herself, changing her old feelings of lack of self-worth to those of self-love and appreciation. Her preference was to do these affirmations on a regular basis in front of a mirror. Within six months her cancer had gone and she went on to live a long life.

Can we deliberately enhance immunity?

Can we enhance the immune system and make it work even better? Does the immune system have intelligence? The answer to these questions comes from ground-breaking research by Robert Ader.

Ader gave rats water flavoured with saccharin and simultaneously injected them with the drug cyclophoshamide. This drug induced vomiting and triggered immune suppression. The rats soon learned to avoid the water. But there was a surprise to follow: when later these rats were given only the flavoured water to drink, they still developed nausea and vomiting, and immune suppression.[6] Some of these 'conditioned' rats died after drinking it, although saccharin in unconditioned rats has no harmful effect. The rats were reacting to a stimulus in the same way as Pavlov's dogs.

Medical psychologist Manfred Schedlowski has used the same principle in reverse in transplanted animals and has successfully increased survival time. He later used it as an adjunct to treatment in patients receiving transplants, boosting the effects off immunosuppressive drugs by 20-40%.[7] He used a mixture of strawberry milk, green colouring and essential oils with immunosuppressive drugs. After conditioning, this mixture alone had 60-80% of the effectiveness of the drugs.[8] There have been positive results in small-scale trials with ADHD, psoriasis and SLE.[7] The method is called 'placebo-controlled dose reduction' (PCDR).

Dr Herbert Spector gave mice a chemical to stimulate natural killer cells whilst at the same time exposing them to the smell of camphor. After a few weeks, he found just the smell of camphor would trigger an increase in natural killer cells. He then implanted tumours into the mice and two of the animals rejected their tumours without any other treatment.[9]

Other experiments by Reginald Gorczynski using skin grafts again found immunity could be enhanced in a similar way, by what was called non-specific, linked stimuli.[10] Clearly the immune system can be trained to up its game. This is good news for anyone with a serious disease.

Putting it into practice

But how can we put this knowledge into practice? Clearly the immune system can up-regulate or down-regulate in response to specific linked stimuli. All that is required is to find a way to increase immunity and then link it to a memorable stimulus. After repetition, the stimulus alone should boost immunity.

Producing a stimulus is relatively easy: an unusual taste or smell or a very specific sound are examples, and the more unique the better. But how can we deliberately enhance our immune system?

Many of the techniques discussed earlier in this book, such as visualisation (page 131), meditation (page 128) or any positive emotions, have been shown to enhance immunity. If these techniques are being used regularly, it makes perfect sense to link them with a specific stimulus, perhaps an unusual but easily recognisable line of music or a unique smell. This is similar to the NLP (neuro-linguistic programming) technique of 'anchoring'. It is also the basis of many TV advertisements where pleasant scenes or music are linked subconsciously in the mind of the viewer to a commercial product.

Putting it into action

1. First choose a stimulus. It could, for example, be pressing your left middle finger and left thumb together, or sniffing a bottle of spice with a distinctive smell.
2. Repeat a series of affirmations that resonate with you. For example: 'My immune system is healthy, all-powerful and relentlessly effective.'
3. Wait until you start to feel the positive emotions that are prompted by the affirmation, and then squeeze the finger and thumb together or smell the spice. As the feeling wears off, stop the squeezing/smelling. The strong emotions may only last seconds, initially.
4. Then you repeat: 'I give thanks for my unlimited healing capacity.' As you feel the positive emotions that arise from this, again press/smell.
5. Then say: 'Nothing can stand in the way of my healing.' Do the same.
6. 'I heal with remarkable speed and efficiency.' Same again.
7. 'My health is unlimited and ever-improving. I will not accept illness.' Same again.
8. Then imagine yourself in vibrant good health, for instance running on a beach. Press/sniff again once you get the positive feelings.
9. Imagine yourself after being cured, perhaps exclaiming: 'It's a miracle. It's a miracle.' Press/sniff again.

Another option once you find you are staying in a positive state throughout the affirmations is to do steps 1 to 9 whilst playing some rousing music.

After using these techniques regularly, just squeezing the same fingers, sniffing the spice or listening to the music will stimulate the positive response. It will need reprogramming from time to time to keep up the intensity.

We know from NLP that the best time to introduce the stimulus is when the positive emotions or the sense of relaxation are reaching or at their maximum. In other words, once the stimulus has been linked with an immune-boosting activity (say visualisation) by repetition then just playing the music or smelling the odour should be enough to trigger an immune-boosting response. The advantage of this is that immunity could be enhanced far more often.

Although this is a novel idea, there seems nothing to lose, especially if immune-boosting methods are already being used.

Psycho-spiritual strategies

A major illness brings life into sharp focus. It brings up issues of life and death; it brings up issues about the meaning of life. Major illnesses typically deepen the spiritual connection. Not surprisingly, psycho-spiritual methods feature strongly in the stories of survivors.

However, this is a difficult area to study. Religious organisations often regard the study of spiritual issues as irreverent, almost heretical, as if it is 'putting God under the microscope', and scientists have often stayed well clear of this controversial area for fear of ridicule.

All the same, clear evidence of the link between health and spirituality has been emerging for decades. Those who go to religious services have a survival advantage. They regularly live longer than those who don't and this increase is not small, in fact averaging seven and a half years,[11] comparable to the benefits of not smoking.[12] They are half as likely to be admitted to hospital. Those who regard themselves as spiritual live longer as well.[13]

Over 1200 studies exist which link prayer and intention with health and longevity.[14] Prayer is a difficult area to study because many people pray, or are prayed for, when they develop a serious disease. However, research with non-human subjects, such as fungi, plants and bacteria, can resolve these difficulties, allowing much greater precision and scientific accuracy. The Spindrift organisation has done decades of laboratory research ᴜ.. healing thoughts and prayer, mainly on botanical subjects. Rigorous testing has shown an unquestionable effect on these organisms.[15] Other studies have even explored which type of prayer works best: directed (asking for a specific outcome) or non-directed (for instance, asking for the highest good). Both work, but non-directed works two to four times as well.[15]

Even how we think of God makes a difference. Patients with AIDs who believed in a friendly God lived longer than those that believed in a judgemental God. The deterioration of essential helper T-cells occurred twice as fast in those who believed in a judgemental God.[16]

Other spiritual practices have been found independently to benefit health. Meditation is an example, but so are acts of altruism. Those who took part in voluntary work had higher immunity and reduced mortality, and the more they did the greater the benefits.[17] Forgiveness is another area linked to health benefits.

Certainly prayer has proved an important strategy in survivors. Many have used a combination of meditation, visualisation and prayer. When survivors were asked by Hirshberg and Barasch to list which activities helped them most, they listed the following: prayer (68%), meditation (64%), exercise (64%), guided imagery (59%) walking (52%), music/singing (50%) and stress reduction (50%).[18]

As the scientific data accumulate, it becomes increasingly difficult to keep spirituality out of medicine. There is something of real significance going on here.

Asking for help

Einstein said that he thought the most important question that we should ask is, 'Is this a friendly universe?' There is no doubt that he thought the answer was yes. But the answer has important implications. In a friendly universe we can assume that help is available.

Many survivors have found unique ways to tap into this. On

a more controversial note, we might conclude that, in a friei ɟ universe, all the events in our lives, good or bad, should be in our greater interest. Certainly many survivors have a sense of being bigger than their problem and sometimes that their illness had a positive part in their life plan.

If Einstein was right and we do live in a friendly universe, it follows logically that we can and should ask for and receive help. How people ask this question has varied. Some talk directly to their body or their subconscious mind, whereas others talk to their guides or to God. Either way, this will involve asking and listening to an inner voice. This is best done in a quiet, relaxed state. Many have found this to be extremely valuable.

Good questions are:

'What do I need to do to heal?'
'What do I need to learn?'
'What is this illness telling me?'
'What am I supposed to do now?'
'What is the message this disease is giving me?'
'What has contributed to it?'
'What are you asking me to do that I'm not understanding?'
'Is there anything I need to release?' (such as negative emotions)
'What's stopping my body from healing?'

Sometimes, if the right course is not obvious, you can ask 'Am I on the right track?' and see what message comes back.

A good time to ask is before going to sleep or in a very relaxed state. Be open to any messages that come back, however strange. If answers don't come immediately, expect them later. Be open to any information from anywhere. It could be from an unexpected source: an internal voice, a word from a friend, something you read or a clue from outside.

Here's an example of the unexpected help which sometimes happens out of the blue. Peggy Paul had terminal liver cancer in her early 40s.[19] She had not responded to standard treatments and was despondent. However, she then received a tray with the words 'Don't Quit' inscribed on it and soon after a nurse told her she didn't have to die just because her doctors had labelled her terminal.

Something stirred inside her. By chance she came across the Simontons' work on relaxation and visualisation, and developed her own system which involved visualising her cancer cells as orange food being gobbled up by rabbits (her white cells) and these rabbits then bred rapidly and gorged on the food. She also changed her goals and priorities in life and released a lot of anger and resentment. She got progressively better. After 22 months she was told her cancer had gone.

Help from dreams

Dreams can warn of cancer. These dreams have been reported to be more intense and vivid than usual and are typically accompanied by a feeling of dread. Often the precise location of the tumour has been revealed. Dr Larry Burk, a radiologist, collected dreams of patients with breast cancer and noted the dreamer sensed the dream to be important and this often led to them seeking medical attention.[20] Sometimes dreams can heal or answers have appeared in a dream. Any recurrent or unusually vivid dream is worth taking notice of.

For Sandra Ingerman, a different and novel approach proved the answer. She was suffering from a painful condition resistant to all medical treatment. She prayed for help to come to her in a dream. She did this every night for months but nothing happened. Then one night a good-looking American Indian dressed in jeans visited her in her dream, told her where her problem was and shook a rattle over the affected area. She remembered the pain leaving whilst she was still dreaming. When she woke up the pain was gone and has not recurred in the 10 years that have followed the dream.[21] She has used this technique with many clients since and says the healing dream will eventually come if they are persistent enough.

Although this is a little bizarre, from a purely pragmatic point of view, it strikes me as a fairly simple thing to do and there seems little to lose from trying it.

Forgiveness

Letting go of hatred or resentment is a subject that crops up repeatedly in the stories of survivors. Releasing resentment can produce powerful healing responses. As we have seen, Louise Hay believed cancer was a disease of deep resentment and she saw many cases resolving after releasing this resentment. Evy Macdonald hated her own body and her story of how she forgave herself and her body and went on to recover from motor neurone disease was given at the start of this chapter (page 143).

A study of patients with chronic back pain in 2005 found those who had an inability to forgive had more pain and psychological distress than those who did not.[22]

Resentment, for self or others, may be the single most health-damaging emotion. It's a luxury we cannot afford if we have a serious disease.

Images of love

Shivani Goodman (see Chapter 3, page 118) used a number of techniques to heal herself after the recurrence of her breast cancer. One included imagining her body being suffused by love. She suggested the imagined source could be from someone who loves you dearly, from your higher self or from a cosmic source. This is a novel idea but there is some science to support it.

David McClelland did research on this topic at Harvard. He got his students to think of moments when they felt deeply loved or cared for, or when they deeply loved someone else. He found these thoughts of love did indeed boost immunity and he even noted that this could stop the onset of colds.

Sometimes the effect is more profound, as in the case of a young man with testicular cancer that had spread to his lungs, neck and chest wall. He was given weeks to live. There was no one treatment that definitely led to his spontaneous remission, but he believed it was the love of his wife, his therapist and his support group that made the difference. It was interesting that a turning point was when his therapist deliberately had him re-live the feelings of being loved by his adored grandmother, whilst in a deep hypnotic state.[18]

Louise Hay believed that lack of self-love is one of the key factors in many diseases. She recommended repeatedly saying: 'I love and approve of myself' dozens of times a day, ideally in front of the mirror whilst looking at yourself. This is a very simple strategy but can be very healing (page 369). It is interesting that this was also part of Evy McDonald's strategy during her remarkable recovery from ALS (page 143).

What all this demonstrates is that love, either experienced directly or imagined, has an impact on health. Research validates this. Almost certainly, the opposite is true: violent and depressing films, books or news stories are bad for our health.

I believe this brings us to a conclusion of profound significance. This is that any positive state we bring to mind, whether it is health, love, joy or peace, enhances our immunity. The more intense the state, the better it works, as we shall see in the next section.

Transcendental experiences

We know that 37% of people in the UK and 40% in the USA have had intense transcendent experiences when they have felt that they were much more than their current self. Many describe these as the most important experiences of their lives, but few have talked about their experiences, even to those closest to them. And yet these experiences can be deeply healing.

Sometimes it is difficult to disentangle what is the key ingredient in any recovery. Here I have combined the stories of three cancer survivors who had very similar experiences.[11, 23] It seemed to me that it was the intensity of what happened to them that fuelled their recoveries.

All three used prayer, visualisation and meditation. In all cases this culminated in a mystical experience. In two of the survivors this happened after three weeks of intense meditation, prayer and visualisation. The culmination for all three was an experience such as they had never known before. This they each described as a sense of oneness, a feeling of their bodies being immersed or bathed in waves of exquisite light and being followed by an incredible sense of peace and joy. In each case, their cancer completely disappeared after the occurrence.

Synchronicity

One of the things that struck me most whilst reading the accounts of survivors was how often happy coincidences took place. This is what we mean by 'synchronicity'. It could be being in the right place at the right time, help occurring out of the blue, or receiving useful information unexpectedly. It could be a hunch, an impulse, or a new idea. It was almost always helpful. Often these happenings were quite bizarre – such as a particular book falling off a shelf in a library and turning out to be just the book the survivor required, or a book opening on just the page they needed. Louise Hay put her trust in the process of life and a supportive universe and the right therapist appeared. It seems that once someone has made up their mind to find a solution, then some sort of help often follows.

Other considerations

Inconsistent results

To sum up: we have a wealth of data showing that the mind has a profound influence on the outcome of any serious illness. Sometimes the effects can be astonishing, including the reversal of cancer. But the results can also be inconsistent. So, what's going on?

One study gives us some of the answers we need. Twenty-two patients with advanced cancer in Canada were offered a one-year course of meditation, relaxation and mental imaging. Nine (41%) of the patients became highly involved with the methods. All but one (88%) were in complete remission with a good quality of life two years later, and two (22%) remained in complete remission for seven years, an incredible statistic for cancer of this severity. In contrast, eight of the patients showed little application. Only one of this group lived for two years (12%).[24]

The message here is simple. Sure, the techniques can work, but they need persistence, determination and an unwavering belief to make them do so. Reversing cancer is always going to be tough.

I am not sure that many people have the belief and dedication necessary to make these mental techniques effective and I think it would be unwise to use these methods as the sole strategy to heal a major disease. I believe they work optimally when combined with dietary and detoxification therapies. This conclusion (that using multiple methods works best) is backed up by research, which we will investigate in more detail in the last chapter (page 327).

Both mental and spiritual techniques use similar processes: they aim to produce positive states or to remove blocks to health. The difference with the spiritual methods is the supposed access to higher realms and the insights this brings. This help might be impossible to get elsewhere. It is uplifting to think you have friends in high places, especially ones who already know the solution to your problems. Many survivors have vouched for the usefulness of this approach.

Remember, these mental techniques cannot be divorced from what is going on in the mind during the rest of the day, when not meditating, visualising or releasing negativity.

To illustrate this, Deepak Chopra tells the story of a young woman with metastatic breast cancer which had spread to her lungs. After using meditation and other natural therapies her cancer miraculously cleared. However, she remained extremely fearful about having a recurrence, lapsed into a downhill cycle after further conventional treatment and eventually died.[18]

This illustrates part of the problem with mental techniques; they don't work well when accompanied by a persistent state of negativity, such as constant anxiety about the illness.

Creating health: the downside

The idea of creating your own reality is topical and ultimately empowering, but it does have a downside which deserves comment. One concern is that it can also make people unnecessarily anxious about their own negative thoughts. One way to deal with this is to remember positive thoughts are more powerful than negative ones and to use affirmations such as: 'My body only responds to positive suggestions' or, when persistent negative thoughts come up, firmly say to yourself 'reject'. Also remember, negative thoughts are absolutely inevitable in a serious illness.

Another downside is that sometimes people can blame themselves for creating an illness and this adds to their difficulties. This should never happen.

I don't believe people should ever feel guilty or personally responsible for creating their illness. Illness is never created at a purely conscious level. In fact, I wonder if illness isn't sometimes brought on for altruistic (at an unconscious level) rather than negative reasons. Certainly anyone who unexpectedly finds a new breakthrough with a major illness can potentially have a huge beneficial effect on mankind which goes way beyond their individual struggle. Though this is speculative, it does mean we need to very careful about making judgements about the reason an illness developed in the first place.

I certainly feel extremely grateful for the discoveries made by survivors. They are now sharing their experiences with us; ones which have come at huge personal cost. From their experiences we have gathered vital new knowledge, knowledge that we might otherwise never have known, not least their revelations about the nearly limitless capacity of the human body to recover from almost any disease. They have shown us what is possible. They are true pioneers who have given us hope and encouragement and given medicine valuable new ideas, even if acceptance has at times been painfully slow. They deserve enormous credit.

In addition, fascinating data on morphic fields suggest that a change in an individual creates a change in the species (see Chapter 11). In other words, the breakthroughs and successes of survivors make it easier for others to heal from similar conditions. We will look at this later.

Positive thinking: the downside

Is there a downside to positive thinking? With a serious illness, a period of grief and despair is almost inevitable. To ignore this would be to detach ourselves from our own deepest feelings, both positive and negative, and from our authenticity and vulnerability. Blocking this grief can lead to the negative feelings becoming stronger. Being able to sit with these feelings, and to observe and accept them, will help to release them. I think the trick is to somehow acknowledge the feelings but not get stuck in them and to eventually move through them.

There is another downside to positive thinking. Sometimes we can ignore our own intuition, overriding it with positive thoughts, when a negative feeling is warning us not to go down a particular road. The cost of ignoring these danger signals can potentially be large, leading us to choose or to be pushed into a treatment that simply isn't right for us.

Summary of the power of the mind

We now know more about the mind than ever before. I was astonished to find how much we do already know and how great an influence it has on healing. I also wondered why doctors were taught so little about this. Yet no one can doubt that changes in thoughts and emotions create changes in the body: changes in its biochemistry, its immunity and its gene expression. Data from placebo-controlled research has verified that the body has its own substantial pharmacy which can be harnessed by the conscious and subconscious minds. Perhaps most importantly, data from research on stress and the relaxation responses have confirmed that the mind can aid or impair healing.

There is so much we can do to improve health and much of it is within our power. Relaxation, positive affirmations, altruism, prayer, imagining great health, gratitude, laughter, spirituality and positive beliefs all push the body in the direction of health and healing, boosting immunity and changing gene expression. This knowledge has been known for some time but has not been fully assimilated by mainstream medicine. Not all these methods are right for every person, but, as knowledge grows, they will surely be used more and more. They are here to stay. What we can say confidently is that the power of the mind has been seriously underestimated.

However, survivors have understood the significance of this unique asset for a long time.

The starting point has nearly always been a belief that recovery is possible and then having the persistence and determination to make it happen through the inevitable downturns. Perhaps the most important message survivors have given us is that the mind is powerfully creative, and by fixing our vision on healing and health rather than on disease, we can modify the outcome of an illness.

A variety of other techniques have been used with success by survivors, including visualisation, meditation and affirmations. Some are exceedingly simple to use, such as asking for healing during a dream. Here knowledge is power.

Many survivors were curious about the meaning of their disease and many changed their lifestyles accordingly, sometimes following their dreams and passions, and sometimes releasing negative emotions and beliefs. Releasing resentment proved crucial for some.

Many survivors have emphasised the importance of their spiritual beliefs. I think it is worth keeping an open mind, whether you are a believer or not. Let's assume that Einstein was right and we live in a friendly universe, one which not only holds the solutions to our problems but wants nothing more than to help us. Think of this as an immense resource at our disposal. Many survivors can vouch for this approach. Look for synchronicities. Be open to answers.

I think the best way forward is to pick one or two methods that gel with you and concentrate on these. One interesting piece of research on mental health was shown on BBC's *Trust me, I'm a Doctor* in November 2017. They found many methods helped but if we enjoy using a method, it is far more likely to work for us. If any of these techniques don't feel right, then don't use them; there are plenty more. At the same time, repetition and persistence are often needed and will pay dividends.

However serious an illness, our minds are an asset waiting to be put into use on our behalf.

Part III
Minimise toxicity

Chapter 6

Toxicity and health

The Precautionary Principle: Where there are threats of serious and irreversible damage, lack of scientific certainty, shall not be used as a reason for postponing cost-effective measures to prevent environmental degradation.
United Nations Environmental Program (UNEP), 1992

The next three chapters look at the often ignored issue of toxicity. I believe we cannot truly understand health and healing without some insight into this increasingly important topic. Take the following story.

Nancy Sokol Green, author of *Poisoning Our Children*, described how she developed multiple symptoms, including lactating breasts, vaginal bleeding, sweating, dizziness, burning feelings throughout her body and weakness.[1] She saw 23 doctors and received 16 different diagnoses but none could find the cause of her problem. Typically, the drugs given to her made her worse. Eventually she saw an environmentally trained doctor, who finally asked her the right questions. Slowly it dawned on her that she had been poisoned by her own home. The house that she had been living in for the last two and a half years had been sprayed with pesticides twice monthly throughout that time, and on the last occasion she had stayed indoors all day recovering from surgery.

Her doctor arranged to give her a series of sauna treatments. Unfortunately her experience with these was far from pleasant. She excreted a yellow and orange sweat laced with the pesticide responsible for her illness. It was now being excreted out of her body through her skin, causing as many problems coming out as it had done going in. She experienced a variety of unpleasant symptoms, such as nausea, blurred vision and swelling of the eyelids. The smell of pesticides being sweated out of her body was enough to cause allergic symptoms in other people having therapeutic saunas, and eventually she collapsed.

She continued to use saunas for 23 days but was unable to complete the programme. All the same, she felt much better but remained highly sensitive to chemical odours, such as those from paint, cleaning materials or even her neighbours spraying next door. The only way she could manage these symptoms was to change her lifestyle dramatically so as to avoid toxic materials.

Her experience illustrates perfectly both the difficulty in diagnosis with chemical toxicity and how an initial toxic exposure can leave a person sensitive to both the same chemical at much lower doses and also to low levels of other chemicals. This is known as the 'spreading phenomenon'.

What is causing the epidemic of cancer, neurological and autoimmune disease that we are seeing today? Could toxicity be the culprit? Let's look at the facts, which I believe speak for themselves. If toxicity is the major cause, then this must be crucial information for both disease prevention and for those dealing with a serious disease.

If you put a frog in a pan of hot water it will jump out. Put it in a pan of cold water and boil it very slowly, then the same frog will be boiled alive. Something similar occurs when we are being poisoned very slowly, in gradual small increments, by toxic chemicals. And what is worse, the true cause then escapes recognition.

Hippocrates thought there was a cause for every disease and that the cause could be found in the air, water or food. No doubt if he had been practising today it wouldn't have taken him long to uncover evidence supporting his theory. Maybe he would have been shocked at the sheer scale of the contamination of our bodies and of our planet. Perhaps he would have wondered why so much of this evidence had escaped the notice of the medical profession.

We can only speculate, but he did have a suggestion. He observed that the body could restore itself to health once the right conditions were present. As we have seen, this astute observation is correct and, in proposing it, he proved himself to be way ahead of his time. Furthermore, this idea is very relevant to the cure of many of today's diseases, for once toxicity has been removed, the body can begin to heal.

Here we are delving into the hidden world of chemical toxicity, a subject that few people and few doctors understand. What we do know for certain is that environmental factors are of huge significance. It is well established that these are responsible for 85 to 90% of cancers and they play a major part in many other diseases. Numerically, environmental factors far outweigh genetic factors in importance and yet receive far less attention. Even more significantly, understanding environmental risks gives us much greater scope for preventing disease, and for anyone with a serious disease, understanding toxicity can make a major difference.

I would like to bring this hidden world of toxicity to light, to show how chemicals have infiltrated every part of our world and have contaminated the bodies of every species on the planet.

You might argue that you don't need to know this. Some people have a philosophy of 'what you don't know about can't hurt you'. Unfortunately, when it comes to chemical toxicity, this is a mistake. What you don't know can make you very ill indeed and, if you are unlucky, might just kill you. And we are not talking about small numbers of deaths.

Devra Davis, Director for the Center of Environmental Oncology at the University of Pittsburgh, is one of the world's leading experts on the epidemiology of cancer. She has estimated that, if we had acted on what has long been known about the industrial and environmental causes of cancer from the beginning, then at least a million and a half lives could have been saved.[2] She has amassed an impressive amount of evidence backing up this statement in her book, *The Secret History of the War on Cancer*. Sadly, we are still not acting on this, and if we should cast our net wider to include other serious diseases, then the numbers of people affected would reach tens of millions.

We often underestimate the dangers of chemical contamination because its effects are so subtle. Toxicity builds up very slowly. Chemicals are so much part of our everyday life that they go by unnoticed. They rarely cause immediate symptoms. It is when they accumulate to a degree that overwhelms our body's capacity to remove them that we become ill.

Most people suffering from a serious disease today are suffering from what could be called a 'modern disease' – what is being described in the current virus pandemic as 'underlying health problems'. Cancer and heart disease are the two most common causes of death today. (The main killers in 1900 were infections, including tuberculosis.) In 1900, cancer and heart disease accounted for less than 4% of all deaths; they now account for 65%. Genetically we have not changed, but the diseases we have developed have.

I have noticed that many survivors of chronic and serious illnesses have been quick to understand the importance of toxicity and have made drastic changes in their environment. They have led the way, changed their lifestyle and restored themselves to health. In essence, they have taken heed of Hippocrates's advice that the body can heal once the environment becomes healthy.

Toxicity in the 21st century

Certain groups of people have always been exposed to toxicity. Felt-hat workers in the 19th century, after years of inhaling mercury, became 'as mad as a hatter'. Workers in dye factories in the 1940s, exposed to benzidine, developed bladder cancer in large numbers. Asbestos is yet another example.

The difference today is we are all being exposed to chemical pollution; this has been increasing exponentially since World War II. However, in the last two decades we have been increasingly exposed to yet another major environmental threat: electro-pollution.

There is something disturbing about the type of chemical pollutants we are exposed to. These are synthetic organic chemicals. Most of these are derived from petroleum or coal, which means they originated in living organisms millions of years ago. You might well ask why chemicals derived from natural sources should be a concern. The answer is two-fold. Firstly, these chemicals and their breakdown products are similar enough to our bodies' own chemicals to create biological reactions in us; in particular, they mimic our hormones. Secondly, they are different enough that our bodies have great difficulty excreting them. Typically, they accumulate over time.

To illustrate the problem, consider the female hormone oestradiol. (Oestradiol is the strongest and most abundant of the three naturally produced oestrogens found in women and is vital for ovulation and the menstrual cycle.) It acts on hormone receptors and is then efficiently cleared from the body within 30 minutes.[3] However, there are many chemicals that can mimic oestrogens. These include a common group called 'organochlorines', which attach to these oestrogen receptors in the same way. Furthermore, the quantity needed to cause problems is very small. Measurable biological effects occur when just 0.1% of receptors are occupied.[4] This effect is important, but far more important is the fact that these chemicals stay on the receptor, typically accumulating over time and remaining biologically active for decades.

In fact, it is this very quality of stability which makes these chemicals attractive to manufacturers while making them so dangerous to our bodies and allowing them to stay inside us for long periods. Not all chemicals are long-lived, but many are, and this means that they build up gradually as we age. This is a completely novel threat, one we have never had to adapt to before, and, as we shall see, it is a huge test for our already overloaded detoxification systems.

It is worth getting some idea of the scale of the problem we face. Since the end of World War II, 70,000 new chemicals have been produced and five more are added to the market every day. In the USA, by 1978, 100 trillion tons of toxic waste had been dumped, enough to fill a highway to the moon 100 feet (30 metres) wide and 10 feet deep (3 metres).[2] That's a lot of toxic waste, and since 1978 it has been increasing relentlessly. The amount of chemicals produced has doubled every seven to eight years, with a 100-fold rise in two generations.[5]

The world's annual output of chemicals has increased from 1 million tons in the 1940s to 600 million tons today. Each year, industry releases a further 10 million tons of chemicals into the environment, or 310 kg per second. A new chemical is added every 20 minutes. It is inconceivable that these massive increases could happen without significant impacts on our health.

Many of these chemicals take hundreds of years to break down, if they break down at all. It has been estimated that it would take between 30 and 2500 years to reduce the chemical burden on the planet by 1%.

Half of these chemicals are released into the air. However, eventually they must land and this is where problems really begin. It is not just that they don't break down where they land; something has happened that no one anticipated:

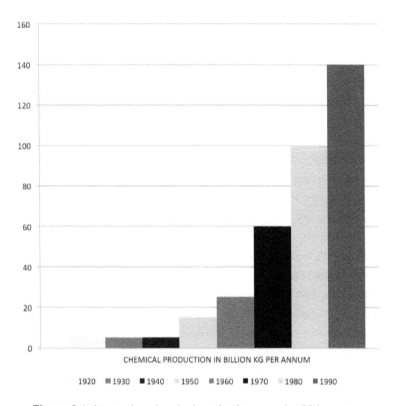

CHEMICAL PRODUCTION IN BILLION KG PER ANNUM

1920   ▦1930   ■1940   ▧1950   ▦1960   ■1970   ▧1980   ■1990

Figure 6.1: Increasing chemical production over the 20th century

bioaccumulation. Chemicals concentrate as they go up the food chain. For instance, the American Environmental Protection Agency (EPA) has discovered that dioxins landing in water concentrate in fish at levels 159,000 times higher than those in the water.[6] Levels of PCBs and DDT in North Pacific dolphins are found at concentrations between 13 and 37 million times higher respectively than in the water.[7] Chemicals concentrate as they go up the food chain and come back to us in a highly concentrated form. And we too concentrate pollutants as we age. No one expected this and it was not the only unforeseen surprise with chemicals.

What about safety testing? You might well ask. In fact, only about 7% of chemicals have been adequately tested for safety, only about 1.5-3% of chemicals have been tested for carcinogenicity, with 43% having no safety data at all. A study by the National Research Council in the USA in 1997 found 70% of large volume chemicals (in other words, those we are most likely to come in contact with) lacked minimal toxicity data. There were no data on reproductive damage in 57% of cases, no data on neurotoxicity in 67% and no data on immunotoxicity in 86%.[8] Less than one 1% of chemicals have been tested for their effect on the developing foetal brain.

In Europe, 21% of the highest volume chemicals have no safety data and 86% don't have enough data for a basic safety assessment.[9] Half of the top 20 chemicals in the Toxic Releases Inventory (1997) are suspected neurotoxins and nearly two billion pounds (c. 1 billion kg) of these found their way into the air, water and ground in the USA in 1997.[10] Chemicals are typically not tested for their effect on immunity, on neurological function or for psychological effects, even though these effects are known to occur. Perhaps the only thing we can be absolutely certain about when it comes to chemicals is our ignorance about their dangers.

As science has progressed, an unmistakeable trend has emerged: many chemicals have been found to be far more toxic than we originally thought. Take the toxicity thresholds for vinyl chloride, ethylene dichloride and six chlorinated solvents. These were progressively lowered from the 1960s to the 1980s as new knowledge became available. These revisions have been considerable, usually reducing the safe limit between one half and one tenth.[11] The acceptable level for lead in 1968 was 80 mcg/ml (that is, 80 micrograms per *millilitre*); thresholds gradually changed to 60, 40, 35, 25 and then 10 mcg/dl (that is, 10 micrograms per *decilitre* - 100 times greater volume) as new knowledge emerged.[12] Now it is believed there is no safe level.

Recent animal studies have found we have underestimated the neurotoxicity of lead, mercury and PCBs by 100 to 10,000 times.[13]

What we do know is that about 5-10% of all chemicals are carcinogens. This was the figure found when the National Toxicity Program tested 400 chemicals in 1956.[14] The International Agency for Cancer Research came up with a slightly higher figure of 11% when they tested 1000 chemicals and found 110 were carcinogens.[15]

What is the effect of exposing whole populations to huge quantities of carcinogenic and neurotoxic chemicals? We can guess. We might logically expect to see large increases in cancer and neurological disorders, and this is precisely what we are seeing: huge rises in cancer and in serious neurological diseases such as Parkinson's and Alzheimer's disease. Tragically, these just happen to be the diseases which fill us with the most dread.

For the moment, let's just note that we are producing increasing volumes of chemicals, most are far less safe than originally thought, safety testing has been minimal and cancer and neurological disorders have increased in parallel with their rise.

Given those facts, how many toxic chemicals are we all exposed to each day? Let's take a look and follow a typical couple, the Joneses. What is their daily toxic exposure and what diseases does that put them at risk of? And how could they reduce their exposure.

A day in the 21st century

Mr Jones's day

For Mr Jones, his day starts when he wakes up and goes to the bathroom. The high electromagnetic field (EMF) from his electric razor and the small dose of fluoride he absorbs from his toothpaste are the first stresses recorded by his body. The fluoride is a potent enzyme blocker, disrupting some of his enzymes and displacing some of the iodine he needs for his thyroid gland to work optimally. He might be surprised to hear that half a tube of his toothpaste contains enough fluoride to kill a small child.

Driving to work, he is faintly aware of the odour of plastic coming from his new car. This characteristic new-car smell is caused by a concoction of chemicals, especially vinyl chloride (banned in some countries), but also solvents including xylene, styrene, benzene and an assortment of other chemicals. Symptoms such as headache, eye and throat irritation and neurological symptoms are a recognised hazard for new-car users and more likely to happen if they use their car a lot. He will inhale these highly reactive chemicals 'out-gasing' from the car's plastics whenever he is driving, and levels will remain hazardous for six months.[16]

If he had researched the subject he would have found levels of toxic chemicals inside new cars often exceed safe levels. He might have wondered what these could do to him. A little bit of knowledge of toxicology would tell him that the main hazards are likely to be firstly, cancer; secondly, brain and neurological effects, such as loss of concentration, memory disturbance, poor co-ordination, mood disturbance and irritability; and lastly, eye and lung irritation. This trio of unpleasant results is characteristic of many of the chemicals we meet in everyday life. Styrene and benzene cause all three problems, whereas vinyl chloride is merely a carcinogen and neurotoxin.

Fortunately, Mr Jones has no symptoms, but by the time he smells the chemicals they will have already arrived in his bloodstream en route to various organs of his body. Altogether, 20% of these chemicals will end up in his brain, 15% in his liver and another 10% in his bones, though amounts can vary. They will join other chemicals which have been accumulating each and every day he has made this journey and there they are likely to remain.

However, these are not the only chemicals his body is busy

dealing with. As he enters a traffic jam he absorbs a variety of pollutants, including polyaromatic hydrocarbons (PAHs) from the outside air. These pollutants also cause cancer, they too can damage the nervous system and they too can cause eye and lung irritation. However, whereas most chemicals are toxic at parts per million (this quantity is so small it is equivalent to one minute in a two-year period), PAHs are toxic at parts per billion (equivalent to one second in 32 years) and perhaps parts per trillion. Furthermore, with this particular chemical there comes another hazard: molecules of it can stick to his DNA, forming 'DNA adducts' causing mutations in his genes. Higher levels of PAH adducts are found in those with lung cancer than in those without.[17] However, it is not just the danger to him that might worry him most. These genetic changes can be passed on to his children, increasing their risk of cancer. And PAHs are far from the only chemicals with this capability.

The pollutants in the air attach to tiny particulates. His lungs are cleverly designed to filter out natural-sized particles, but particulates produced by car engines and industrial processes are so small that they easily by-pass this protective mechanism. From there they make their way into his bloodstream and to the organs and cells of his body. It's just as well that he doesn't know that higher levels of particulates in the air are associated with higher levels of heart attacks, strokes and lung cancer.[18,19] For he has no choice but to inhale them.

He stops at a petrol station, noting the familiar smell of petrol whilst he refills his tank without realising he is absorbing a small dose of another carcinogen, benzene, which adds to the chemicals already accumulating in his body and brain. The knowledge that there is a higher rate of Alzheimer's disease in those working in industries exposed to benzene, toluene, solvents and phenols would not reassure him.[20] Almost certainly, he has taken in all of these today and his day has only just begun.

He works in a new, modern office, complete with computers,

plastic-based appliances, man-made worktops and new carpets. Dioxins and PCBs are released from the electrical appliances, inks and plastics and various volatile organic compounds (VOCs) and pesticides are emitted from the new carpets. Other toxic chemicals, such as formaldehyde, hexanes, trichloroethylene, toluene, phenols, and benzene, outgas from various fittings in the office; most of these are carcinogens. The ozone from the printers is not a carcinogen but amplifies the effect of other carcinogens. The copiers emit trichloroethylene, which causes a range of neurotoxic symptoms: poor concentration, cramps, poor coordination and fatigue. While waiting for his computer to load he absent-mindedly puts his memory stick in his mouth unaware that he is absorbing highly toxic beryllium from the metal.

Later he goes to the toilet and washes his hands using a soap dispenser and absorbs a small dose of parabens, an endocrine-disrupting chemical known to damage male reproductive functions, plus the antibacterial agent, triclosan. This compound can be contaminated by dioxin, a potent carcinogen. Far from protecting us against bacteria, triclosan is a major contributor to bacterial resistance as it contaminates over half our water supplies.

During his coffee break, Mr Jones drinks from a polystyrene cup; his body takes another hit from yet another small dose of carcinogen, this time styrene. As the day is cold, the windows in the office are closed and the levels of chemicals in the room rise as do the levels in his body. During summer the windows are open, but this is little consolation as out-gasing of chemicals can increase up to 400% when conditions are hot. He is unaware of his body's attempts to keep him safe, but his body is already transferring these chemicals to the safest place it can find: his fat cells. Unfortunately, this includes his brain and nervous system.

His body tries to keep him safe by exhaling some of the chemicals. He would be surprised to know that these are present in high enough concentrations to be measured in his breath. (A study by Wallace et al of residents in the USA found 89% had benzene in their breath samples, 93% had perchloroethylene and 29% had trichloroethylene.[21]) His body was never designed to deal with so many chemicals; there are just too many, the hits are coming too quickly and his nutrient reserves are too low to fully protect him.

The quantity of chemicals he is taking in is small, but each day the tally is accumulating. If his body could speak, it would say, 'Stop, there's more than I can cope with – get me out of here'. Chemical exposure can be tolerated year after year but then suddenly a disease appears, as if out of the blue, when the body can no longer handle it.

During his time at work he keeps his smart phone in his pocket and his body is receiving a steady stream of microwave radiation, damaging his sperm. Other electrical equipment produces yet more electromagnetic radiation, adding to the load. His body responds to the electromagnetic fields (EMFs) by releasing stress hormones.

Besides cancer, neurological disease and respiratory irritation, chemicals are producing another important and disturbing effect: endocrine disruption. Mimicking his natural hormones, many of the chemicals he has been exposed to attach to his hormone receptor sites, scrambling normal messages. They also block hormones such as testosterone and thyroid hormones. At the same time, levels of synthetic oestrogens are rising, creating a double hazard of blocked male hormones and increased female hormones. His energy level, his libido and his risk of hormone-related cancers are slowly but surely changing, and in a direction he would not want.

He spends the rest of his day at work and then travels home and his body insidiously amasses more of the same toxic chemicals he met on his journey in.

Chlorinated chemicals deserve a special mention; Mr

Jones has already absorbed several of these, including PCBs, dichlorobenzene and trichloroethylene, during the day. The American Public Health Association (APHA) has stated that virtually all chlorinated chemicals cause one or more of the following major toxic effects: suppression of immune function, reproductive dysfunction and infertility, endocrine disruption, carcinogenicity and developmental impairment.[22] But perhaps the major reason for concern is that they resist breakdown, and typically remain in the body for decades.

On his return home, his body gets a little help. He goes to the gym and the exercise makes him sweat. The sweating releases many toxic substances from his fat cells, flushing them out of his body. The sweating also depletes him of important protective nutrients, particularly magnesium and zinc. These are essential for detoxification. On finishing his workout, some of the sweat on his body, complete with toxins, starts to be reabsorbed but a quick shower washes most of them away.

Soon Mr Jones starts to feels better. However, someone in the changing room is using an air-freshener and soon the air is filled with a pleasant-smelling chemical odour as he inhales and absorbs more toxic chemicals: some that he has met before – formaldehyde, styrene, toluene, benzene and phthalates – and some he has not met before today, such as ben-naphthalene and P-dichlorobenzene. These have endocrine-disrupting properties.

Mr Jones has a drink of water from a plastic bottle which contains small amounts of phthalates that have leached into the water – yet another chemical, yet another carcinogen, yet another endocrine mimic, all destined to accumulate within him.

He comes back and this time has a nutritious meal with plenty of fruit and vegetables, allowing him to replace some key nutrients, such as magnesium. For every toxic chemical his body has dealt with today, he has used up one molecule of adenosine triphosphate (ATP) and of one of glutathione. He needs the ATP for energy and the glutathione for detoxification, and badly needs more of both. Sadly, even the nutritious food is adulterated. The pesticide residues in the milk, meat, fruit and vegetables get absorbed, adding to his total load of toxic chemicals.

After dinner he works on a refurbishing project in one of the bedrooms of his house. Here he is exposed to a complex combination of glues, paints, latex from old carpets, and particle board. These produce a variety of volatile organic compounds (VOCs) and soon he is inhaling and absorbing them. These VOCs will mostly be formaldehyde (this is another carcinogen and is found in chipboard, plastics and carpets) and solvents (from the glues and paints), but also benzene, another carcinogen. The higher quantity of chemicals emitted and the smaller space within the bedroom combine to make the toxicity far more potent than in his office. Again they will be disseminated to various organs of his body. They have an affinity for fat, so again they will target his brain and nervous system. It is no surprise to find these chemicals have been associated with that typical trio of side-effects: cancer, neurological disturbance and eye and respiratory irritation. In addition, some of the chemicals, such as the glycidol from the epoxy resin glues, can attach themselves to his genes, altering his gene expression and, potentially, the genes of any children he might have in the future.

Mr Jones doesn't know that house painters have high rates of multiple sclerosis, myeloma, and bladder and kidney cancers or that over half of those who work with solvents suffer from mood disturbances and depression or about the recognised association between solvent exposure and the risk of developing an autoimmune disease. He might be alarmed by the fact that there is a 95% increase in myeloma in painters.[23] He has no idea that VOCs decrease testosterone, cause infertility and reduce sperm counts. (In women, VOCs alter hormones and increase the risk of miscarriages and can trigger congenital abnormalities. His wife has been helping him on some days but fortunately she's not pregnant.) He has never been told that parental exposure to paint, solvents, pesticides and petroleum products has been associated with higher rates of brain tumours and leukaemia in their children.

Eventually he goes to bed. He enjoys having sex and absorbs the last carcinogen of the day – 2-mercaptobenzothiazole (MBT), which seeps silently into his body through his condom. It is linked with bladder, bowel and blood cancers.

At last he rests; it is time for his body to recuperate from the toxic assault of the day and to start the recovery process. However, he leaves his mobile phone on charge through the night and his body now has to deal with a continuous pulsed microwave radiation, subtly impairing his body's ability to repair itself.

Mrs Jones's day

Mrs Jones's day is different. First, she flosses her teeth. Little does she know that the floss contains perfluoroalkyl substances (PFASs) known to cause cancer, thyroid disease and birth defects. These chemicals have been found to be toxic at unbelievably small concentrations (between 1 part per billion and 60 parts per trillion) and can accumulate within the body.

After she gets up, she has a shower. This refreshes her but she inhales a small dose of chlorine. The cosmetics she uses after her shower are absorbed directly through her skin and wetting agents within them ensure that they travel easily to the various organs in her body. They are principally made from solvents and hence are toxic to her nervous system. She has no idea that 125 chemicals allowed in perfumes can cause cancer, others can cause birth defects and many are hormone disruptors. The perfume she is using, as with nearly all perfumes, contains toluene, a neurotoxic agent and carcinogen. It is a major ingredient of solvents and glues. Many perfumes contain phthalates, (sometimes up to 10%), another hormone disruptor, and another probable carcinogen. They are also a cause of premature puberty and birth defects in animals.

The dyes in her make-up are probable carcinogens, as is butylhydroxyanisole, the preservative in the make-up. Her nail varnish and hair spray give her further doses of phthalates, and the toiletries she is using, like her cosmetics, expose her to a group of chemicals called parabens, also endocrine disruptors. It's just as well she doesn't know that women working in nail salons in the USA have eight times the incidence of brain tumours. She is unaware that 60% of the substances she puts on her skin will be absorbed into her body. She is yet to get out of the house, but her toxic load is escalating at an alarming rate.

During Mrs Jones's short drive to work in an older car, she absorbs fewer pollutants than her husband. She works as a teacher in a new-build school. The new furnishings, carpets and various fittings give off the same chemicals as are found in her husband's office, and they, too, will be building up in her body causing a similar array of problems. For her, there is a further consideration. Some chemicals, like benzene, are known to cause birth defects and others are hormone disruptors which can impair her fertility. She is hoping to become pregnant next year.

During pregnancy she will unload a significant quantity of her body burden of accumulated chemicals into her unborn child. This will be good for her health but bad news for her developing baby; she would be shocked to know that she will simply be shifting the toxins out of her body into that of her foetus. She will transfer even more if she chooses to breast-feed. The more she accumulates, the more she will pass on. The unluckiest child will be her first-born; he or she will receive the highest dose of pollutants. Then her toxic load will come down. Further children will receive less, but their chemical load, derived from their mother in utero, from her breast milk together with dioxins and phthalates that seep from disposable nappies, mean their toxic load will vastly exceed that of past generations.

Mrs Jones's school uses wi-fi. For the next few hours she will be exposed to microwave radiation. Swedish studies have found those exposed to EMFs have higher rates of birth defects. She goes home to eat as she has the afternoon off. For lunch, she microwaves some food. During microwaving bisphenol A (BPA), another 'endocrine mimic' thought to increase the risk of breast cancer, leaches from the plastic around the food. From the milk carton she receives another small dose of BPA. The cheese has been wrapped in plastic. Phthalates, another endocrine disruptor, as already described, from the plastic wrap have seeped into the cheese adding ever so slightly to her chemical load. Small amounts of polyfluoroalkyl substances (PFASs) leach from food wrappers into her food. Her risk of hormone-related cancers, neurological diseases, fertility problems, polycystic ovary syndrome, miscarriages and birth defects are all subtly increasing by the day.

After lunch, Mrs Jones does some cleaning. The chemical compounds she uses contain a mix of those familiar poisons: formaldehyde, toluene, butane and xylene. We already know the hazards. These enter her body through two main routes: the skin and respiratory system. The hand wipes and the disinfectant she uses both contain quaternary ammonium compounds ('quots'), known to cause infertility and hormone disruption in animals.

Later in the afternoon she has her hair dyed. She has no idea that the chemicals used for this can cause leukaemia, lymphoma and bladder cancer. She stops at the shops and uses her credit card. A little BPA on the receipt finds its way into her body through her skin.

She comes back and does some cooking using a Teflon pan. The perfluorinated chemicals released are toxic and bio-accumulative and known to damage the female reproductive system; they are another cause of bladder cancer. Animal studies have linked Teflon exposure with autoimmune disease.[24]

She takes several long phone calls using the DECT (cordless) phone in the hallway. This phone gives her a double dose of microwave radiation, both through the phone and through the base unit. No one has told her that using a DECT phone for five minutes or more causes changes in brainwave activity and blood flow to the brain.

She has the same meal as her husband, with the same mix of positive and negative effects. Her sleep is less restorative than it should be due to the combination of microwave radiation from her husband's charging mobile and the DECT phone by her bedside.

The Joneses' day in summary

This is a normal day in the life of the Joneses. They have received multiple and repeated hits from carcinogenic, neurotoxic and hormone-disrupting chemicals. Through food, through drink, through breathing, through the skin, these chemicals have relentlessly found their way into their bodies, outside their awareness and without their consent. The Joneses are oblivious to the time-bomb ticking within them and that each day it rises inexorably.

Let's compare this experience with a couple living a century earlier. A person would have been exposed to virtually none of these hazards, and in those days cancer, heart disease, dementia and arthritis were rare.

The above account demonstrates three major problems with chemicals: carcinogenicity, endocrine (hormone) disruption and neurotoxicity. Let's look at each of these further.

Chemicals and cancer

What do we know about chemicals and cancer? The Mount Sinai Study found that the average person had an average of 53 carcinogens within them.[25] However, the true amount is likely to be much greater (see later). The fact that cancer has increased, decade by decade, in parallel with increases in chemical exposure (and at the very time when smoking has been going down), suggests that cancer and chemical exposure are intimately linked. But does the evidence fit with this hypothesis?

The first strand of evidence is the simple observation that many chemicals have been responsible for clusters of cancer. There are many examples: lymphoma in Iowa from drinking water contaminated with dieldrin,[26] childhood leukaemia in Woburn, Massachusetts, due to water contaminated with chlorinated solvents,[27] high rates of non-Hodgkin's lymphoma in Finland from water contaminated with chlorophenols,[28] increases in leukaemia in New Jersey from volatile organic compounds in the water[29] and cancer clusters in Bynum, North Carolina, from water contaminated with industrial and agricultural chemicals.[30] Any medical statistician will tell you that it is incredibly difficult to prove statistically that local clusters of cancer cases are due to any one toxic substance, so the fact that so many clusters have been found, all linked to specific chemicals, suggests this is likely to be the tip of one very large iceberg.

Let's add the well known fact that chemicals are used deliberately to trigger cancer in experimental animals and also that studies of wildlife have found that cancer in wildlife is closely associated with industrial pollution.

Another strand of evidence is that many chemicals are known carcinogens. I noted previously that about 10% of all chemicals are carcinogens.[14,15] What this means is that there are thousands of carcinogenic chemicals in common use, even though only a handful, about 200, are officially listed as such.

Another piece of the jigsaw comes from looking at different countries. Altogether 50% of cancers occur in the 20% of the world that is most industrialised. There is a similar association within countries. The highest mortality from cancer in the USA has been found in the counties with the most chemical industries.[31]

There is also an association between cancer incidence and the number of waste sites in different counties in the USA.[32, 33] Add to this the fact that numerous studies have shown higher cancer incidence in both industrial workers and populations living in polluted areas.[2]

The evidence that chemicals are a major cause of cancer comes from a multitude of different sources and is now very strong indeed.

One day an enlightened government might take action to reduce the massive carcinogenic load we all now face. However, it is unlikely to happen any time soon. In the USA, there have already been 64 Bills to ban toxic chemicals, all rejected following lobbying by industry. Much the same has happened in Europe. Everyone has witnessed how the tobacco industry successfully and persistently blocked measures to reduce smoking for decades, and sadly the same has happened with the chemical industry.

However, the data are certainly powerful enough for individuals to start taking action themselves and to start reducing their chemical load wherever possible. A very good reason to do this is that most of these chemicals carry multiple health threats, not just cancer, as we shall see.

Fat-loving chemicals and the nervous system

We have already noted that between 25 and 50% of chemicals have been found to be neurotoxic in various studies. Some, like pesticides and herbicides, are designed to damage the nervous system. Most chemicals are 'lipophilic' – that is, attracted to fatty tissue. Here they will be stored and this fatty tissue includes the brain and nervous system.

So, the first questions to ask are:

Are we seeing any increase in diseases linked to our fat stores?

Are we seeing increases in cancers of those parts of the body with a high fat content?

The answer is unequivocally, yes. Some of the steepest rises in cancers have occurred in organs with the highest fat content, including the breast,[34] brain[35] and bone marrow,[5] involving cancers such as myeloma.

The next question is:

Are we seeing increases in neurological diseases?

The answer is again unequivocal. Alzheimer's disease has increased massively in nearly all developed countries over the last few decades: a major study found increases of 20% (defined as substantial) to 1200% in western countries between 1979 and 1997.[36] Environmental causes were postulated to be responsible. During the period from 1955 to 1986, deaths from Parkinson's disease increased by 411% and during a nine-year period between 1977 and 1986, motor neurone disease increased by 328%. Multiple sclerosis has shown large increases, with one study finding a five-fold increase in the 35 years up to 1999.

At the other end of the age spectrum, we have seen large increases in recent decades in brain disorders, including autism, ADHD and learning disorders, to the order of 200-1700%. However, such associations are only one type of evidence. There are other clues.

Individual studies on children exposed to PCBs, heavy metals and dioxin have shown behavioural disturbance, learning problems and cognitive defects, suggesting neurological impairment. Over 100 studies have linked pesticide exposure with Parkinson's disease (see later) and pesticides have triggered individual cases of multiple sclerosis. Multiple sclerosis sufferers have been found to have more than double the quantity of organochlorine pesticides in their bodies and five times more synthetic chemicals than those without the disease. An epidemic of MS in Florida in the 1980s was found to be triggered by toxic debris containing high levels of lead and mercury.[37] Alzheimer's disease is commoner in those who work with organic solvents, toluene, phenols and benzene,[38] and higher levels of heavy metals, including mercury and aluminium, are found in the brains of those with Alzheimer's disease.[39, 40] The risk of the deadly neurological disease amyotrophic lateral sclerosis (ALS – a form of motor neurone disease) was found to be increased five-fold by exposure to pesticides in one study[41] and the risk was increased 600% from exposure to the banned pesticide cis-chlordane. We can clearly see from this evidence that chemicals have been linked in a variety of different ways to many neurological and behavioural disorders.

However, it seems to me unlikely that any of these diseases would be linked with any single chemical or even one group of chemicals. The effect on disease is more likely to be related to the total body burden of pesticides, heavy metals, organochlorines and other chemicals.

Problems are likely to happen once the body's detoxification system becomes overwhelmed, and keep in mind that most of these chemicals are persistent and bio-accumulative, as mentioned, and our individual capacity to break them down varies widely. This means the danger increases as we age, unless we do something about it.

So here we can see the beginnings of a solution. This solution is two-fold: to reduce the total load of chemicals and to enhance the detoxification process. This strategy, as we shall see, is one that many survivors are well aware of and one we will discuss later. In the longer term, we need to stop producing persistent, bio-accumulative chemicals and find safer ones.

To sum up then: the neurological system is peculiarly vulnerable to chemical exposure, probably because most chemicals are lipophilic (attracted to fat). One study found the average person had stores of 62 chemicals that were toxic to the brain and nervous system (the Mount Sinai Study[25]). If you have a neurological disease, these facts are something you need to know.

Endocrine disruption

Many chemicals, as mentioned above, are endocrine (hormone) disruptors (in addition to being carcinogenic and neurotoxic) and this effect can occur at very low levels of exposure, sometimes at parts per trillion and far below levels generally regarded as safe.

In the early 1990s, scientists around the world made a series of disturbing discoveries that were completely unanticipated. They found out that many chemicals had the ability to mimic natural hormones, and worryingly they could do so at extremely low levels. Not surprisingly, the foetus was at the sharp end of this danger and had a 'window of vulnerability', when most at risk.

It started with a series of seemingly disparate and unrelated observations from across the world. In the UK, a third of male fish were changing sex and taking on bizarre appearances. At the same time, biologists found feminised eels in the Seine in France. In Florida, male alligators were found with low levels of testosterone and high levels of oestrogen whilst female alligators were developing micro-penises. Gulls were noted by zoologists to be indulging in same-sex mating and were spending less time protecting their nests. Lethal viral epidemics in seals and dolphins were found to be due to immune system defects and, at the same time, seals were noted to have a high incidence of tumours and abnormalities of the uterus and fallopian tubes.[42]

A disturbing pattern was appearing in a variety of species in the natural world, involving dramatic genital changes, changes in sexual behaviour and abnormalities of reproduction. Anything that had the capacity to create changes of this magnitude was surely able to have equally damaging effects on the human race – but was there evidence for this?

Chapter 6

Human studies soon started to accumulate. Infertility increased by 25% between 1982 and 1995,[43] but perhaps the most worrying feature was that younger couples (those under 25) were those most affected. Sperm counts were also dropping and a much publicised review of 61 studies in 1992 found a 50% drop in sperm counts over five decades, between 1938 and 1990.[44] This was backed up by a further review of 101 studies in 2000.[45] Research in Scotland found those born in the 1970s had a 25% drop in sperm count compared with those born in the 1950s.[46] It should have been the other way round. This decline has been found in America and Europe, but not in non-western countries.

A study of sperm counts in the USA found men in rural Missouri had half as many active sperm as their counterparts in urban centres. A follow-up study pointed to the cause: the Missouri men had far higher level of pesticides in their urine and those with the highest levels had the worst sperm quality.[47] A study of healthy sperm donors found an inverse relationship between organochlorines in the semen and sperm counts.[48] Solvents, pesticides, glycol ethers and heavy metals were also linked with low sperm counts.

However, it wasn't just reproductive health that was being compromised. In the western world, hormone-related cancers, such as breast, testicular and prostate cancer, were escalating, with a doubling of testicular cancer over 25 year in the 20-30-year age group. At the same time, there was an epidemic of early puberty in girls in Puerto Rico and the USA. In the USA, breast growth became so common in young girls that it was considered almost normal in coloured girls of seven and white girls of eight. Disorders of genitalia in male infants (including a deformity of the penis called hypospadius, and undescended testicles) were showing large increases. Diseases such as polycystic ovary syndrome are showing similar upward trends, with a probable doubling in 30 years.[49]

Scientists began to put the pieces of the jigsaw together. The

189

first clue was the discovery by Drs Soto and Sonnenschein that an ingredient in test tubes, p-nonylphenol, was responsible for an unexpected proliferation of breast cancer cultures in their laboratory.[50] This chemical was acting as an oestrogen mimic: it promoted cancer-cell growth. Other scientists found that polycarbonate lab flasks, which contained bisphenol-A (BPA), the world's most widely manufactured chemical, could do the same.[51] Further discoveries followed: for instance, alkylphenols produced from the breakdown of detergents in rivers were causing feminisation of male fish.[52]

What was disquieting about these findings was the fact that so many of these chemicals, once considered safe, were now being shown to have major biological effects, including the proliferation of cancer cells. And these chemicals were everywhere.

In the Arctic, those species higher up the food chain found themselves most affected. Polar bears and some whales had such high levels of toxicity that they would otherwise be categorised as toxic waste.

Yet more evidence came from studies on human fertility. Toluene, perchlorates (from Teflon pans), styrene and solvents were linked with reduced fertility in females, whilst perchloro-ethylene, chlorinated hydrocarbons, formaldehyde, solvents and pesticides were linked with miscarriages.

The mechanisms are still not fully understood, but an example is instructive. Many chemicals cause a double hit for the male: they act as an anti-androgen, blocking the male hormones, and at the same time they are oestrogenic. The commonly-used pesticide atrazine is a good example: it increases conversion of testosterone to oestrogen, so causing an unpleasant combination of de-masculinisation and feminisation.

However, what concerned scientists particularly was just how minute were the quantities that were capable of causing these disturbing consequences. It had been known for many years that key traits in the personality of rats, such as aggressiveness and dominance, were determined by their position in the womb.[53] The reason is well understood: the different locations of the offspring within the womb subtly alter their exposure to oestradiol (see above), which determines the diversity of their personalities, and this in turn has a beneficial effect upon the species.

However, the difference in hormone levels that each foetus is exposed to depending on location in the womb, is miniscule – only 35 parts per trillion. Incredibly, these tiny differences in hormones had a major effect on their developing personalities. Could something similar be happening to our children?

Scientists in Rotterdam postulated that minuscule doses of artificial hormone-like chemicals could change the personality of children whilst in the womb. They measured levels of PCBs and dioxins in the final month of pregnancy in mothers and also in the umbilical cord and breast milk. The level of exposure was within normal levels for the population, but girls exposed to slightly higher levels of PCBs were more likely to play with guns, cars and machines and indulge in rough and tumble play. Boys exposed to slightly higher levels of PCBs were more likely to prefer dolls, dressing up and tea sets and avoid getting dirty. The researchers concluded that minute amounts of chemicals were indeed altering gender-related behaviour in both boys and girls. These unbelievably small amounts were able to scramble sexual and gender orientation.[54]

The message coming through loud and clear from a multitude of studies was this. Low levels of chemicals found at what are called 'environmentally relevant' levels (this is scientific-speak for those levels found routinely in the general population) are capable of altering hormones, causing changes in gender-related behaviour, damaging reproductive function and stimulating hormonally-responsive cancers. The World Health Organization has described the effects of endocrine-disrupting chemicals on health and fertility as a nightmare waiting to unfold.[55]

Our exposure to chemical toxicity is now vastly higher than

we have ever experienced before. This increase has paralleled the rise of many 'modern' diseases. We now know that many of these chemicals are carcinogenic and neurotoxic and can be endocrine disruptors, though these are by no means their only harmful effects.

It might seem that the hazards we are now exposed to are overwhelming; there is simply so much toxicity coming from so many sources. However, it is now time to look for solutions. The following chapter looks at ways to reduce our exposure to toxicity while Chapter 8 explores some powerful ways to help release chemicals from our body and hence to reduce our total load of toxicity. Both strategies can help return the body to health.

Chapter 7

Reducing exposure to toxicity

Man did not weave the web of life; he is merely a strand of it. What he does to the web he does to himself.

Chief Seattle, 1854

As described in Chapter 6, evidence has been amassing from a multitude of sources, and for a considerable time, of something we hoped never to hear. The chemicals that we are using on a daily basis are damaging our health and our environment in far more dangerous ways then we could ever have imagined. We have created a nightmare scenario: the diseases that terrify us most are showing some of the steepest rises and our newborn children are bearing the brunt of this toxic assault. In this chapter I will look at ways of reducing exposure to toxicity.

Apart from chemicals, there are three other ways that toxicity can affect the body. One is old and two are very new. We will start with the oldest.

The toxic mouth

I attended a medical conference in 2016 which included some memorable case histories. I listened to these stories in amazement. There were several of complete recovery from rheumatoid arthritis and one from motor neurone disease. The latter is normally regarded as a death sentence, and a particularly unpleasant one at that, and recovery is virtually unknown. The treatments were complex and usually involved patients having nutritional infusions. However, the turning point in all these cases was the removal of dental materials, including fillings, crowns, implants and root canal fillings. These patients had been tested for and shown to have toxic or allergic reactions to dental materials, including mercury, titanium, nickel and stainless steel. Once these had been removed, recovery followed.

At least for these patients, their dental work had been the major causative factor in their illnesses.

Amalgam fillings and mercury

Perhaps the most toxic dental treatment is amalgam fillings. These are equivalent to putting a hazardous waste dump into our body, which slowly seeps toxic metals over time. Amalgams are 50% mercury, 35% silver and 13% tin.

Even in the modern world, surrounded as we are by so much toxicity, few substances are as dangerous as mercury. Although some people are far more susceptible to its dangers than others, there is no safe level.

Mercury attacks the nervous system and can cause visual changes, hearing loss, incoordination, memory loss, changes in mental function and neuropathies. However, mercury can also cause symptoms in almost any part of the body, with effects on the cardiovascular, respiratory and endocrine systems. J Levenson lists over 100 different symptoms.[1]

The bottom line is that with any chronic disease, mercury needs to be considered; this is especially true for diseases of the nervous system. Unfortunately, deciding if your fillings are part of your problem is far from straightforward, but the most important thing is to consider it. However, frequently it is overlooked.

Amalgam fillings are so toxic that when not in our mouths

they are treated as toxic waste. They are kept in unbreakable, sealed containers, handled with a 'no touch' technique. Amalgam scrap has to be stored under water and areas where amalgams are used are required by law to have annual tests to measure mercury vapour – hardly the safest material to put in the human mouth, you would think. In fact, the evidence that it is unsafe has been accumulating for decades.

Mats Hanson collected 13,000 papers, published between 1965 and 1991, on mercury toxicity.[2] This sheer weight of evidence has led some countries, including Sweden, to ban amalgam fillings and many others to recommend they should not be used in children or in pregnant women. However, in spite of these major concerns, amalgams are still widely used.

Amalgam fillings are allowed because of a basic misunderstanding by dentists. They are considered to be inert – in other words, dentist believe that once a filling has been placed in the mouth then the mercury stays in place, causing no danger. Unfortunately, this is untrue.

Here is the evidence. Mercury vapour is detected in the mouths of all those with amalgam fillings, and it vaporises 24 hours a day. Chewing increases the levels six-fold, and this elevation continues for 30 minutes after chewing and then declines over the next 60 minutes.[3, 4] Both brushing and grinding the teeth produces large increases in mercury vapour. The concentration of mercury vapour in the mouth in those with multiple fillings is typically high enough to close down a factory. The amount of mercury vapour depends on the number of fillings.

On insertion, an amalgam is 52% mercury, but after five years this has reduced to only 27%, and after 20 years the amount is only 5%. You might ask where all this mercury has gone. The answer is that it has spread throughout and poisoned other parts of the body. Also, the amount of mercury found in our organs correlates with the number, size and position of the amalgam fillings.

Canadian researchers confirmed as much by putting fillings

labelled with radioactive mercury (Hg203) into the mouth of sheep.[5] After a month, this mercury had accumulated in the sheep's jaw, liver, kidney, gut and brain, with high levels in the glands (pituitary, adrenals, thyroid and ovaries). This research was criticised in some quarters because sheep chew in a different way to humans. Researchers then repeated the experiment on a monkey.[6] The result was broadly similar, with spread of mercury after one year to the jaw, liver, kidney, brain and glands. We can be sure this pattern occurs in us as well.

As always, the foetus is at the sharp end when it comes to toxicity. Mercury levels in the brain, liver and kidney of the foetus correlate with the number of fillings in the mother.[7]

Unfortunately, the roof of the mouth is very close to the base of the brain. It is therefore hardly surprising that the amount of mercury in the brain correlates with the number and size of amalgam fillings.[8, 9] Patients with Alzheimer's disease have higher amounts of mercury in their brains[10] and rats exposed to mercury vapour develop changes similar to Alzheimer's disease,[11] suggesting it is a causative factor.

Mercury destroys nerve cells, and the idea of using a material that continuously releases a poison with such destructive potential strikes me as madness.

Unfortunately, removing amalgam fillings is not without its problems. Drilling amalgam fillings can vaporise mercury, producing more toxicity in the short term. Removal should be done only by an expert dentist with a good understanding of specialist techniques, such as using rubber dams. Often deciding whether to remove the amalgams is a difficult decision and will depend on the illness. It will require tests of mercury load and mercury sensitivity. Suffice it to say that fillings contribute significantly to our toxic load and it is always worth considering their contribution to any illness, especially neurological illnesses like multiple sclerosis.

Tom Warren's recovery from Alzheimer's disease is discussed

in Appendix II (page 376). Although his treatment was complex, one of the issues he faced was mercury toxicity and he decided to have his amalgams removed. He described how, the moment his final amalgams were removed, he felt his brain change and he began to recover.

Unfortunately, other types of fillings, although safer, are not without their problems. There is a basic concept in environmental medicine: any foreign material can cause harm once implanted into the body. For example, titanium used in hip transplants can cause cardiac arrhythmias, as can methylacrylates from dental glues. Silicon implants can trigger autoimmune disease. Porcelain crowns contain arsenic and other toxic materials, and white fillings are made from plastics which are endocrine disruptors. Most dental sealants and the resins used in white fillings contain BPA, another endocrine disruptor. However, amalgam remains, far and away, the most toxic dental material. Never let it into your mouth.

Another dental procedure with the potential to cause chronic disease is root canals. A root canal can be used to save a tooth. The idea is to remove the root tissue, seal it and then sterilise it. In reality, the procedure cuts off the supply of blood, oxygen and the nutrients. This lack of oxygen and the destruction of the normal cleansing system together allow bacteria to change their metabolism from aerobic to anaerobic. This switch can lead to the production of toxins potent enough to trigger the onset of degenerative disease.

The dental researcher Dr Weston Price (see page 27) spent 25 years investigating root canals in the early part of the 20th century. He became puzzled by a woman who developed severe arthritis and was confined to a wheelchair. He suspected this was related to her root canal treatment and removed hers. The arthritis dramatically improved and she was able to walk without a stick and even do fine needlework. However, Weston Price was a great scientist and didn't stop there. He followed up with further experiments to clarify what had happened.

Firstly, he implanted the extracted tooth from the patient beneath the skin of a healthy rabbit: it too developed severe arthritis and died 10 days later. He took the study a step further. He ground up, filtered and sterilised the teeth, to remove any bacteria, and injected tiny amounts of this material into yet more rabbits. They also died. He had elegantly proved that it was the bacterial toxin, not the bacteria, from the root canal that was creating the disease.

Finally, he injected rabbits with teeth containing root canals taken from patients with no health problems and found that the rabbits usually stayed healthy.

In summary, he neatly demonstrated that root canals can bring on a degenerative disease in a susceptible person by creating an environment that released bacterial toxins. He also established that this outcome was not invariable. Some people have enough compensatory mechanisms to remain healthy in spite of root canal fillings. However, it was impossible to know this in advance.

Weston Price's research has never been disproved. Instead, it has been ignored. This means that having a root canal filling is a lottery and a lottery that could cost you your long-term health.

There are other options to root canals. If the tooth is still alive, then a vital nerve cap with Mineral Tri Aggregate can be effective, though few dentists are familiar with it. If the tooth is dead, then extraction may be the better option.

There is a basic problem with dentistry: placing foreign materials in the mouth inevitably creates the potential for health problems, particularly when metal is put in the mouth and interacts with living tissues.

There is a further but less common problem: electric currents in the mouth. These are produced between metals placed in the mouth (usually amalgam fillings). These can be up to 2-3 microamps. This is a thousand to a hundred thousands times greater than the brain's natural current. Although this is outside the scope of this book, let's note that it can cause a range of symptoms from pain to loss of consciousness.

For these reasons, it is best to keep dental work to a minimum and, where possible, use non-metallic materials. For instance, it is best to avoid bridges or crowns that contain metals and instead to use composite materials or porcelain.

Electro-pollution

A significant new hazard has appeared in our environment. Before we have understood or adapted to the dangers posed by chemicals we have added yet another major hazard. This is electromagnetic radiation.

The change in electromagnetic radiation is mindboggling. Compared with the lives of our grandparents, this has increased a hundred million-fold. What's more, in the last 15 years, the quality of this electro-pollution has become more aggressive and dangerous. This change is due to microwave electro-pollution. It is everywhere: from mobile phones to phone masts, from smart meters to wifi. And yet we are basically electrical organisms designed to respond to the tiniest of electrical currents and constantly interacting with subtle natural electromagnetic fields (EMFs). Our bodies' electrical fields are now being overwhelmed by EMFs seven million times stronger.

In 2011, the World Health Organization (WHO) took the major step of classifying mobile phones as possible carcinogens because of the increased risk of glioma – cancer of the glial cells in the brain, that is, a form of brain cancer. Not only are EMFs a significant threat to health in their own right, but they also have the capacity to interact with and amplify chemical pollution.

Overhead power lines, electricity substations and electricity in homes were the first types of electro-pollution to affect us. As is so typical of environmental hazards, it took decades to identify the danger. Although electricity had been used from the 1920s, it was not until 1979 that Wertheimer and Leeper showed that childhood leukaemia was higher in children living in homes next to transformers.[12] Multiple studies have since confirmed this link between high electromagnetic fields (EMFs), such as from transformers and power lines, and childhood leukaemia.

Those who work assembling televisions and radios have a 290% increased risk of leukaemia and brain tumours.[13] Electrical workers also were also found to have a higher risk of motor neurone disease.

A 10-year review, the California EMF Project, concluded that power lines and EMFs were probable causes of childhood and adult leukaemia, adult brain tumours, breast cancer, spontaneous abortions, infertility and motor neurone disease.[14] Other studies have shown links, in those living near power lines or occupationally exposed to EMFs, to Alzheimer's disease.

However, before we had any chance to heed this warning, we jumped in with both feet, exposing ourselves to a new and far more disturbing type of EMF – namely, microwave radiation. There is now an extensive medical literature showing that this new type of radiation damages DNA, causes cancer and endocrine disruption, is associated with neurological degeneration and neuro-psychiatric effects, lowers fertility and creates oxidative stress.

Disturbingly, animal studies have shown that some of these effects, such as infertility and brain damage, become irreversible with increasing exposure. Major disturbances of heart rhythm, cardiac arrest and mycocardial infarction have been noted with EMF exposure.[15, 16]

Unfortunately, the official safety (ICINIRP) guidelines are designed only to protect against the heating effects of microwaves. Indisputable and disturbing evidence of biological effects unrelated to heating have been disregarded.

The BioInitiative reports of 2007 and 2012 by leading experts in the field recommended precautions against EMFs at exposures well below current guidelines.[17] Guidelines vary hugely: safety limits in Switzerland and Russia are 100 times stricter than in the UK.

The parts of the body which are most vulnerable to EMFs are the neurological system, heart and testicles. Numerous human and animal studies have confirmed neurological damage, including changes in memory, cognitive function and damage to the blood-brain barrier.

With regard to the testes, EMFs have been found to promote all stages of cancer development. This was noted by the ECOLOG report from the ECOLOG Institute in Hanover which reviewed 220 research papers in 2000.[18] Other studies have linked EMFs with suicide and depression.[19]

Findings from rodent studies, such as early onset dementia and irreversible infertility at relatively low levels of EMF exposure, are deeply worrying. A catastrophic crash in collective brain function and plummeting fertility are the chilling vision of some experts in the field. The new 5G network, if introduced, would make this even more likely. The fact that we are already seeing this happening, with studies showing major reductions in sperm counts, (known to be affected by mobile phone radiation[20]) in several technologically advanced countries, adds to the concern.

Swedish oncologist, Dr Lennat Hardell, has found a 5% increase in brain tumours for every 100 hours of mobile phone use, an 8% increase for every year of mobile phone use and a 280% increase after 10 years.[21] Mobile phone use increases the risk of gliomas two-fold and acoustic neuromas three-fold. For gliomas, the risk is greater for teenagers and young adults. High users of mobile phones have a 50% increase in salivary gland cancer.[22]

A major concern is the vulnerability of unborn babies to EMFs. Children born to mothers using mobile phones in pregnancy are 80% more likely to have behavioural problems and 35% more likely to be hyperactive. However, these dangers can be expected to increase as mobile phone usage increases and newer phones carry ever more information and hence ever more toxic EMF pulsations.

Other symptoms noted with mobile phone use include memory loss, twitching, dizziness, headaches, fatigue and poor concentration.

Mobile base stations are another hazard. Reports have found a four-fold increase in cancer in populations living within 350 metres of a mast in Israel and a 10-fold increase in cancer in women.[23] These cancers were more aggressive than usual. Those living within 400 metres of base stations in Germany had a three-fold increase in cancer.[24] In Poland, those exposed to microwave radiation similar to a base station were found to have a 10-fold increase in leukaemia and a six-fold increase in non-Hodgkin's lymphoma.[24] Another report found a 59-fold increase in depression and a 40-fold increase in fatigue, plus an increase in epileptic attacks.[25] CancerWatch reported on a block of flats in Canada with 32 radio and TV dishes on the roof. They reported that 80% of the residents had developed cancer. Today, most mobile phone masts are being hidden and are difficult to spot.

If 5G comes into force it will require 500 base stations per square metre with no informed consent. This could make the difference between life and death for anyone with cancer living within the beam of one of these mobile transmitters.

Interactions

As we now live in a world with both chemical and electromagnetic pollution, an intriguing question is whether the two interact. This is especially important for those trying to recover from serious illness, but it is relevant to us all. Have we evidence that one augments the other?

For many years it has been noted that there is an association between heavy metal accumulation and autism. It is thought that autistic children have a defect in methylation, with an inability to excrete heavy metals, such as mercury. Treating these children with chelation to remove the heavy metals can be an effective, if somewhat controversial, treatment. However, doctors and therapists using this treatment started to notice an unusual pattern. Older children were not excreting heavy metals in the same way as younger children and often failed to respond to treatment. One of the therapists, Tamara Marica, met up with George Carlo, an epidemiologist and expert in EMFs, and they both wondered if EMFS could explain this.

They set up an experiment with a 10-year-old boy with autism who had failed to respond to any treatment to see if this was true.[26] They created a programme which reduced toxicity and made his home EMF-free. It worked. At last he started excreting heavy metals. He told them 'the noise has gone in my head' and he started speaking for the first time and his autism started to reduce.

They followed this up with a further study of 20 autistic children.[27] This was less demanding in that the children were only kept in an EMF-free environment for four hours, two to three times a week. But it was enough. After three months they began to clear heavy metals from their bodies; this happened spontaneously without chelation.

This fits well with current scientific research which shows EMFs can damage the blood-brain barrier, allowing toxic substances to enter the brain. It gives further credence to Hippocrates's hypothesis that if we can remove all obstacles to health, then the body will ultimately heal. More importantly, it suggests electro-pollution increases the toxicity of chemicals, something with implications for the health of everyone on the planet.

For many people in today's world, the combined toxicity of electro-pollution and chemical contamination is proving too much for their overstressed bodies.

Nanoparticles

Many people now know something about the dangers of chemicals. Increasingly people have concerns about electro-pollution. But few know anything about nanoparticles.

Nanotechnology is a billion-dollar industry and we are being exposed to it on a regular basis. This new and disturbing invention presents us with yet another unknown hazard and again one that we've never faced before.

However, nanotechnology is here to stay. Basically, materials like carbon can be cut into minute pieces about the size of a virus. A nanometre is a billionth of a metre and a nanoparticle is usually between 1 and 100 nanometres (nm). For comparison, a cold virus would be about 25 nm and a red blood cell would be 7000 nm in width. As with so many environmental hazards, we are being exposed to unknown risks before a proper assessment of their dangers has been done.

One area that we do understand is particulates. Studies of air pollution have made one fact abundantly clear: the smaller the particulate, the more dangerous it is.[29] This is because the smallest particles can travel straight through the lungs and into the bloodstream and hence into the cells and organs. This happens because they are too small to be picked up by the lungs' protective mechanisms. The smallest particles also have the greatest surface area and hence carry more toxic chemicals on their surface. The same is true of microplastics which now exist in large amounts in the air we breathe.

Nanoparticles are a lot smaller than those linked with air pollution so they enter the body with ease.

It has been shown in animal experiments that the blood-brain barrier is no obstacle to these particles and they can accumulate in the organs, including the liver, spleen, kidney and brain.[30] For instance, mice that ingested copper nanoparticles developed severe organ damage whereas similar microparticles (which are a thousand times larger) had no effect.[30] Nanoparticles have been found to contaminate fish, passing inside their brains and causing an illness similar to Alzheimer's disease.

A sensible step is to avoid them. The three most likely places we come into contact with nanoparticles are in clothing, in food containers and in cosmetics. Worryingly, medical dressings are another source.

Clothing: Nanoparticles are widely used in clothing. They are added to the surface of the clothes to make them resistant to stains, water and static. These layers will be only a few atoms thick. The problem is that this is enough to allow absorption into the skin. The nanoparticles in clothes are typically released after one or two washings and are likely to be taken up by other clothes, adding to the potential for absorption into the body. Watch out for the label 'silver technology', especially on socks; this usually means treatment with nanoparticles. Feet sweat a lot and this allows easy absorption of nanoparticles. Other labels to regard with suspicion are 'antibacterial', 'odour-eliminating' and 'hygienic' for silver nanoparticles and 'sun-protection' for titanium nanoparticles. Nanoparticles released from washing are a hazard to fish and are known to cause congenital deformities in some species.

Food containers and some fridges and freezers use silver nanoparticles for their antibacterial properties. Unfortunately, the risk from nanoparticles far exceeds the danger from the bacteria they are being used to treat. The body has developed mechanisms to fight bacteria but has no known mechanism for dealing with nanoparticles.

Cosmetics are another source of nanoparticles. A survey in 2006 by the Environmental working Group found nearly 20,000 products using ingredients of nano-size and nearly all were unlabelled. One group of nanoparticles is called fullerenes, which are used in face creams. They have been found to cause brain, liver and skin damage in cell cultures after two days of exposure when used at only 50 parts per *billion*. Sun creams often contain titanium dioxide nanoparticles and these again can find their way into the body's organs with unknown effects. Products labelled as containing fullerenes, micronised titanium dioxide or micronised zinc oxide, micronised quartz silica and nano zinc oxide are best avoided as they will all contain nanoparticles.

At the moment we cannot really assess the dangers of nanoparticles. What we do know, whether we are talking about particulates, microplastics or nanoparticles, is that the smaller the size, the more dangerous. Nanoparticles look to me like a risk too far in a world already overwhelmed by toxicity. It would therefore seem prudent to avoid nanoparticles whenever possible.

Sources of toxicity

So what are the principal causes of toxicity and how do we avoid them? The following section describes the main ones. It covers toxicity in food, water and the air we breathe. It also looks at the risks from pesticides, clothing, personal-care products and many other everyday products. Again, I would stress we are not looking to completely avoid them for this would be impossible, but simply to keep toxicity to a level where it doesn't overwhelm our body's ability to maintain health.

Reducing toxicity in food

Never before has food contained so many toxic substances such as artificial flavourings, emulsifiers, stabilisers, preservatives and thickeners. Over 90% of artificial flavours are synthetic, usually derived from petroleum or coal tar. Some food chemicals, such as citrus red, are suspected carcinogens.

Synthetic flavours are favoured by the food industry because of their stability, but with this stability come two twin dangers: biological activity and resistance to breakdown and hence the ability to accumulate in the body. Environmental physicians have known for decades that many colourings cause hyperactivity and behaviour changes in children, and recent work has confirmed this.[31]

Apart from the 1500 flavours that can be added, food typically also contains other contaminants, such as pesticides and hormones. (Hormones are banned in meat in the EU but 30% of meat imported to the UK comes from countries where no ban exists.) Processed foods are typically high in chemicals and just avoiding foods with a list of chemical ingredients on the label will take you a long way.

The fat of animals and fish can be high in chemicals as chemicals accumulate in the fat as it is part of the body's storage system. PCBs and dioxins have been found to be highest in dairy produce, processed foods and meat in that order. The most dangerous substances we regularly come in contact with are heavy metals and pesticides. It makes sense to reduce our exposure to both.

Heavy metals

Of heavy metals, mercury is the most toxic as I have said. Apart from dental fillings (see page 198), the other major source is fish, particularly large fish, such as tuna and swordfish. Mercury can also be found in some paints and tattoo inks.

Pesticides

Would you take an apple, spray it all over with fly spray until it was glistening with chemicals and then eat it? Probably not, but in reality that is what most of us do. Even if we wash our fruit and vegetables, it only helps a little as the pesticides are absorbed deep inside them.

Pesticides are designed to destroy the nervous system, to

damage reproduction and to kill. We are the collateral damage. Hard evidence is mounting of increasing problems with human reproduction and neurological diseases.

We take in 150 mcg of pesticides every day and many of these residues accumulate within us over time. The European Food Safety Authority (EFSA) tested 84,341 food samples in 2015 and traces of one or more of 774 pesticides were found in 97.2% of these, although most did not exceed the legal limits.[32] As mentioned in Chapter 2, there are more pesticide residues in meat, farmed fish and milk products than on fruit and vegetables. This may explain why pesticide residues in the breast milk of vegetarians are about one third to a half of those of non-vegetarians.

One purpose of this chapter is to highlight dangers that otherwise might not be expected. Many people might be surprised that the most heavily contaminated food we eat is farmed salmon. The UK Pesticide Residues Committee in 2001 found 99% of farmed salmon had pesticide residues (as compared with 24% in wild salmon).[33] The dichlorvos used to kill the sea lice in farmed salmon is linked with testicular cancer. In one survey by the US Environmental Protection Agency, Scottish salmon were found to have such high levels of PCBs, dioxins and pesticides that they recommended eating it no more than once every four months.[34] Pacific salmon had much lower levels of pollutants.

I was surprised to find that lamb often contains high levels of pesticides.

Breads, especially fruit breads and malt loaf, have been found to have significant pesticide residues in 78% of samples.

Half the pesticides used on arable land are used on vineyards. Tests on a range of wines found 240 different chemicals present. Half of wines contained pesticide residues.

Fruit and vegetables with lower levels of pesticides include bananas, asparagus, avocados, broccoli, cauliflower, sweet corn, kiwis, mangos, papayas, pineapples and peas. The bottom line is that every non-organic fruit or vegetable you eat comes laden with multiple pesticide residues. This is likely to be higher in imported foods. They often contain banned chemicals (which, ironically, we may have exported to the countries from which they came).

Pesticides, health and the environment
To illustrate the dangers of pesticides it's worth taking a look at farmers. They typically live healthy lifestyles; they are usually non-smokers and get plenty of exercise and fresh air. You might expect them to have excellent health, but this isn't the case. They have higher rates of myelomas,[35] lymphomas,[36] leukaemias[37] and other cancers than non-farmers. They also have higher rates of asthma.[38] A study of farmers' children in Minnesota found elevated rates of congenital defects[39] and, like asthma, rates were highest where most pesticides had been used. The deteriorating health of farmers is a warning to us all. Farmers, however, are not the only ones affected. It is well-established that pesticides are a cause of Parkinson's disease. Two meta-analyses[40, 41] and the largest cohort study done[42] have found a consistent raised risk of Parkinson's disease with pesticide use.

But do pesticides increase the risk of other neurological diseases? A study in Spain showed those living in districts with high pesticide use had, as expected, significantly higher prevalence of Parkinson's disease compared with those districts with lower use, but they also found higher rates of multiple sclerosis, Alzheimer's disease and suicide, and for males, higher rates of neuropathies.[43] This finding should come as no surprise. Studies by the US Department of Health on rats exposed to pesticides found changes in the brain similar to those found in epilepsy, MS, Parkinson's' disease and Alzheimer's disease.

MS patients have been found to have more than twice the level of organochlorine pesticides in their bodies compared with controls. Sufferers from chronic fatigue syndrome have been found to have twice the level of pesticides in their blood.[44]

In fact, symptoms from pesticide exposure are predominately neurological. They can cause ataxia (balance problems), paraesthesias (numbness and tingling), inability to concentrate, memory loss, fatigue, anxiety and depression.

Major neurological diseases are serious enough, but they are not the only concern. A systematic review of the medical literature found a consistent link between pesticide exposure and the development of many cancers, including those of the prostate, kidney, breast, pancreas and brain, as well as non-Hodgkin's lymphoma and leukaemia.[45]

Several studies have noted increases in childhood leukaemia[46] and childhood non-Hodgkin's lymphoma[47] in homes where pesticides were used. Exposure to pesticides is also a known risk factor for non-Hodgkin's lymphoma in adults, with a two- to eight-fold increase in this disease.[48, 49] Mothers using garden pesticides or living within a quarter of a mile of agricultural crops have higher rates of birth defects.

In laboratory animals, at least 23 pesticides can cause breast cancer. Organochlorine pesticides are about 50% higher in the blood and fat of those found with breast cancer.[50, 51] Many people are unaware of the dangers of flea collars on pets, which contain concentrated pesticides. These are highly toxic and best avoided.

In America alone, 1.2 billion pounds of pesticides are sprayed on food and only 0.1% of these chemicals reach the insects they are intended to kill.[52] The rest poisons the earth. The half-life of some pesticides can be 50 to 75 years, although organo-phosphates typically have a short half-life.

Because of this, contamination of groundwater is now becoming a major environmental threat. One estimate for the cost of cleaning up the groundwater in the USA was $8 billion every year.[53]

An impending catastrophe is the loss of biodiversity, now threatening bees and other pollinating insects. The cost of wiping out bees and having to pollinate by hand, something that has now already occurred in parts of China and the USA, has been estimated at £1.5 billion annually in the UK alone. One in five insect species have already vanished from the UK in the last century. Future generations will shake their heads in disbelief at our short-sightedness, when the cost to our health, our wildlife, our planet and, not least, to future generations, is so astronomical. They are unlikely to excuse us for their legacy of a poisoned earth. The answer is to eat organic where possible.

Safe as houses

How safe are we, relaxing in our own home? Half a century ago homes were built largely of natural materials. Chemical exposure within these homes was virtually non-existent. Today, the situation is very different and homes have changed beyond all recognition. Now levels of toxicity indoors far exceed those outdoors.

Occupational disease, as always, is a clue. Carpet workers have higher rates of cancer, especially leukaemia, and house painters have high rates of multiple myeloma and other cancers.[54] The reason is due to 'outgasing'. The bad news is we are all exposed to hundreds of airborne pollutants in our homes and often this exposure is all day long. In the last 20 years there has been a more than five-fold increase in the use of chemicals in building materials.

One study found that the level of pollutants present in indoor air at three different locations (including one within a mile of a major source of industrial pollution) was two to five times higher than the air breathed when sitting outdoors, in the gardens of the same houses. A British study in a rural location in Avon found pollution was 10 times higher indoors than outdoors.[55] This study found 200 indoor chemicals in the air, of which 80 were known to be harmful.

Nowadays most materials in the home are synthetic and the

majority outgas toxic chemicals. This means that, whilst relaxing at home, we are constantly inhaling chemicals, including carcinogens. For example, many substances, including chip-board, carpets, adhesives, synthetic furnishings and furniture, outgas formaldehyde and many others outgas VOCs. Paints can be a major source. Homes with higher levels of VOCs are linked with childhood asthma. Brominated flame-retardant chemicals, now found in most furniture, are an increasing source of toxicity.

To reduce toxicity in the home, think where the greatest danger lies. Carpets are a good place to start; they are major contributors to formaldehyde and benzene in indoor air and outgas up to 200 VOCs. Generally more colours mean more formaldehyde (formaldehyde, a known carcinogen, is the commonest chemical we are exposed to). Outgasing is at its maximum when carpets are new but they outgas sizeable amounts of VOCs for up to three years. Old disintegrating carpets are also dangerous. Carpets also contain significant pesticide residues. Where possible, remove carpets. If you are buying a new carpet, make sure the area is well-ventilated. Avoid wool carpets as these are routinely treated with pesticides. Buy carpets with latex-free backing and use nails or gripper strips instead of glues when putting them down. Dispose of decomposing old carpets and those with latex backing.

In an experiment done on American TV, mice were put in a jar containing pieces of carpet. All the mice were dead within 24 hours, poisoned by chemicals released from the carpet.

Paints are a major source of chemical toxicity. A study from Johns Hopkins University found 300 toxic chemicals and 150 carcinogens may be present in paint. The VOCs in paint can easily reach 100 times the safe levels.

The most dangerous way to paint is by spraying. VOC-free, low-VOC and no-VOC paints and water-based paints are safer and are now available, although there is still no set standard on these. Paint strippers can contain methylene chloride, which is highly toxic with similar effects to carbon monoxide. Vinyl and self-stick wallpaper will also outgas high levels of chemicals.

A general rule is new furniture is more toxic than old. Formaldehyde levels have been shown to triple on bringing in new furniture. The answer is simply not to buy too many new materials for one room at once, especially if it is a room where you spend a lot of time. Keep windows open whenever possible after introducing them. In the bedroom, it is worth considering an air purifier which can remove outgasing chemicals. These should have an HEPA (high-efficiency particulate air) filter, which removes most of the toxicity from the indoor air.

Indoor plants, such as spider plant, drachea, Boston ferns, chrysanthemum and English ivy, can also reduce toxicity, albeit slightly. The Boston fern is the most impressive detoxifier of all: it is able to detoxify 1000 mcg of formaldehyde in one hour. In addition, there is now a much wider range of environmentally-friendly products.

Dust easily enters the house, becomes airborne and is then inhaled, adding yet more pollution to the home. Scientists at George Washington University found 45 hazardous chemicals in samples of house dust, including carcinogens and chemicals toxic to the immune, respiratory and reproductive systems.[56] This situation can be prevented by a combination of measures such as using a vacuum cleaner with an HEPA filter, ventilating rooms, opening windows and removing shoes before coming into the house.

Activities such as sanding or cutting chipboard or medium density fibreboard (MDF), will release more formaldehyde and other chemicals. This is better done outside, (or using a mask if that's not possible). Adhesives and glues also outgas multiple harmful chemicals. Avoid these if possible. Epoxy resins contain the endocrine disruptor bisphenol A. They also contain glycidol, which is highly reactive and can attach to DNA. Pure silicon, silicon rubber glue and water-washable wood glue are safer options.

A useful tip is that water-based products are safer, including water-based paints, stain removers and cleaning products. Environmentally-friendly products are becoming increasingly available. For instance, computers and monitors with the TCO 95 eco-label have limited amounts of brominated flame retardants.

Sometimes non-chemical toxicity from moulds can be a potent source of toxicity and this is usually associated with damp areas (although treatment is outside the scope of this book).

Outdoor pollution

Although indoor pollution is usually the greater danger, outdoor pollution has also increased. People exposed to outdoor particulate pollution, as in cities or near industrial complexes, have higher rates of heart disease and lung cancer.[57] Simply driving a car increases exposure to particulates. According to the World Health Organization, one in eight deaths worldwide is caused by air pollution.[58] In the UK, the figures are 29,000 deaths per year (according to the Committee on the Medical effects of Air Pollutants in 2013) and one in 11 of all deaths (nearly half that for smoking and twice the rate for alcohol).

Particulates are the most dangerous components of air pollution, followed by nitrogen dioxide. However, there is increasing concern about levels of microplastics in our air. The major source of particulates is from cars, but paints, perfumes and fragranced products are now a significant part of outdoor pollution.

Higher rates of cancer are found around oil refineries, power plants and smelting plants.[59] Professor Knox found childhood cancers were up to 12 times more common around chemical and oil installations, incinerators and bus stations.[60] Incinerators simply take waste and turn it into micro-particles, thereby forcing us to inhale our own waste. This is like land-filling the sky with toxic particulates. Our waste simply becomes part of the air we breathe and then part of our bodies. In reality, it is difficult to avoid outdoor pollution today unless you live away from polluted areas, industrial complexes and incinerators.

Hair dyes, cosmetics, aerosols

Many people use organic food when they can and try to avoid chemicals in food. However, few understand the toxicity of cosmetics. The average person absorbs about 0.5 kg (5 lb) of chemicals each year through cosmetics, and the average woman eats the equivalent of five lipsticks a year, yet cosmetics are not routinely assessed for toxicity.

With cosmetics, the absorption of chemicals is mainly through the skin, but absorption through the lungs occurs as well. These routes are considered more dangerous than intake through the gut because they bypass the liver's protective filters.

Put another way, if you wouldn't eat it, it's a mistake to put it on your skin; either way, it goes into your body.

Hair dyes have been shown to increase the risk of non-Hodgkin's lymphoma[61] and leukaemia.[62] One study found 20% of all non-Hodgkin's lymphoma was due to hair dyes, especially dyes of a darker colour. Those containing para-phenylenediamine (PPD) are especially hazardous. Permanent hair dyes may be associated with a doubling of the risk of bladder cancer. A safer alternative is using vegetable-based dyes or henna hair colourings. Taking extra doses of antioxidants, such as vitamin C and alpha lipoic acid, before dyeing hair may give protection. Tattoos can also be toxic and often contain phthalates.

Perfumes are some of the most toxic pollutants in the environment. They are mainly made with solvents and 95% are derived from petroleum. Many chemically sensitive people typically react to perfumes and this is a clue to their toxicity. Only 20% of perfumes have been tested for safety. They cause a wide range of symptoms, and it will be no surprise to discover they are characteristically neurotoxic. They contain toluene and often phthalates and toxic metals. The most dangerous time to use them is in pregnancy as it can adversely affect foetal development and cause genital deformities.

We already know that one of the best clues to toxicity is occupational exposure. At a hearing in 1989 on such, there were numerous reports of asthma, memory loss, balance problems and serious disorders of the nervous and respiratory systems in those who worked with perfumes. An analysis of 2983 chemicals used, found that 884 were toxic, 218 caused reproductive abnormalities and 146 were carcinogens.[63]

An easy step to improve health is to stop using aerosols, including air fresheners. These products produce fine droplets coated with chemicals. These are readily inhaled, allowing easy access to the bloodstream and then elsewhere in the body. They typically contain toxic chemicals, such as formaldehyde, naphthalene and the solvent P-dichlorobenzene, none of which you would want inside you. They all depress the central nervous system and use of air fresheners can trigger or worsen depression and asthma. Other ingredients have unpleasant properties, including 'musk ambrette', which can cause testicular atrophy and citral, which can cause prostate enlargement. It's the familiar story of chemicals: hormone disruption, neurotoxicity and cancer. Perfume sprays and, to a lesser extent, hairsprays, give a double whammy of absorption through the skin and the lungs. This is bad news.

Cleaning products typically contain a multitude of toxic chemicals, such as benzene, toluene and xylene. It is fairly straightforward to change these to natural products, such as vinegar, lemon juice and sodium bicarbonate, or to buy environmentally friendly products. Chemical carpet cleaners are definitely something to avoid as they outgas toxic chemicals. Steam-cleaning is a simple, safe alternative. Soap dispensers and detergents often contain parabens, triclosan and other unwanted chemicals – use natural, unscented soaps instead.

Fluoride is a powerful enzyme inhibitor and is best avoided in toothpaste. Other products to keep clear of are deodorants that contain aluminium, a metal which will be absorbed into the body. Natural alternatives are available.

One simple tip is to avoid products containing 'fragrances', a group of up to 4000 chemicals. The rule is, if it smells, don't use it. In fact, by the time you smell it, the chemicals have already entered your bloodstream. (Natural essential oils such a lavender are a different matter.)

The long chemical names in many of these products can be confusing. One helpful clue is to look out for any chemicals with 'chlor' or 'fluor' in them, such as vinyl chloride, perchlorethylene and perfluoroctane sulphonates (in Scotchguard). Virtually all of these are toxic. What is more important is that they are bio-accumulative – in other words, they don't break down in the body or the environment. Similarly, watch out for the seemingly innocent label 'parfum' on cosmetics and toiletries. This label means it could contain any of a hundred hazardous and persistent chemicals.

Chemicals in clothing

Compared to the dangers from pesticides, cosmetics and the outgasing in our homes, the dangers from clothing are relatively small. The main risk is absorption of chemicals through the skin. Much of today's clothing is made from nylons, acrylics and especially polyester, and these will release chemicals. This will include the common carcinogen, trichloroethylene, used as a mothproofing agent. Trichloroethylene is a known cause of leukaemia and has been associated with learning disorders, cancers and neuropathy. Cotton/polyester combinations mean formaldehyde is being used as does 'water-resistant', 'water-repellent', 'crease-resistant', 'permanent press' and 'polyester/

cotton'. This chemical will be released more readily when hot, such as during ironing.

Be wary of dry cleaning, which uses formaldehyde, trichloroethylene and perchloroethylene. These continue to outgas from the dry-cleaned clothes and can cause memory loss, cardiac arrhythmias and mood swings.

Like clothes, bed sheets also stay in contact with the skin; they can be changed from synthetic to cotton (ideally organic). Most mattresses contain pesticides but safe alternatives exist.

Probably the most sinister development with clothing today is the addition of nanoparticles.

It is obviously not possible to suddenly change a whole wardrobe, but it is possible to gradually switch to more natural materials, such as cotton. Washing clothes before using them for the first time is a good idea as it removes some of the chemicals.

Chemicals in water

Occasionally, the solution to toxicity can be easy. Fortunately this is true for water. One of the most useful steps anyone can take is to buy a water filter.

Tap water contains vast quantities of chemicals. Pesticides and fertilisers dumped on the land end up in the water, as do household and industrial chemicals, heavy metals and solvents, together with pharmaceuticals at concentrations similar to pesticides. A ground-breaking study by the Ralph Nader Study Group, after reviewing 10,000 documents acquired through the Freedom of Information Act, found 2100 chemicals in USA drinking water, many of which were carcinogenic.

A third of our water in the UK comes from waterways where, as has already been noted, one third of male fish are changing sex due to oestrogenic chemicals. If our water can cause such profound changes in fish, we can be sure it's harmful for us. For those with hormone dependent tumours (breast, prostate and ovarian cancers), reducing this risk is crucial.

Chapter 7

Today more chlorine than ever is added to water to compensate for the nitrates and phosphates from fertilisers. However, chlorine reacts with organic matter and other chemicals to form toxic products called 'disinfection by-products' (DHPs). This innocent-sounding name hides the fact that they are considered probable carcinogens. Over 20 studies have linked chlorinated water to cancer, especially to cancer of the bladder[64] and rectum,[65] but also of the brain, pancreas, kidney and stomach. It is interesting that the cancer risk correlates with the amounts of DHPs in the water and, in the case of colon cancer, with relatively small increases.

Another hazard in water has recently come to light. A study found 83% of tap water samples in the USA contained microplastics. It was estimated that we consume 3000-4000 microplastic particles per year. Like particulates, these carry a cocktail of chemicals and additives.

Having a bath or shower exposes you to the same chemical cocktail. One study in 1966 found that after taking a 10-minute shower or bath, the subject's breath had elevated levels of VOCs. These had been inhaled from the hot water. The exposure was equivalent to that from drinking 2.2 litres (4 pints) of water.[66]

Chemicals can be removed from water using three main systems: reversed osmosis, distillation and using carbon filters. Reverse osmosis is the most effective way of removing pollutants but also the most expensive. Even this method is not entirely free from problems due to the amount of plastic piping which can itself release chemicals. Distillation is useful but does not remove all VOCs. For most people, the easiest way forward is to use a carbon filter. These can be used in a jug, but a system where water is purified before it comes out of the tap is generally preferable. (Many jug filters are made from polycarbonate plastic which leaks bisphenol A into the water). Carbon filters typically remove chlorine, pesticides and organic chemicals, but not fluoride or nitrates.

Cooking utensils and packaging

Endocrine-disrupting chemicals ooze out of plastic wraps and food containers. Although this is not a big issue for the majority of people, for those with hormone-dependent cancers, such as prostate, ovarian or breast cancer, and other hormone-related disorders (endometriosis, polycystic ovary syndrome), it could be. These substances act like a fertiliser, stimulating cancer growth.

Foods wrapped in plastic contain significant residues of phthalates, a known endocrine disruptor and carcinogen. This can occur even when the plastic is not in direct contact with the food. The solution, where possible, is to not wrap food in plastic and also to avoid microwaving food in plastic, (which causes migration of chemicals into the food). Two situations are especially problematical with plastic: firstly, when they are in contact with fatty foods such as meat, dairy, yoghurts, cakes and pastries; and secondly, whenever heat is involved, as with microwaving.

Canned foods usually have linings containing a plasticiser, BPA, which has been found to seep out of the container into the food. As canned foods have a long shelf life, this leakage can be large and at high enough levels, to cause cancer cells to divide. BPA also leaches out of polycarbonate bottles given to babies. The label PC7 is a clue to this danger and warns that BPA is present. Bottled water, especially if left in the sun, can be an important source of endocrine disrupting chemicals. Typically, hard plastics contain BPA whilst soft plastics contain phthalates. Both are endocrine disruptors.

Cookware and food containers also release toxic chemicals; sometimes it is worth changing them. Top of the list would be aluminium cookware. Aluminium levels are higher in people with Alzheimer's disease and cooking in aluminium pans is a significant source. Fizzy drinks in aluminium cans are another important source, as are deodorants (see page 187).

Very high on the list would be Teflon non-stick cookware as these release a group of particularly unpleasant pollutants called perfluorinated chemicals (PFCs). These are carcinogens and can cause birth defects, but a particular concern, as with many fluorinated and chlorinated compounds, is they are virtually indestructible, building up in the body and in the environment over time. Perfluoroakyl chemicals are found in the blood of 98% of USA citizens.[67]

Stainless steel cookware is better but can be a source of cadmium and nickel. Ideally, use cast iron products. Ceramic, glass and enamel containers are also good, but even some ceramic cookware contains heavy metals, such as cadmium.

Electromagnetic fields (EMFs)

We are, as discussed earlier, being exposed to ever more powerful and dangerous EMFs. Completely avoiding them is impossible but we can steer clear of the most problematical sources. Many people spend nearly two-thirds of their life in two places: in bed and at work. If we reduce exposure in these two places then we can reduce the risk considerably.

Microwave exposure comes from four main sources:
1. mobile phones
2. digitally enhanced cordless technology (DECT) phones
3. wifi systems and smart meters
4. mobile phone masts.

1. Mobile phones

The most hazardous source of EMFs for most people is their mobile phone, and with each generation of phones, the danger increases. The more information they carry, the greater and more irregular the electromagnetic pulsing they produce and the higher the risk to health. The risk has gone up exponentially with each change of network (2G to 3G to 4G to 5G).

For anyone with cancer, carrying a mobile phone could prevent recovery due to its ability to block DNA repair and cause DNA degradation. In fact, mobile phones can trigger cancer themselves. There have been 38 recorded cases of breast cancer in women who kept their mobile phones in their bras. I wouldn't be surprised if men carrying mobile phones in their trouser pocket have developed prostate and rectal cancers for similar reasons, but this would be less likely to be picked up. To my way of thinking, this is a risk you simply can't afford if you have cancer.

Over 90% of studies show mobile phones create oxidative stress in the body. The significance of this is that it will aggravate virtually every known chronic illness and reduce the chance of a recovery.

The smarter the phone the more dangerous it is. If left on standby, a phone will be producing almost continuous irregular nanosecond pulses in vast numbers. These have been unequivocally shown to damage basic cellular mechanisms.

However, if the wifi on the phone is switched off (go to settings and switch it off) then pulsed waves are massively reduced. This largely limits the negative health effects to the period when calls are being made and avoids exposing parts of the body to continuous harm.

Even then precautions are necessary. Keep calls short. Most mobiles will allow you to forward a call to a landline. If not, use in loudspeaker mode or with an air-tube headset. EMF radiation can be 100 times stronger just before and during the time of connection, so waiting until you are connected before holding the phone close helps reduce exposure; this only takes 5 seconds but protects against a microwave hit to the brain. Exposure is greatly increased when making calls from cars, trains etc as the phone continually searches for connections. In poor signal areas, the transmission power can go up by a thousand-fold. Exposure is also higher inside buildings.

2. DECT phones
DECT phones cause changes in brainwave activity and blood flow in the brain within five minutes of use. These phones act like a mobile phone mast in our homes, constantly radiating the house with microwaves. They can be replaced with an analogue phone, although these can be hard to find, or an ECO-DECT-Plus cordless phone. These don't send out microwaves when not in use.

3. Wifi and smart meters
When it comes to wifi, cables are a safer alternative or, failing that, switch the wifi off at night. Avoid sitting near the router. This is often situated close to the computer and is another source of EMFs. The closer you are to it, the bigger the impact. Smart meters, installed to monitor electrical use, can be regarded as similar to wifi. They emit yet more microwaves 24 hours a day, adding to the load of electromagnetic smog, and are best avoided.

4. Phone masts
If possible, make sure you don't live near a mobile phone mast, but remember they are usually well hidden. The dangers of masts are considerable (see above) but will greatly increase with 5G which will have multiple small transmitters. If you can't avoid living near a mast, there are protective measures you can take, although they are complex.

5. Other sources of EMFs
In addition, take care with laptops with wifi connections. Avoid using these on laps as microwave radiation to the genitals becomes inevitable; instead, keep the wifi switched off. The radiation produced is less when run on battery.

Keep the bedroom as free from EMF exposure (and other toxicity) as possible. The bedroom should be an oasis away from the toxicity of the world. Remember Hippocrates's adage that the body will heal once given the right conditions for health. The body does much of its healing at night; this is a crucial time to be free of electro-smog.

EMF monitors are available. They can rapidly identify areas of high EMFs within a house and tell you if your sleeping area is safe. I was impressed to find how much EMFs were reduced on my laptop by switching it to flight mode.

The brain is very sensitive to EMFs, especially to microwave frequencies. Probably the worst thing you can do is charge mobile phones near the bed. Charging phones give off strong microwave emissions. Even having a mobile phone on standby will give intermittent microwave emissions at full power, depending on the local signal strength. Some phones, including some iPhones, give off radiation even when switched off. Keep them out of the bedroom.

Bedside light and clock radios should be as far away from the bed as possible. Electric clocks give off high EMFs at up to five times the safe level and are best placed at least a metre from the bedside. Bedhead lights also give off strong fields and are best avoided. Ideally, avoid metallic headboards and beds with metal frames as these can concentrate EMFs. Never use electric blankets whilst in the bed as these produce very strong EMFs. If you use them to heat the bed before going to bed, then switch them off at the mains before sleeping.

Other electrical devices in the home create electromagnetic fields. Cordless devices tend to give off the highest EMFs and hairdryers and electric razors give off very high fields. Fortunately, they tend to be used for short periods of time and the field drops off rapidly with distance from the body.

Microwave ovens also give off high magnetic fields which can extend for a metre beyond the microwave; they alter proteins within food. Microwaved food causes different biochemical changes in the body compared with foods cooked in other ways. If the meal is microwaved, leave the food for a few minutes after cooking as, during this time, the food will continue to give off radiation and contain harmful free radicals.

In the kitchen, other appliances to avoid include magnetic induction hobs, although these are not in common use. The motors in cooker hoods can also give off high EMFs.

It is worth giving some consideration to lighting. Transformers used in fluorescent lighting, halogen lights and dimmers can create powerful EMFs. High EMFs can be found around plasma screen TVs, extending for up to six feet. Underfloor heating can create high fields and faulty wiring can increase EMFs by up to a thousand times.

Summary

We are now being exposed to a bewildering array of toxic chemicals and more recently to increasingly dangerous types of electro-pollution. Chemical contamination is detectable in the bodies of every species living on the planet and now every person carries a significant body burden. Even by the time of birth, the toxic load has become serious, and this contamination accumulates throughout life. The properties of many of these chemicals include carcinogenicity, neurotoxicity and endocrine disruption.

The safety of most chemicals is impossible to determine because of factors like the cocktail effect, lack of long-term safety testing, differences in individual susceptibility, the effects of early exposure and the fact that endocrine disruption can occur at unbelievably tiny concentrations. Regard all chemicals as potentially hazardous. Electro-pollution, especially microwave electro-pollution, has been added to the toxic equation and evidence suggests it amplifies chemical toxicity.

Protecting ourselves from this toxicity is not easy as chemicals are everywhere. However, what is absolutely clear is the need to decrease the total load of chemicals, to decrease our ongoing daily exposure and to enhance our ability to get rid of them. It is well worth knowing where the greatest dangers come from. Fortunately, many of the changes needed to protect ourselves are fairly easy to put into place.

Measures to reduce exposure through food include eating organic food, not using or microwaving in plastic containers and avoiding processed food with its long lists of chemical names. A water filter will quickly reduce chemical exposure from water. For airborne exposure, avoiding aerosols and air fresheners, using water-based or VOC-free paints and reducing furniture and fittings which outgas will help. Consider using an air purifier. For exposure through the skin, reduce or use safer cosmetics, perfumes and toiletries, replace chemical cleaning products and use more natural products.

We will discuss measures to remove toxins in the next chapter.

Reducing toxic exposure at night is critical as this is when much of the body's healing takes place. This can be done by making the bedroom as uncontaminated as possible and making it free from electro-pollution.

For those with hormone-dependent cancers, keeping exposure to endocrine-disrupting chemicals down to a minimum makes absolute sense.

The aim is not to do all of these things. Life is complicated enough already. But each step taken will lighten the load until it reaches a tipping point at which the body can heal. Each step makes healing illness that bit easier.

Chapter 8

Releasing toxicity

This study confirms that even before birth, a child is exposed to hundreds of chemical compounds, many of which could harm the child's health and development. This provides the opportunity for irreversible effects to occur during critical windows of development.

Statement of Scientists and Paediatricians after EWG study of body burden at birth, 2005

For many diseases it will be difficult to find the cause and recover without a good understanding of toxicity. Take the following case. Dr Patrick Kingsley recalled asking a cancer patient about previous toxic exposure. She eventually remembered working in a small kitchen when she was younger. It had been infested with cockroaches and a pest control company was called in. Then, every month for two years, they sprayed the kitchen with an unpleasant, smelly chemical. She later contacted five of the six people she had worked with at that time. Two had died of cancer, two had developed multiple sclerosis and one had developed chronic fatigue syndrome, yet all had remained unaware that it had been these chemicals that had most likely destroyed their health.

Dealing with toxicity

Every living organism on the planet now has industrial poisons in its body and this includes us humans. How can we protect ourselves?

The first step is to reduce our exposure as explained in the last chapter. The second step is to release as much of this toxic material as we can; we are going to explore this in this chapter. There are three major ways of doing this:

1. sweating them out (either with exercise or saunas)
2. fasting
3. enhancing the detoxification process, mainly by ensuring we have adequate nutrients on board.

However, before we look at these let's first discuss why releasing these chemicals is so vital for our health.

Other associations

Although we have looked at the link between chemicals and cancer, neurological disease and endocrine problems, these are far from the only problems. Some chemicals can impair immune function,[1] some can alter behaviour,[2] some attach to genes[3] and some can lower intelligence.[4]

There is a significant connection between chemicals and autoimmune diseases, such as systemic lupus erythematosus (SLE), scleroderma and rheumatoid arthritis. These diseases have become far commoner in the last 50 years and now affect one in nine women in the UK. Occupational exposure is always a clue and people who work with chemicals are at greater risk of these conditions. A long list of chemicals has been shown to trigger different types of arthritis and connective tissue diseases. Chemical exposure is also known to increase the rate at which the body forms auto-antibodies.[5]

The boomerang effect

For years we have dumped chemicals carelessly into the environment in the belief that they would simply disappear. But they haven't. They have come back to bite us. They have become incorporated into our bodies. Biopsies show that dioxins, PCBs, xylene and styrene were found in the fat of 100% of Americans tested. PCBs can now be found in all species studied including those living in deserts, the arctic circles and the deepest oceans. I like to think of this as the first rule of toxicity:

Whatever we put out into the world sooner or later comes back and becomes part of our bodies.

And thanks to bio-accumulation, these chemicals often come back in a more concentrated, and therefore potentially more dangerous, form. The result is we all have a body burden of chemicals.

A study by the Mount Sinai School of Medicine in 2003 tested healthy volunteers for 210 chemicals and, on average, found 167 chemicals in each person. There were, on average, 52 carcinogens, 62 chemicals toxic to the brain and nervous system, 55 chemicals associated with birth defects, 77 chemicals toxic to the immune system and 77 toxic to the reproductive system.[6] Other studies in Canada and Europe have given similar results.

Another study found that we are routinely exposed to 65 carcinogens in food, 40 in water and about 60 in the air we breathe.[7] However, we know this number is an underestimate as it includes only those chemicals that can be measured. To give some idea, studies of populations in the USA and Canada have found at least 190 organochlorine residues in their bodies. This is just one group of chemicals and the US Environmental Protection Agency has estimated the average adult American's body has accumulated about 700 organochlorines that have not been identified.[8] The number could be far greater. This means we are likely to have thousands of chemicals in our bodies, many with toxic effects that are hardly understood.

This body burden is like filthy water or sewage surrounding the cells of our body. We hope our bodies can still keep functioning under this load, but no one knows at what point they will be overwhelmed.

As we have seen, most chemicals get stored in fat, including the brain and nervous system. In addition, they attach to and damage cell membranes, which also happen to be composed of fat. Unfortunately, healthy cell membranes are critical for good health. The chemicals don't stay in the fat permanently but are periodically released to be detoxified; this release can cause damage to cellular mechanisms. Importantly, this toxic load accumulates with age.

There are many reasons to think this toxicity is playing an important role in many of today's chronic diseases. The corollary is that reducing the toxic load can be critical to recovery from these diseases.

The polluted foetus

If the first rule of toxicity is worrying then what I call the second rule is alarming:

> *Whatever chemicals are present in the body of the mother will be delivered straight into the body of the foetus (and breast-feeding infant) where they will concentrate further.*

We think of apex predators as being on top of the food chain and at maximum danger from bio-accumulation. However, even higher in the food chain are the foetus and breast-feeding infant. The reason is that any toxicity present in the mother will be concentrated in her unborn baby. This is true for the majority of chemicals studied. We know that the chemical load within a baby correlates with the total amount of persistent contaminants that the mother has built up in her fat cells during her lifetime.[9]

The foetus is uniquely vulnerable to toxic chemicals. It has no fatty tissue during most of its time in the womb and so no place to store these chemicals. They are therefore sent to the only fatty tissue available: the brain and nervous system. In addition, the foetus has a very limited capacity to detoxify chemicals, and many of these, especially endocrine disrupters, can be far more toxic during a critical window of time, especially between the eighth and 12th weeks of pregnancy.

Defects affecting the brain and nervous system, such as neural tube defects, have been found to be increased in those living near toxic waste sites. We don't, however, need to live near such a facility to experience this problem because, as the studies described above show, mothers possess their own toxic waste dump and will offload some of this on to their hapless offspring during pregnancy.

A major study in 2005 found an average of 200 industrial chemicals and pollutants, (out of 413 tested) in the umbilical blood of 10 randomly chosen babies. These included 180 carcinogens, 217 chemicals toxic to the brain and nervous system, and 208 that can cause congenital defects and abnormal development in animals.[10] A statement by scientists and paediatricians said the report raised issues of substantial importance to public health, showed up gaping holes in the government's safety net and pointed to the need for major reforms in the nation's laws to protect the public from chemical exposure.

The bottom line is that today, by the time any baby is born, its body is already contaminated. The US Cancer Prevention Coalition has found a child's lifetime safe toxin level is reached by the time it is 18 months.

Breast milk should be the greatest gift a mother can give for the future health of her child, but things are not so simple today.

In the USA, studies have shown that 90% of samples of breast milk contained a disturbing 350 chemicals.[11] Breast-fed babies take in more contaminants during this time than at any other time during their lives and breast milk has now become the most polluted food on the planet.[12] Bottle-fed babies have their own problems: endocrine-disrupting chemicals can leach from bottles and this process is accelerated when the bottles are heated.

We have lost a very basic freedom: the right to have a child with an uncontaminated body and the health consequences are unlikely to be minor. For example, one study estimated that 5% of babies born in the USA had been exposed to sufficient pollutants to affect neurological development.[13]

There are, however, two other hazards that await the youngest members of our society. These were surprises that again no one anticipated. They are potentially even more serious, highlighting just how little we know about chemicals and how their dangers have been grossly underestimated.

Trans-generational toxicity

A deeply worrying piece of research found that chemical toxicity doesn't just affect the exposed individual but can damage future generations. Scientists at Washington State University gave pregnant rats a fungicide, vinclozalin, and a pesticide, methoxyclor. Altogether, 90% of these rats developed reproductive abnormalities. Then something completely unexpected happened. Three generations of the male rats from this bloodline, who had never been exposed to these chemicals, developed reproductive abnormalities (low sperm count and increased rates of infertility).[14]

These transgenerational, or 'epigenetic', effects have now been shown to occur with a variety of chemicals, including DEET, permethrin, phthalates, BPA, nicotine and tributyl tin – all chemicals in widespread use. An added concern is that these effects can occur at miniscule doses and at levels currently regarded as safe.

This new research tells us that chemical contamination has the potential to damage not only exposed individuals but also their offspring, even if the offspring have zero exposure.

This research is yet to be fully assimilated by the scientific community but is a warning that we need to drastically reduce our exposure. An alarming thought is that even if we could somehow remove all the toxic chemicals from the world today at a stroke, it would take six generations before we would be free from the adverse effects.

Early exposure primes disease later

Sometimes early exposure has no immediate impact but leads to devastating consequences in later life following re-exposure. In one study, mice were exposed to two pesticides (maneb and paraquat) in the first 20 days of life;[15] this caused no immediate, apparent harm. However, when these mice were re-exposed to the same pesticides later in life, the consequences were major. They developed a 70% reduction in motor function and a progressive Parkinson's disease of mice. The researchers concluded that early exposure to pesticides can trigger later neurodegenerative disease on re-exposure.

We know the same occurs with cancer. Exposure to a number of carcinogens in the foetus or infancy, including PAHs and nitrosamines, has been found to increase the risk of cancer to a greater degree than exposure later in life.[16, 17]

The risk from chemicals is falling disproportionately and unfairly on the youngest members of our society.

The cocktail effect

Chemicals have given us yet another unwelcome surprise. It is known as the 'cocktail effect'. Chemicals are tested for safety one at a time, but this is not what happens in reality. Just as mixing drinks is usually not a good idea, mixing toxic chemicals in our bodies is not a good idea either.

As mentioned in Chapter 6, numerous studies have found that combinations of chemicals are more dangerous than single chemicals and sometimes vastly so. For instance, one study found that animals exposed to a combination of 16 organochlorine pesticides plus lead and cadmium at 'safe doses' developed impaired immune responses, altered thyroid function and altered brain development in response to the combination.[18] Rats exposed to a 'safe' dose of the pesticide chlordecone and a low dose of carbon tetrachloride had a 67 times higher chance of dying than if exposed to the carbon tetrachloride alone.[19] These studies show that the so-called 'safe level' of a chemical is all but irrelevant.

Sometimes the extent of this amplification can be extra-ordinary. A study of the oestrogenic effects of pesticides published in *Science*, found combinations of pesticides could increase toxicity by between 500 and 1000 times.[20]

The Soil Association found that the number of pesticides has increased greatly from 1.8 in 1966 to 32.6 in 2015 (on leeks and onions) with similar rises on other crops.[21] The potential for dangerous and untraceable increases in toxicity is all too obvious.

We can sum this up as telling us that allowing combinations of chemicals into the human body uninvited is madness. We simply have no idea what the consequences will be. It' doesn't take a genius to realise that it won't be good news.

Removing toxicity

I think all this data tells us we need to reduce toxicity as much as possible. However, the sheer number of chemicals, their unfamiliar names and the range of hazards all make this a complex subject. However, imagine for a moment that you were being poisoned and this was going to rob you of your health, your vitality and possibly your life. How would you act? Surely you would try to prevent it?

Well, the truth is that you are being poisoned slowly, perhaps not deliberately, but certainly systematically and in multiple ways. But you *can* make changes, and because toxicity accumulates slowly, time is on your side. You can gradually put solutions in place.

The basic problem is this: if we accumulate toxic substances faster than we eliminate them, we end up with polluted bodies and more at risk of disease. The speed at which we accumulate poisons and become ill depends on our genes, our nutrition and the efficiency of our individual detoxification system.

Individual differences in detoxification can be critical. There is, for example, a ten-fold difference between individuals in the breakdown of the carcinogenic substance PAH benz(a)pyrene,[22] and a 150- to 450-fold difference in how we respond to airborne particles.[23] Other studies have found an 85- to 500-fold difference in detoxification, metabolic activity and DNA repair in 95% of the US population.[24] A chemical that might be safe for one person could be highly toxic for another. This is why a person can inexplicably develop cancer even when they appear to be living a healthy lifestyle. None of us can be complacent.

The first point to consider is toxic load: this is the amount of toxicity accumulated over a lifetime. The sources are not always obvious. They can include exposure from chemicals in the home, the garden, the loft, occupational exposure, home renovations or visiting the dentist. Position in the family can be important as first children are likely to start their life with a higher toxic load than later children. The amount of toxicity is also affected by factors which naturally reduce it, such as exercise, good diet and genetic differences.

Reducing the toxic load does not mean removing all toxicity; this would be impossible. It means reducing the total load to a point at which the body can heal.

The second point to consider is the daily toxic exposure and what can be done to reduce it. The section, 'A day in the 21st Century', in Chapter 6 (page 173) gives some idea of where these risks originate as does Chapter 8.

Reducing the toxic load

It is interesting that there is no medical specialty which deals with detoxification, and in my experience doctors rarely consider toxicity. It is an important blind spot in medicine but, to be fair, doctors are hampered by the absence of any readily available test for toxicity. Our bodies, however, are not stupid. It is for good reason that the liver is the largest internal organ and a major portion of our genetic material is given over to dealing with toxicity.

Our goal is to assist this detoxification process, both by reducing the intake of toxic substances and by accelerating the elimination of chemicals within us.

Smell

Let's note that we have a warning system for toxicity. It is our sense of smell. The stronger the smell coming from a plastic or of a fragrance, the more likely it is to be toxic. Synthetic fragrances are a major warning sign. Notice that smell of a new car or TV, the odour of a new-build house or carpet shop or furniture showroom; these are signals that you are absorbing chemicals and often something toxic. Your nose can be a valuable asset.

Environmental control units

Nothing demonstrates the principle laid out by Hippocrates better than Environmental Control Units. These are buildings that are free from the toxicity of the modern world: they are made from wholly natural materials and all air coming into the building is filtered. Patients who visit these units are given a limited range of organic and uncontaminated foods. Here, patients can be successfully treated for a variety of diseases, such as asthma and arthritis, but also a wide range of ailments, including many that conventional medicine is presently unable to help. (Sadly, no environmental control units exist in the UK, only the USA).

The late Dr John Mansfield, an allergy specialist, described his experience visiting an Environmental Control Unit in the USA and watching patients with severe arthritis and a variety of other illnesses recovering after fasting at the Unit. He witnessed patient after patient becoming virtually free of symptoms after five to six days.[25] What surprised him most was that the staff at the Unit had become so accustomed to these miracles that they no longer seemed impressed by them.

For me, Environmental Control Units rank as one of the greatest medical advances of the 20th century, but sadly few doctors have heard of them.

Releasing toxicity

Exercise and saunas

Sweating is one of the principal methods for removing toxins. It follows that any exercise which makes us sweat will make a difference. This may turn out to be one of the biggest benefits exercise can give us. Keep in mind that sweating can also reduce nutrients, especially magnesium, so a good diet is also important. For people with chronic illness, exercise is not always an option.

One alternative is saunas. Their use was pioneered in Environmental Control Units. Dr Rea and colleagues did a study of 210 patients with chemical overload, treating them with saunas once or twice daily for one month. This led to a 63% reduction of toxic chemicals in their bodies and a 30% improvement in symptoms.[26] Nancy Sokol Green's story, described in Chapter 6 (page 165), is a good example; it proved to be the turning point in her illness.

Firemen are typically exposed, on a regular basis, to a wide range of toxic and carcinogenic chemicals. These can cause bizarre symptoms, predominately relating to the brain and nervous system. Sauna treatment has successfully been used to clear chemicals from their bodies.

Dr Sarah Myhill has estimated, after doing before and after toxicity tests on patients, that 50 saunas reduce the toxic load by 50%.[27] If you use saunas, it is crucial to shower after to wash away the toxins on your skin, otherwise they will be reabsorbed. The towels used also needed to be washed regularly.

High temperatures from conventional saunas can release chemicals into the bloodstream. Sometimes this leads to unpleasant symptoms. An alternative solution is a far infrared sauna (FIRS). FIRS has been extensively researched in Japan and China; it has also been found effective in reducing toxicity in electrical workers. Sweating is not necessary for FIRS to work. Far infrared heat will penetrate one and a half inches into fatty tissue, stimulating the release of stored toxins. It also improves lymph and blood flow. It induces these changes at lower temperatures than conventional saunas, making it safer and more comfortable. Keep in mind that drugs can be sweated out too, so for those on medication this needs care. Some FIRS machines have the advantage of being small, inexpensive and easily transported.

As with exercise, water and various minerals are lost whilst sweating, so drink plenty of water and replenish with vitamins and minerals.

Fasting

When animals become ill they typically fast. They do this until they begin to recover. Fasting has been used by naturopaths for decades to treat a wide range of diseases and to detoxify the body. It is cheap and easy to do. Fasting involves stopping all food and keeping to drinks; these can be either water or fruit and vegetable juices. Fasts can last from one to many days. These juices ideally should be organic as juicing will concentrate pesticides as much as nutrients. Juice fasting is like having an infusion of nutrients and enzymes. Fasting also makes the body more alkaline, known to assist healing.

To understand the benefits of fasting, it is worth retelling the fascinating story of Professor Arnold Ehret. Born in Germany, Ehret developed a kidney condition called Bright's disease when he was in his early 30s. This was at the beginning of the 20th century and he was pronounced incurable. He was told his condition was terminal. In a desperate search for a solution he visited 24 physicians, which virtually bankrupted him. Worse still, none were able to help him. However, he was not a man to give up. He explored conventional medicine, vegetarianism and naturopathy, taking courses in all of these plus various other therapies. His curiosity knew no bounds.

His efforts eventually paid dividends. After fasting on nothing but fruit, he noticed his health begin to improve. He started fasting for progressively longer periods and experimented with different fasting regimes. He eventually did a mammoth 49-day fast. His health went up in leaps and bounds, and he made a full recovery from his illness.

But then something unexpected and remarkable happened. He found he had reached an entirely new level of health and vitality, far surpassing the best health he had ever known before. He expressed it like this: 'an indescribable feeling, never known before, of better health came to me, with more vital energy, better efficiency, more endurance and strength and a great joy and happiness just to be alive'. On one occasion he walked for 56 hours without sleep after a seven-day fast and on another occasion took an 800-mile bicycle ride with a trained cyclist and surprised himself by being the stronger of the two.

Curing the Incurable

Professor Ehret is far from the only survivor of a serious illness who has astonished himself by not only recovering but by also taking health and vitality to new levels.

What is so extraordinary about this story is that most people would assume that such long periods without food would be barely tolerable. Surely it would lead to exhaustion and illness. Ehret describes the opposite: as his fasts continued and became longer he developed increasing vitality. For instance, he describes feeling sharper and better after a 20-day fast than after a five-day fast.

He realised he had stumbled upon one of the greatest secrets of health and, in his own words, found one of the most effective methods of healing for almost any disease.

He was so excited about his discovery that he started doing public lectures and fasts. This, in turn, led to many people seeking his help. At his sanatorium in Switzerland he treated thousands of people, including many thought to be incurable, often with great success. He did this for 10 years before his untimely death from an accident. He believed good health was simple: we need good quality food and we need to remove accumulated waste by fasting. He felt that what was not simple could not be the truth.[28] His story gives further credence to Hippocrates's hypothesis that the body has the ability to heal once the right conditions are present.

Ehret would start his patients on a 24-hour fast. People typically felt worse during this time. They would often develop headaches, excess mucus and dizziness. He noted something of importance: this short fast was a good indicator of the body's toxicity. Those with the most severe symptoms were usually those needing fasting most, but they were the very ones who needed to approach fasting cautiously and start with short fasts. He would gradually increase these and vitality would typically return.

He found most people needed periodic fasting for about three years to cleanse their bodies and to become well again. He observed that, during these treatments, patients would sometimes excrete drugs through the skin, sometimes drugs

240

that had been taken 10 to 40 years before. Nancy Sokol Green experienced the same phenomenon. He also observed that as they became less toxic they would sweat less.

He kept experimenting with his regime and eventually developed what he called the 'mucus-less diet healing system'. A similar approach was used by the renowned naturopath Otis Carroll, who used fasting and his own method of hydrotherapy to cure people with a variety of different illnesses. He lived in the same era as Ehret and, like Ehret, cured himself from a major illness early in life, in this case 'arthritis'.

I would have some reservations about using these longer fasts today. Ehret lived at a time when the world was far less toxic. There were then no pesticides and few synthetic chemicals. Even a short fast today can release a considerable quantity of toxins, especially in the first day or two, and needs to be done with care and often with nutritional supplementation. A fast for a day gives a useful idea of the toxicity of the body, as mentioned. Only then should fasts get longer. The book *7-Day Detox Miracle* is a good guide to how to proceed in the modern world. This book describes how fasting can be combined with supplementation to heal many diseases.[29] Another good source of information is *SuperJuice Me* by Jason Vale who uses 28-day juice fasts, as described in Chapter 2 (see page 79).

Hearing about fasting was a revelation to me. Here was a simple method that costs next to nothing, with vast potential to heal many of the diseases we are faced with today, and yet one that most doctors had never heard of. The lessons learned the hard way by Ehret remain as true today as they were at the turn of the 20th century. Detoxification, through fasting, is a simple and effective way of restoring the body to health.

Research on fasting
There has been a spate of research on fasting in recent years and it has confirmed its many benefits: it increases energy production

by the mitochondria,[30] improves immunity,[31] speeds up toxin removal (nine times faster for arsenic,[32] for example), steps up antioxidant production, reduces inflammation,[33] reduces cancer recurrence (with nightly fasting of greater than 13 hours),[34] causes sick cells to die and stimulates neuron growth.[35]

Sadly, this crucial and ground-breaking information has been largely overlooked by modern medicine despite this being a time when it has never been needed more.

Oil pulling and Epsom salts baths

Oil pulling has been controversial. It is an ayurvedic method that has been in use for centuries. The theory is that most toxic chemicals are 'lipophilic' – that is, fat-soluble – and hence get pulled into the oil.

The method involves holding a tablespoonful of olive oil (or coconut or other oil) inside the mouth for about 10 to 15 minutes. During this time the oil is thought to pull fat-soluble chemicals out of the body and into the oil. After the time is up, the oil can be spat out (not swallowed) and the mouth rinsed. Done regularly, this simple method is reputed to reduce toxic load, although there is little research on its effectiveness. It is also thought to prevent bacterial decay in the mouth and keep the teeth white.

Hot baths with Epsom salts (magnesium sulphate) are in a similar category. There are few studies on this approach, but it has a long history of clinical use. These baths allow the absorption of magnesium and sulphur. To be effective you need at least 250 grams of Epsom salts (that is enough to fill a medium-sized mug) and you need to stay in the bath for at least 20 minutes to absorb it. Don't use soap or shampoo – or at least not until the end.

Soluble fibre

Adding soluble fibre to food reduces toxicity. Soluble fibre includes oats, brown rice, barley, lentils and many fruit and vegetables (wheat bran is insoluble fibre). Concentrated sources of soluble fibre include psyllium husks and pectin. It is important to drink plenty of water with soluble fibre. It reduces the level of nearly all toxic chemicals taken in through the gut, including heavy metals and pesticides. It binds to them, allowing them to be excreted. It is worth knowing that it also binds to medicines and supplements, so take these at least 30 minutes after the fibre.

Enhancing the detoxification system

The body has two choices when faced with a toxic chemical. It can either store it or detoxify it. Storing it usually means transporting it to the fat cells. There it will remain until the body is ready to remove it. The other alternative is to detoxify the chemical within the cells.

It is worth understanding a little about this process, even though there is a bit of biochemistry. It will then become more obvious how detoxification can be improved.

There are two phases of detoxification. Phase 1 can be regarded as the basic phase and for many chemicals this might be all that is needed. Phase 2 can be regarded as the back-up system to help when Phase 1 is underperforming, but it is also used for complex chemicals.

The aim of Phase 1 is quite simple: it is to convert any unwanted chemical into a less toxic one. The way it works is to convert the chemical into an alcohol, then into an aldehyde, and then into an acid. Then it can be excreted in the urine. So far so good, but this system can malfunction. Each step of the pathway needs both nutrients and enzymes to work optimally. A deficiency in either will cause problems. For instance, to convert the alcohol into the aldehyde requires zinc, and to convert the aldehyde into the acid requires molybdenum.

If too many chemicals are being processed through Phase 1,

or a key nutrient is missing, then a back-log of by-products will occur. Unfortunately, the by-products can be more toxic than the original. This happens surprisingly often. For instance, low levels of molybdenum can lead to a build-up of aldehydes and this build-up in turn leads to the production of chloral hydrate. This causes a 'spaced-out' or drunk feeling. For people with toxic and environmental problems, this is a common symptom.

Another group of toxic by-products can be produced when both Phases 1 and 2 are overloaded, and these are called epoxides. They are highly reactive, damaging chemicals. They can trigger cancer, impair immunity and alter genes.

The aim of Phase 2 is also quite simple: it is to attach the toxin to another chemical which makes it safer and more easily excreted. This involves conjugation – the process of attaching the chemical to an amino acid or a protein. The most important pathway involves glutathione, a highly versatile molecule, which can attach itself to many different chemicals. This pathway is critically important, being responsible for about 60% of Phase 2 detoxification reactions.

Unfortunately, an excess of chemicals can deplete glutathione levels. This molecule can be recycled but needs magnesium, vitamins B2 and B3, and selenium to do so. Deficiencies of these are all too common and will reduce available glutathione. Magnesium is critical for detoxification but some surveys have found levels to be low in up to 80% of the population.

Other pathways in Phase 2 include conjugation with the peptides glycine and taurine, and also sulphation, glucuronidation, acetylation and methylation. The sulphation pathway has a lower capacity than others and is especially prone to breaking down. Faults in this pathway are known to occur in autism, Parkinson's disease and Alzheimer's disease.

Metallothioneins are proteins that are essential for removing heavy metals, such as lead, cadmium and mercury. They are rich in cysteine, a sulphur-carrying amino acid. What this means is that a good supply of sulphur-containing foods is essential for the detoxification of heavy metals (see below).

Problems with the glycine pathway can occur from overload with benzoates, the principle source of which are being soft drinks. This creates further difficulties in breaking down other toxic chemicals, such as toluene, which use the same pathway.

As with Phase 1, it is easy to see that a deficiency in a key nutrient (such as molybdenum), or an excess of a harmful product (such as benzoates), can cause the detoxification process to malfunction. Too many chemicals can do the same: for example, the acid-blocking drug cimetidine can block excretion and increase the toxicity of some pesticides. A further problem is that Phase 2 is not always able to keep pace with Phase 1 and this too leads to increased toxicity.

We are now not only living in the most toxic environment the human race has ever experienced but, at the same time, we are living on a more nutrient-depleted diet than ever before. It is a dangerous, and sometimes deadly, combination.

Amino acid deficiencies that can impair phase 2 include deficiencies of glycine, taurine, glutamine, arginine and ornithine.

So how we can aid the detoxification process and make it function better? The first step is to avoid overloading it. This means reducing our exposure to toxins and drinking more water, which dilutes them.

The second step is to ensure that we have adequate nutrients on board. Numerous studies have found nutrient deficiencies in the standard western diet, partly due to depletion of minerals in the soil. This is why good nutrition is so critical to detoxification, but supplementation also makes sense (see Appendix III), particularly at times of toxic overload. B vitamins, magnesium, zinc and selenium are some of the more important ones.

Here are some examples of foods which contain key nutrients.
- Magnesium can be found in green vegetables, seeds and nuts

- Zinc can be found in oily fish, seeds and nuts
- Molybdenum can be found in red cabbage, beans and buckwheat
- Selenium can be found in brazil nuts and also in alfalfa and mushrooms
- Sulphur can be found in onions, garlic, watercress, asparagus, turnips, eggs and fish
- Cysteine can be found in eggs, onions, garlic, brazil nuts, asparagus and sunflower seeds
- Glutathione can be found in fruit and vegetables
- Glycine is in meat, fish, almonds and walnuts
- Taurine can be made from cysteine.

Iodine

Iodine deserves a special mention in the context of detoxification. Due to the increase in halogens in the environment, iodine is easily displaced from the body. Halogens include fluorides (toothpaste, PFAS, Teflon, drugs), chlorine (tap water and chlorinated chemicals) and bromides (flame retardants, personal care products). Conversely, having enough iodine helps displace these toxic compounds. Iodine is important for the thyroid and other glandular structures, including the ovaries and breast. It is crucial to brain function and is thought to protect against hormone-dependent cancers. This is another critical nutrient and iodine deficiency is widespread. It is very safe and was given to vast numbers of people after Chernobyl, with positive results. It can be found in fish and kelp. A good and cheap supplement is Lugol's 12% Iodine.

Summary

Chemicals can produce a mesmerising variety of toxic effects. We are all exposed to too much toxicity, with too many chemicals stored in our bodies. Genetic differences mean a particular chemical can be a thousand times more dangerous for one person than another. Mixtures of toxins produce unquantifiable dangers. It makes sense therefore to help our bodies as much as possible, as they struggle with a greater toxic load than at any time in our history. We need to both reduce our exposure and to boost our ability to release toxins. Methods that help the latter include sweating (exercise, saunas), fasting and taking in sufficient nutrients.

Practical steps to reduce toxicity

Here are some changes that can help:

Easy changes to make

- Avoid using aerosols and air fresheners
- Avoid fragranced products
- For smokers, avoid smoking in the house
- Remove shoes before walking through the house
- Microwave (if you must) in ceramic or glass containers
- Avoid using pesticides in the house
- Avoid farmed salmon
- Don't charge mobile phones in the bedroom whilst sleeping
- Say no to amalgam in fillings (and sometimes root canals)
- Wash new clothes before wearing them
- Use your sense of smell to alert you to chemicals

Moderately easy changes to make

- Use a water filter
- Eat mostly organic food
- Exercise often – ideally enough to cause sweating
- Bath with Epsom salts
- Increase iodine intake (which displaces brominated, fluorinated and chlorinated compounds)

- Use oil pulling (see page 242)
- Use cables instead of wifi and/or switch wifi off at night
- Switch mobiles off when not using them – use like an answer phone or switch wifi setting to 'off' when not needed and especially at night if you have to keep your phone on
- Don't keep mobiles next to your body when switched on
- Avoid permanent hair dyes
- Don't wrap foods in plastic
- Avoid plastic water bottles
- Take breaks every three-quarters of an hour whilst painting, ideally going outdoors
- Keep perfume use to a minimum and avoid perfume sprays
- Avoid chemical carpet washes
- Be cautious of products containing fluoride, parabens and/ or triclosan
- Be wary of chemicals with 'chloro' or 'fluor' in the name
- Be suspicious of labels such as 'stain-resistant', 'water-resistant', 'water-repellent', 'crease-resistant'
- Change to natural soaps, cosmetics and cleaning products
- Leave a newly painted room unoccupied for a few days
- Avoid products with 'silver technology' or 'nanoparticles' on the label.

Somewhat harder changes to make

- Don't put anything onto your skin that you wouldn't eat
- Make the bedroom as free of toxins as possible with as few electric appliances as possible
- Change DECT phones to analogue phones
- Fast on a regular basis
- Use a sauna or FIRS (far infrared sauna) machine
- Use an air purifier in the bedroom or in rooms where there

is much outgasing from carpets, paints and furnishings
- For smokers, stop
- Use water-based solvents, paints and cleaning products
- Avoid pesticides in the garden
- Use supplements which enhance the detoxification process including: B vitamins, magnesium, zinc, selenium, molybdenum and iodine.
- Avoid dry cleaning where possible
- Add soluble fibre to your diet
- Clear toxic products and any 'smellies' from the house

More complicated changes to make

- Avoid soft furnishings containing stain repellents and flame retardants
- Reduce the amount of carpeting and plastic floorings
- Change pans from non-stick or aluminium to cast iron
- Change food containers from plastic to glass or ceramic
- Remove amalgam fillings

Part IV

Maximise your energy

Chapter 9

How energy can heal

There are more things in heaven and earth, Horatio, than
are dreamt of in your philosophy.

William Shakespeare (*Hamlet*)

Healing with energy

In the 1980s a Chinese national badminton champion called Feng
Jian, aged only 21, developed lung cancer. Standard treatment
was surgery, followed by chemotherapy and radiotherapy. Even
with this he knew his prognosis was poor. He decided against
conventional treatment and instead elected to visit a teacher of
Guo Lin qigong.

Qigong can be roughly translated as energy work and typically
involves exercises to increase a type of energy within the body
called *qi*. *Qi* is considered by Chinese medicine to be the life force
that maintains the health of the body. This particular form of
qigong was specifically designed for cancer.

It had been developed by a lady called Guo Lin after she
developed metastatic uterine cancer. Given only months to live
and having had two major, but unsuccessful, operations, her
doctors told her there was nothing more they could do. She
was to prove her doctors wrong, living for another 20 years
and eventually dying from an unrelated cause. After recovery
she established the Beijing Ba Yi Lake Cancer-Resistant Paradise

to make this type of cancer treatment available to others. It is said that over a million cancer sufferers in China now use these exercises. Many stories of miraculous recoveries exist and over 90% are said to improve. Even those who eventually succumb to cancer are said to do so more comfortably using the therapy. As expected, with any type of treatment, relapse can occur if the exercises are stopped.

Feng Jian did his exercises diligently, sometimes for 12 hours a day. He combined these with good diet and rest. Within days he started to feel better; 10 months later his x-rays showed complete clearance of his tumour. Twenty years later, he remained well, a remarkable statistic for someone with lung cancer.

In China, people can either go to a western-style hospital or have traditional Chinese Medicine (TCM). Even though *qigong* is probably the oldest healing method in China, the majority of Chinese, at that time, would not have chosen TCM if they had cancer. However, this one high profile case changed the minds of the Chinese people about the traditional approach. It also changed the minds of many western-trained Chinese doctors.[1]

Two things strike me about this story. One is that lung cancer is extremely difficult to treat by any method, responding poorly to conventional treatment (the five-year survival in the UK is 16%). Anything that cures a disease as lethal as this warrants investigation. The other point is more extraordinary. The cancer was treated by manipulating energy, and, more strangely, by manipulating a type of energy the existence of which is not even recognised by western medicine.

What is energy?

This implies energy is important. It suggests that its significance in health and healing has been overlooked. So, it is energy and its impact on health that we are now going to investigate.

Instinctively we know that there is some link, some connection, between energy and health. We can sense it. When our health is good we feel full of energy and when our health is poor our energy plummets. We all want energy; we feel wonderful when we have it. We are drawn to people with it. Our energy is giving us a message about our health. But what exactly is energy?

Einstein said that all matter is modified energy and all matter radiates energy. If so, this means that our bodies are modified energy and all diseases must involve an alteration in this energy. The cure too, in some form, must involve a transformation in that same energy. The great scientist Tesla, the inventor of the electric motor, alternating current, fluorescent lights and wireless transmission, understood this. He said that 'Once science stops thinking in purely physical terms then in one decade it will make greater strides forward than it has in the last century'. Medicine should take note.

New treatments using energy are emerging. Energy psychology is an example. Dawson Church has claimed that energy psychology rivals any discovery in the last few centuries in terms of the alleviation of human suffering.[2] What is exciting about some of these therapies is they have shown us that the body can sometimes heal at astonishing speed. Nevertheless, energy medicine is in its infancy, it is poorly understood and much of what we know is incomplete. Perhaps the biggest obstacle is our inability to measure it. Be that as it may, we cannot leave it unexplored. There are many methods of healing involving energy, they are available to everyone, and they can make a difference to the outcome. I will give examples.

The links between energy and health are not new. For thousands of years physicians in China understood that a form of energy called qi or chi flows through our bodies and they considered this flow was essential to health. They believed that blockage of the flow of qi created disease and they developed ways to nurture and increase it. This basic understanding led to the development of numerous methods of healing the body, including acupuncture, *t'ai chi* and *qigong* designed specifically to balance and help the flow of *qi*.

Western medicine is one of the few medical systems that has no concept of energy within the body. In the words of Nobel laureate Albert Szent-Gyorgyi: 'In every culture and in every medical tradition before ours, healing was accomplished by moving energy.' This observation of energy flow is certainly not unique to Chinese medicine. It is intriguing that there are people, often known as 'sensitives', who have the ability to see energy, both within and around the body, and to detect diseases. They have confirmed that the energy channels they can see are the same as those originally mapped out by ancient Chinese physicians. And now new scientific data have verified many of their findings.

A surprising observation is that disturbance of the energy field precedes disease rather than the other way around. This has important implications. It means finding ways of identifying and correcting energy disturbances before they manifest could prevent disease. Also, it follows logically and crucially that healing must start with a change in the body's energy.

We now have good data to show that these energy fields exist both inside and outside the body, confirming both the observations of 'sensitives' and the knowledge of traditional Chinese physicians. But there are other forms of energy. There is electricity. Our bodies cannot function without it. All chemical reactions in our bodies are powered by electricity. Its vital role in our bodies is poorly understood and it is often in the areas where knowledge is lacking that the biggest breakthroughs come. There are other forms of energy too: the energy of thought and the energy of healing. We will explore these too.

There is, however, another important aspect of energy: it carries information. This brings us to perhaps the greatest mystery of all. If we could solve this one then medicine could make one of those huge strides forward, hinted at by Tesla.

Chapter 9

Why do diseases persist?

The mystery is this: why do diseases persist? In other words, why does the body continue to build diseased tissues and organs? Let me explain. It has been estimated that the body replaces itself every seven years. For instance, the stomach lining replaces itself every five days, the red blood cells replace themselves every four months, the brain every two months and the liver, every three to 18 months. The skeleton replaces itself every 10 years. We don't know what controls this incredibly complex and elegant process, but clearly some mechanism or organising field must oversee it.

Think about it – why should any disease that has lasted for longer than a few years (or even a few months) continue to exist? Surely by then the body or organ should have renewed itself completely and returned us to good health? The disease should have disappeared and the diseased tissue should have been substituted with healthy tissue.

Of course, we know this doesn't happen. Unfortunately, as the body is renewed, so is the disease. But the key question is, why? Why doesn't the body simply rebuild itself, disease-free? Surely this would be a far better and simpler option. It built the body disease-free in the first place so it must know how to do it. But for some inexplicable reason it recreates disease.

In other words, the fault in many illnesses is at the level of the organising field or blueprint rather than within the cells, organs or genes. The fault is in the body's programming; it is in the body's information system. If this is where the problem lies, then this must also be where the solution lies.

The approach of mainstream medicine has always been to deal with the disease at the physical or cellular level, but a purely physical approach has limitations. The perfect approach would be to understand and correct the blueprint. And the blueprint is information, a form of energy.

Now, if the body is reproducing defective cells and producing diseases because of some error in its organising intelligence, how can we correct this? The Norwegian writer Marit Jarstad gives us a clue. She had suffered from chronic hepatitis for 25 years. She spent three months in hospital at the onset of her illness. She was aware of the puzzling fact that all her liver cells replaced themselves every three to 18 months. She spoke to her nephew, a medical student at the time, and asked him why the illness was perpetuating itself. Her nephew thought the question was interesting and suggested that perhaps the images of the disease were being passed from the old cells to the new. He further suggested talking to her liver to see if it would change. So, for three months, every morning, she spoke to her liver saying: 'All is well, there is no danger anymore.' She realised this was an odd thing to do but after several weeks of repeating it she suddenly began to feel better. Blood tests would later confirm that the hepatitis had indeed left her. The disease never returned.[3]

Doctors who saw her following this told her that perhaps she had never had the disease in the first place, for they could find no signs of it, or even evidence that it had ever existed. This disbelief by the medical profession after recovery from serious illness is a story heard all too often by survivors; one that causes immense frustration. She was by no means the first to get better only to be told that she had never had the disease in the first place.

In a sense her method was deceptively simple, but all the same it did something fundamental: it changed the internal programming of the liver cells – it changed the blueprint. And this is far from the only example. Of course, this strategy may not necessarily work for other diseases or other people, but the fact that it could work at all is immensely important, and it brings us to another interesting question when it comes to treating a disease. Is the treatment being aimed at the physical disorder or is it being aimed at the underlying blueprint?

Brendon Bays's story, described in Chapter 5, is another

example of changing the blueprint (see page 145). Once she had found and healed a traumatic memory her tumour rapidly resolved.

Energy and health

However, let's go back to energy. What exactly is it that we are feeling when we say we are full of energy and how can we enhance it? Most people have noticed that exercise increases energy, as does good sleep, enjoying ourselves, new surroundings, sunlight, a sense of purpose or passion, good company, meditation, being in nature and a good dose of laughter. Not surprisingly most of these factors have independently been found to enhance health.

Energy also gives an important clue to whether an illness is improving. For instance, in a healing crisis, which often happens before recovery, symptoms often become more marked but energy typically remains high. An increase in energy is a good pointer to recovery.

Some have postulated that these factors increase the vibration and energy of the body and the higher this becomes the more resistant we become to disease. Survivors of serious disease have not been slow to investigate these. Observing what boosts our energy gives us a major clue to healing the body.

More widely-known forms of energy

For this book, I have divided energy, somewhat arbitrarily, into more and less widely-known forms. Of course, this will almost certainly change over time and less widely-known forms are by no means less important when it comes to healing. In this chapter, I will look at the better known forms.

Imagine for a moment that you could buy a drug, a drug that was powerful enough to do all the following: strengthen bones, reduce fractures by 25%, reduce falls, strengthen muscles even without exercise, prevent tooth decay, boost the immune system and reduce the risk of heart diseases. Furthermore, it could lower blood pressure, increase heart output and lower both cholesterol and blood sugar. Additionally, it could reduce the risk of many cancers, including those of the breast, colon and prostate cancer. It could also help in a wide variety of other conditions, including back pain, psoriasis, multiple sclerosis and diabetes.[4]

Of course, no drug has benefits that can remotely approach these. However, there is something that really does deliver these and more. It is a type of energy. And it is free.

This energy is sunlight.

Sunlight

These benefits have been recognised for a long time but have been largely forgotten by modern medicine.[5] In fact, we have been encouraged by modern medicine to fear and avoid the sun, but at the turn of the 20th century the power of the sun was viewed differently. It was beginning to be accepted by medicine as a means to treat serious diseases and with good reason.

One of the most extraordinary displays of healing power I have ever come across are the astonishing before and after photographs of children hideously deformed from tuberculosis (TB) of the spine and bones.[4] The treatment they were given was heliotherapy (which simply means healing with sunshine). This treatment was developed by Dr Auguste Rollier and used in his clinics at the turn of the 20th century. It involved progressive exposure to sunlight.

At this time TB was common. Dr Niel Finsen had already received the Nobel prize for discovering that TB of the skin (lupus vulgaris) could be successfully treated with ultraviolet (UV) light. Then, as his ideas expanded, he developed a preference for using sunlight.

Rollier was a surgeon but he became disillusioned with the poor results of radical surgery for TB: the gross disfigurement and high mortality. Following the example of Finsen, he developed his own treatment. This involved slow tanning with sunlight in the cool conditions of the Swiss mountains, with exposure to fresh air, good nutrition and exercise. The body was very gradually exposed to sunlight, starting with the feet then working up to full exposure after about two to three weeks. These seriously ill patients needed to be treated with great caution when first exposed to sunlight and cold air. Their tolerance was initially low and this was regularly assessed.

Rollier believed sunlight was fundamental to the cure of TB. However, he treated much more than this and had success with rickets, osteomyelitis, abscesses and varicose ulcers. His 40 years of experience taught him that early morning sunshine was the best (6:00 to 9:00 am), that exposure to sunlight in cool air was better than warm air; short bursts were better than long; and tanning was necessary for recovery.

His methods were slow to be accepted as they turned traditional ideas on their head, but his success was hard to ignore. His work expanded, his clinics became well known and he eventually had 36 clinics operating with more than 1000 beds. His methods were copied by other clinics all around the world. Rollier was a successful pioneer, curing a disease once considered incurable, but his magic ingredient was simple: sunshine. And the sunshine he advocated was morning and late afternoon sunshine.

His ideas were not new. Greek and Roman physicians, including Hippocrates, had advocated sun exposure. The so-called Indian Hippocrates, Charaka, prescribed sunlight for all diseases and recommended early morning walks.

Dr John Christopher, a renowned herbalist, developed a programme for treating his 'incurable patients'. He was known for the saying that there are no incurable diseases, just incurable individuals. He described these methods in his booklet *Curing the Incurables*.[5] He used his regimen for treating serious diseases such as cancer, stroke, arthritis, multiple sclerosis and muscular dystrophy. His system included sunbathing, which started with only two minutes a day and avoided the time between 11:00 am and 1:00 pm. Other components of his program included fresh juices, hot baths followed by cold showers and skin brushing, herbal remedies and castor oil packs. The success rate of his programme was not recorded, but complete healing was not uncommon.

Vitamin D

So, why is sunlight so vital for us? We know it increases nitric oxide (beneficial for the heart and blood vessels) and serotonin (beneficial in depression), but, almost certainly, its major role is in the production of vitamin D. And treatment with high-dose vitamin D may turn out to be the most exciting development in the treatment of autoimmune disease for decades.

We now know that vitamin D is not really a vitamin but a hormone and perhaps the most potent immune modulator in the body, altering nearly 300 genes and regulating thousands of functions in every cell.[6] How much of it do we need?

Many years ago a patient came to see me and told me that his psoriasis had completely disappeared following treatment. This, in itself, was unusual but the circumstances were even more so. It turned out he had mistakenly been taking his weekly vitamin D supplement every day. Fortunately, vitamin D is extremely safe at high dosage. One of the world's leading vitamin D researchers, Dr Michael Holick, has stated that no adverse effects have ever been seen in people taking 10,000 IU daily, even for prolonged periods.[7] This brings me to Dr Cicero Coimbra, Professor of Neurology at the Federal University of Sao Paulo in Brazil.

I have always found the concept of autoimmune disease, in which the body supposedly attacks itself, hard to accept. It seems much more likely to me that something is interfering with the immune system, perhaps a deficiency of a vital substance. Dr

Coimbra believes most people with an autoimmune disease are resistant to vitamin D and need much higher doses than usual. He typically gives doses of 70,000 IU daily, and sometimes 200,000 IU daily. He uses a protocol which includes other supplements, notably vitamin K, and carefully monitors the blood and urine of his patients (see www.coimbraprotocol.com).

He treats many patients with multiple sclerosis and the results have been remarkable.[6] Typically, high-dose vitamin D seems to switch off the disease: patients stop having relapses, and recent lesions (appearing in the previous two years) start to regress. However, this same protocol has been equally successful in other autoimmune conditions, including rheumatoid arthritis, psoriasis, ankylosing spondylitis, vitiligo and Crohn's disease. Most of these patients have already tried standard regimes and, on changing to his protocol, have noticed their energy increased and they had progressive improvements in their symptoms.

Vitamin D also prevents cancer, reduces the likelihood of metastasis, and low levels are predictive of poor survival.[8] Just about everyone with a serious disease needs vitamin D and plenty of it.

Another advocate of sunlight was John Ott. This tireless researcher did much to draw the attention of the scientific community to the benefits of sunlight and to how plants and animals become healthier in natural light. Some of the benefits are shown in the box on page 264.

Individually these findings are not that significant but collectively they present powerful evidence that natural light is vital for good health.

Ott likened lack of full spectrum light to a deficiency of an essential vitamin. He continued to experiment and make discoveries. He found that removing specific light frequencies typically had a negative impact. An example is that continuous exposure to light with a green filter damages the retina in a number of animal species.

Research on sunlight

Here is a selection of the evidence noted by Ott.[9]

- In different experiments, rats subjected to carcinogens and mice of the BALB-C type (these mice are prone to melanoma) both developed fewer tumours and had slower growth rates of tumours when kept under real or simulated natural light compared with those kept under artificial light.

- Another experiment with a C3H strain of mice (also susceptible to tumours) revealed that tumours developed later when kept under natural light as opposed to artificial light.

- Rats kept under fluorescent light tended to be irritable and bite their keepers whereas those kept under natural light were docile and easy to handle. Similarly schoolchildren sitting under fluorescent light were found to become more hyperactive, fatigued and irritable. These features reversed when they were put under natural light.

- Rabbits bred better under full spectrum light which included UV light.

- Fish in aquariums lit by fluorescent light were unable to lay eggs.

However, it was lack of ultraviolet (UV) light which concerned Ott most. It is worth stressing that we are frequently deprived of UV light for long periods of time. Both spectacles and windows filter out most of the UV light. Outdoor pollution has not only progressively reduced available sunlight over several decades but has selectively reduced UV light (twice as much as normal light). Ott found that UV light, though it had acquired a bad reputation, appeared to be essential; plants grew better and rats and mice bred more easily when it was available.

Of course our main concern in this book is recovery from serious illness. Ott provided fascinating anecdotal cases. He described the case of a man in his 70s with terminal lung cancer who was a regular user of sunglasses. Cancer of the lung typically has a poor prognosis, but this man recovered from his cancer once he started living outdoors as much as possible, without his sunglasses, and after reducing his exposure to artificial light. He remained well until his death eight years later from an unrelated condition. Ott also related a similar story of a man with prostate cancer who remained well for three years after recovery but unfortunately gave no further details.

Ott had one other outstanding contribution to make. By an extraordinary coincidence, his own life came to illustrate this beautifully.

Ott developed arthritis of the hip and wondered if lack of sunlight or his own work using photographic lights was contributing to the problem. He tried increasing his exposure to sunlight by walking on the beaches in Florida, but it made no difference. Then by accident he broke his glasses and, by a strange quirk of fate, his spare glasses didn't fit properly. He stopped wearing glasses. Whilst waiting for a new pair, even though it was winter and the weather was cold, he spent most of his time out of doors.

To his surprise, he noticed his arthritis began to improve and he was able to walk without a cane. One day he was able to walk one mile and his hips felt better than they had for three or four years. Encouraged by this he continued to spend at least six hours a day out of doors and reduce his exposure to artificial light, TV and photographic lights. He made another astute observation: his eyes were now becoming less sensitive to light. His recovery continued and x-rays confirmed the improvement in his hips and the previous 30-degree restriction in hip movement disappeared. Later he noted that prolonged driving or prolonged exposure to studio lights or TV caused his arthritis to relapse. Ott had stumbled on a great discovery: sunlight through the eyes was crucial for health.

It is always fascinating when multiple pieces of evidence from a variety of sources point in the same direction. Ott's research, the successes at Rollier's clinics and Christopher's use of sunlight for his 'incurables' all gave evidence that sunlight had remarkable healing powers.

There is surely enough evidence here to conclude that sunlight can and should augment any healing programme used to remedy any serious disease. No wonder animals, like us, love to bask in the sun.

Photodynamic therapy

Before we leave sunlight, let's briefly look at photodynamic therapy (PDT), a promising treatment for cancer. Here substances known as porphyrins are injected into the body; they are taken up selectively by cancer cells. Once exposed to light (usually a red light or laser) they kill the cancer cells but have little effect on normal cells. There are now over 3000 published papers with a recent review[10] on this method of treatment and the agents used are becoming more selective, including newer agents based on chlorophyll. These release oxygen when light is added, leading to cancer cell death within hours. Another researcher, Dougherty, found that patients unresponsive to standard therapy responded to a single treatment of PDT 70-80% of the time.[11] The method has few adverse effects, apart from sun sensitivity, but is largely limited to tumours that can be reached by the light beams. I believe this is an underused treatment with great potential.

Exercise

Let's look at another source of energy. It is interesting to compare it with sunlight. The benefits are wide-ranging and in many ways similar. This form of energy lowers the risk of heart disease, reduces the risk of stroke, leads to better mental health, relieves depression (as effectively as antidepressant drugs), improves memory and mental function, reduces risks of falls and fractures, reduces blood pressure, improves glucose control in diabetes, improves sleep, reduces the risk of gallstones, reduces cholesterol, and reduces the risk of many cancers including those of the colon, testicle, breast, prostate, lung and uterus. It lowers levels of dangerous hormones like IGF-1 (see page 73) and stimulates lymphatic flow. It also stimulates mitochondrial production.

As with sunlight, no drug comes even close to achieving these benefits. Like sunshine, it costs nothing. These benefits come from exercise.

Medicine is prone to fashions. The benefits of sunshine were beginning to be recognised at the start of the 20th century, but this didn't last, even though the evidence is as strong today as it was at that time. The pattern is different with exercise. In the 1950s doctors were just as dismissive about exercise as they are now about sunlight.

It would take an elegant and ingenious study to challenge entrenched attitudes within the profession. Bus and tram conductors proved to be an ideal study group as they could be compared with their more sedentary colleagues, the drivers.[12] Conductors were estimated to climb up to 740 steps a day whereas drivers were seated 90% of the time. Professor Jeremy Morris compared rates of heart disease in the two groups between 1949 and 1950. The results were unequivocal. Conductors had 42% less heart disease, developed heart disease at a later age and were less likely to die suddenly with heart disease.

Other studies mounted up to validate this. Postman showed similar benefits and this varied with their level of activity. Those with the lowest activity had twice the mortality from heart disease compared with the most active. A later study of longshoremen found the same: the most active group had a 30% lower mortality from heart disease and an even greater reduction in sudden death.[13] High bursts of physical activity appeared to protect against sudden death.

Morris now knew for certain that exercise was strongly protective against heart disease but foresaw a problem. He realised many people didn't have the option of an active job. He therefore turned his attention to an office-based group, investigating leisure activities in 16,882 civil servants between the ages of 40 and 64, over an eight-and-a-half-year period. The results were similar: exercise gave substantial protection against heart disease. Those who took vigorous exercise reduced their chance of a heart attack by over 50%.[14] In the long-running Framlingham study the most active group had a 40% reduction in mortality from heart disease compared with the least active. Mortality from heart disease was reduced by both the frequency and the vigour of the exercise.

Strokes showed a similar pattern: a sedentary lifestyle was found to increase the risk of stroke eightfold – higher than the risk of smoking and two to four times the risk of raised blood pressure.[15] However, the most telling evidence about exercise was its effect on longevity.

The College Alumni Health study tracked 50,000 college alumni over four decades and found a direct correlation between amount of exercise undertaken and longevity.[16] This study, which generated over 80 papers, found exercise reduced rates of breast and colon cancer, reduced strokes, increased bone density and improved mood and sleep. In short, exercise reduced the risk of all today's major killers, made people feel better and increased longevity. No medical intervention comes close to having this impact on so many different areas.

But does exercise make a difference with cancer? The answer is yes, both for established cancer and for prevention.

Can exercise help cancer

Exercise has been shown to reduce relapse and mortality rates in breast, colorectal and prostate cancers.

• Two studies have found that women with breast cancer

who did at least 150 minutes of moderate exercise per week (such as brisk walking) had a 40% reduction in both mortality and recurrences compared with women doing less than an hour's exercise a week.[17, 18]

- Just under 30 studies have found exercise reduces the risk of developing breast cancer by 30-40%.[19]
- With colorectal cancer two studies have found that six hours of moderate exercise per week reduced the recurrence rates and mortality by 50%.[20, 21]
- A review of 52 studies found that exercise, in a variety of forms, reduced the risk of developing colon cancer by 24%.[22]
- For prostate cancer, two studies have found that doing three hours per week of moderately intense activity reduced mortality by 30% and disease progression by 57%.[23]

The following story related by a woman described in the book *Healthy at 100* shows how much difference exercise can make in the most serious diseases. In this case exercise was combined with diet.

At the age of 47 she was diagnosed with metastatic breast cancer. The cancer had already spread to her bones and lungs and her situation seemed beyond hope. One day she became fascinated by an event on TV called the Iron Man triathlon. Following this, she started a vegan diet and embarked on a programme of vigorous exercise.

Doctors would have no doubt been horrified by the thought of a patient with bony metastases doing exercise of this severity. Furthermore, no woman had ever before attempted the Iron Man triathlon. She entered every race she could, including a 37-mile run up Mount Haleakala in Hawaii. Her strength increased and the metastases in her bones began to improve. Eventually her cancer disappeared and she managed to complete the Iron Man triathlon six times. Sixteen years later she was well and remained extremely fit.[24]

This story tells us something remarkable about the healing power of exercise combined with an optimum diet and a huge determination to get better.

Meanwhile, another woman, Pat Reeves, was diagnosed with an inoperable brain tumour in 1983 at the age of 38 and given 18 months to live. Deciding not to use conventional treatment, she put herself on a vegan and raw-food diet, favouring sprouting seeds and wheatgrass. Her program included long fasts and she started exercising daily, running 100 miles a week. She made a remarkable recovery but her problems were not over. Ten years later after a period of intense stress she developed an osteosarcoma. Brain tumours and osteosarcomas are notoriously difficult tumours to treat but she stayed positive, returning to her strict diet, intermittent fasting and exercises. In the process she won marathons, triathlons and power-lifting championships, becoming the oldest female competitor to take a record in power-lifting in 2010. She remains healthy today and says that her energy is amazing.[25]

There seems something incredibly life enhancing about testing the limits of our physical ability and these two women are certainly not the only ones to have made this discovery.

The Simontons, who we met in Chapter 4, treated patients with incurable cancer at the Cancer Counselling and Research Center in Dallas, with outstanding results. Of 159 patients not expected to live one year, 18% recovered, 22% had tumour regression and the rest had, on average, double the normal survival time.

The Simontons are best known for their use of visualisation but they also incorporated exercise into their regime. They found that a significant number of their most successful patients kept up a programme of vigorous exercise after diagnosis. They asked all their patients to exercise for one hour three times a week. They found shorter periods had less benefit. Many people might express surprise about terminal cancer patients doing this level of exercise. At Dallas they did far more than most people assumed possible and over half of their incurable patients remained 100% active. A patient with metastatic cancer was able to run a marathon and another with bony metastases did a half marathon.[26] Those that were bedridden imagined doing exercises several times a day for 10 minutes. The Simontons discovered that it was the regularity of exercise that was important rather than the type.

It is intriguing that they encouraged visualisation of exercise when real exercise proved impossible. Is there any evidence that this can make a difference?

The story of Jess recounted in the book *Recovery from Chronic Fatigue Syndrome* gives us a fascinating insight. Whilst suffering from chronic fatigue syndrome (often known as ME) she described her state as one of lying in bed all day, drifting in and out of sleep and taking paracetamol. However, one day she was inspired whilst watching the London Marathon. She decided to make running the marathon her goal and, every day, visualised herself crossing the finishing line and feeling outstandingly healthy. One year later, just as she had imagined, she achieved her goal, running the London Marathon in just over four hours. She combined the visualisation with a raw food diet.[27]

The same book relates the story of Anna Hemmings. Already a champion canoeist, she developed chronic fatigue syndrome in 2003 and felt permanently exhausted, sleeping 13 to 14 hours a day. She was told that her body was finished, due to all the demanding training she had previously done. She was advised she needed to retire from the sport.

Instead she started to vividly picture herself back on the water competing, feeling the fulfilment of winning, having the gold medal round her neck and standing on the rostrum. By 2005 she had indeed become European champion again and later a world champion.

Both of these remarkable women used other therapies in addition to visualisation, but what strikes me is how dramatic their recoveries were and from a condition which is, typically, very challenging to treat. It demonstrates the almost unlimited power of the body to heal and how visualising competing in these races proved a critical turning point.

I would hazard a guess that visualising exercise in this way programmes the body for health, keeping the mind focused on well-being and away from disease. This may be another reason why taking part in races has proved so popular with survivors.

Conclusion

Sunlight and exercise have both been extensively researched and their profound and far-ranging benefits on health are not in question. They can help in almost any condition. Additionally, they are cheap and relatively easy to use. I have classified them as more widely-known forms of energy.

In the next chapters we will turn our attention to some less widely-known forms of energy. Here things become less straightforward but perhaps more interesting.

Chapter 10

Healing, vital force and electricity

It has often appeared, whilst I have been soothing my patients, as if there was some strange property in my hands to pull and draw away from the afflicted parts aches and diverse impurities.

Hippocrates

Sometimes recoveries can seem miraculous. Consider the following story. Rock star, Ronnie Hawkins had been diagnosed with pancreatic cancer. Five doctors had told him they could not cure him and, as is well known, pancreatic cancer has an appalling prognosis.

A gifted young healer named Adam asked if he could try distant healing. Adam had the ability to visualise Hawkin's cancer from a distance. He noted it was the size of a tennis ball and sent Ronnie healing energies on a daily basis from 3000 miles away. Ronnie felt a quivering in his abdomen and started to feel better and the jaundice caused by his cancer improved. Adam then decided to compare Ronnie's pancreas with his dad's and noticed that Ronnie's pancreas was 'blocked'. He treated the blockage and later observed that it had cleared.

After two months Adam could see that the cancer was gone and the remaining tissue was being reabsorbed. A CT scan at that time found that the tumour was less than half its former size. After a further three months the cancer had healed and the CT scan returned to normal. Two months later another scan was normal. Ronnie was declared cancer-free and went back to performing.[1]

Everything is energy

According to physics everything is energy vibrating amidst vast amounts of empty space. Quantum physics tells us that this vibrating energy creates our world and our bodies. These are not solid, but rather a bizarre world of limitless and changing possibilities waiting to be crystallised into one particular version of reality, in line with our intent and our consciousness.

These ideas are extraordinary and many scientists have pondered about their inherent strangeness. Some have said that the conclusions are not only stranger than you think but stranger than you could think. The Danish physicist, Neils Bohr, has said that 'anyone who is not shocked by physics has not understood it'.

Physicists did the equations many decades ago but somehow most of us don't quite believe them. Matter is too solid, diseases too real and too frightening, and our everyday world too concrete. And yet, for anyone one with a serious illness there is something refreshing and exciting in knowing that our world is one of infinite possibilities and that it is far more fluid and changeable than we once thought. So how can we make use of this knowledge?

In this chapter we are moving away from the well researched areas of medicine and into new arenas; in some of these there are good data and in some we are at the edge of the unknown; only time can provide the necessary proof, or not. What we do know is that more and more people are testing the limits of what was once thought possible and coming up with different answers.

Here I will be looking at five less widely-known forms of

energy though I suspect there may be more. I will list what these
are next and then look at each in detail in this and the following
chapter:

1. **Healing energy** is the unknown force which can be
    transmitted by healers. Healing and healers have
    undergone extensive investigation in recent years.
    Although the mechanism of healing remains unknown,
    its effectiveness is not in question. An unusual property
    of this form of energy is that it can be transmitted over
    a distance. Non-local effects of this nature seem bizarre,
    but they are allowed for, and indeed expected, within
    the laws of quantum physics.

2. **Life force energy** goes by different names in different
    cultures, including 'vital force', *chi, qi, ki* or *prana*. It has
    been recognised by ancient systems of medicine for
    centuries. These energies have been reliably seen by
    many gifted 'sensitives'. More recently they have been
    documented by science. For thousands of years, notably
    in China, physicians have successfully healed diseases
    by manipulating this force.

3. **Electromagnetic energy:** The body is an electromagnetic
    organism with its own measurable electromagnetic
    field (EMF) and electromagnetic forces control the
    body's chemical reactions. Outside EMFs can enhance
    or interfere with the body's own EMFs. Considering
    its importance, this aspect of health has received little
    attention from modern medicine.

4. **Thought energy:** Quantum physics is unequivocal here:
    our attention matters; when we give our attention to
    something it alters reality – at least in the subatomic world.

5. **Organising fields:** A further aspect of energy is the
    organising fields or blueprints within and around all
    living beings. These are of paramount importance
    as they control the growth, healing and moment by

moment organisation of the entire organism. It is this blueprint that produces new cells as old ones die but this blueprint also allows diseases to be recreated (as noted in the last chapter). We know very little about this organising field.

Energy and disease

This chapter looks at the first three types of energy. In the first two categories there is clear-cut evidence that they have contributed to the healing of major diseases. For the third, electrical energy, we have less evidence but this section does identify a block to healing that may be far commoner than we think.

1. Healing energy

Some might dismiss the case of Adam and Ronnie Hawkins as anecdotal. That's why the research of Dr Bill Bengston is so ground-breaking. If a disease is universally fatal a control group is unnecessary. Once there are a handful of successful outcomes the odds of this being a chance finding quickly reach millions to one against.

Bill Bengston did just that. He not only worked with a universally fatal disease but he also used a control group. Mice injected with a lethal strain of mammary cancer called C3H/HeHu were used in a series of experiments. The mortality of this cancer is 100%: all such mice die within 14 and 27 days. The scientific literature had previously not recorded a single mouse surviving longer than 27 days. Bengston used 'healing' as his method of treatment. During the 'healing' he did not touch the mice but imagined energy running down his left arm, through the cage and into the mice and then running back through his right hand. He held an intention to heal but aimed for concentrated detachment, just allowing healing to happen with no concern for the outcome.

First he performed the healing himself and then he asked

a group of sceptical students to conduct the healings. The methodology was rigorous, with a control group within the building and another control at a separate location.

The results were unequivocal. The healing cured 87.9% of cancers and what's more this led to life-long immunity. Even if the mice who survived were later injected with higher loads of the cancer, they would recover. More surprisingly, tumours that were implanted from recovering mice into new mice injected with over double the usual quantity of mammary tumour proved protective. These new mice had a 62% survival.

The control groups outside the building all died. Unexpectedly, 69% of the control group within the building survived, almost as if they were picking up the healing energies.

Bill Bengston published his work.[2] His healing powers whilst treating volunteers were investigated using functional MRI (fMRI), heart rhythm and EEG. When he was asked to start healing, the volunteers would develop changes in their brain activity on fMRI. In a similar way their heart rhythms would develop synchronisation almost immediately after healing started and their EEGs would develop a similar pattern to his within seconds.

Bill Bengston could heal people as well as mice and had no failures with cancer unless the subject either failed to complete the course or had been previously treated with radiotherapy or chemotherapy. Those with aggressive cancers and younger subjects healed the fastest. Surprisingly, he had better results with sceptics than believers, who tended to give up if they weren't healed on their first visit.

Let's now go back to the healer Adam and Ronnie Hawkins. This is an example of distant healing. Several meta-analyses have been done on distant healing and the majority show significantly positive results.[3, 4]

What may be more convincing for sceptics is the fact that many were non-human studies on plants, algae, yeasts, insects and mammals, where a placebo effect cannot happen. More impressive is the ability of *qigong* and other healers to alter the very precise rate of decay of radioactive matter, either speeding it up or slowing it down.

One reason to seriously doubt the placebo explanation is that in many cases the patient had been unaware they were receiving healing or positively believed it would not work. The remarkable healer, Harry Edwards, described the case of a man with severe pain from arthritis. The man said: 'I was convinced no one could help me and I came only to please my aunt.'[5] In spite of his open scepticism, Harry was able to treat him rapidly and successfully.

There are many intriguing things about healing. One is brain 'attunement', where brain wave changes occur simultaneously in both the healer and the patient during healing, as noted with Bill Bengston. A study designed by Dr Jeanne Achterberg of South Western Medical School, Dallas goes a long way to establishing scientific proof. She recruited 11 healers from Hawaii who described their method as sending prayers, intentions or good wishes. The healers sent their healing to 11 recipients while they were having their brains monitored by an MRI scanner. There was no contact between the healers and the recipients. At the exact time that healing was being sent, the MRI showed activation in the recipient's brain. The possibility of this being a chance happening and of this occurring at the precise moment when healing was being sent was less than one chance in 10,000.[6]

This was not an isolated study. Robert Beck noted that healers from all cultures seem to change their brain wave patterns during healing. In addition, they are able to transmit their brainwave pattern.[7] Olga Worrall, known for her miraculous healings, was investigated by Dr Elmer Green, using EEGs, ECGs and various monitoring devices. He noted that many patients developed a similar pattern of EEG to Olga at just the time she sent her healing even though Olga was in a different room and had not met the patient.[8] The results on another well known healer, Mietek Wirkus, produced similar results: the brain waves (as shown by EEG) of the healer and of the subject altered at the exact same moment.[9]

Another gifted healer to be evaluated was Ostad Parvarandeh. He was given a photograph of a group of 30 patients whom he had never met and who were being monitored in a separate building 100 feet away. After a long period of normal EEG activity, he commenced healing and 84% of those being treated showed dramatic increases in alpha-wave activity at the precise moment healing began. In another test he was asked to increase brain wave frequency in the subjects. In 75% there was an increase at exactly the same time he started the healing and in the other 25% there was an opposite effect. In yet another test he was able to measurably increase cardiac output and stroke volume in five patients, again treating them from 100 feet away.[10] The odds of all these being chance findings are millions to one against.

Studies like this effectively rule out the placebo response and point to something much more extraordinary – a transmission of energy through space.

The late Harry Edwards was a renowned healer who treated thousands of patients. At one time he was receiving 9000 requests for absent healing every week. He kept extensive records and these revealed that, with healing, over 80% of people achieved easing or improvement of their condition and 30% reported complete recovery.[11]

Reading through the reports is fascinating; they illustrate just how serious many of the illnesses he treated were. Few people go to see a healer for minor problems and most only consider healing once all other options have been exhausted. The speed of recovery was often remarkable. Harry could treat a joint which had been locked for years and have it moving freely in minutes. On many occasions he demonstrated these skills in public. He had great success with spinal problems and slipped discs. These are notoriously difficult to treat with conventional medicine. Perhaps more impressively, he recounted many cases where cancers were cured.

The purpose of this book is to document times when 'incurable' diseases have been successfully treated, to try to understand how this happened and to see if these successes can be replicated. Harry gives evidence of 281 cases of tumours which were either cured or greatly improved after healing by him, often to the amazement of the patient's doctor.[12]

His descriptions of the changes which occurred after healing are just as fascinating as his ability to cure them and give some insight into the healing process. These included severe, almost painful sweating after healing tumours and, in the case of abdominal cancers, very large bowel movements as if the tumour was being expelled from the inside. My impression, after reading these case histories, is that the healing somehow stimulated the body's defences to go into overdrive and remove the cancerous material from the body as rapidly as possible.

Some of the cases recounted were exceptional even by Harry's own high standards. He described the case of a nurse who had suffered for many years from a distorted spine and a deformed chest caused by tuberculosis. Harry was able to rapidly straighten her spine and unlock her chest, leaving friends, who had watched her struggling for years, incredulous.[12]

My own experience as a doctor is that the figures he gives for cures are utterly extraordinary and I don't believe any doctor anywhere in the world could achieve anything remotely resembling his success. Harry wanted the medical profession to investigate his work and expressed his frustration on many occasions at their lack of interest in these well-documented cures.

Healers characteristically learn not to put limits on what can be done, and discount the word incurable. However, they are typically unable to anticipate in advance who can and who cannot be healed or how long healing will take.

When used for a chronic illness, healing often takes time

and the first change is usually a feeling of increased vitality and energy, better sleep and increasing optimism. However, sometimes changes can be rapid. Harry Edwards calls these 'supernormal healings'. His records showed that there were 10,000 'supernormal healings' in a four-year period.[10] Letters were kept so they could be inspected by bona fide researchers. No one currently can explain how the healings occurred. A not infrequent experience at the centre was for healing to take place before the letter requesting healing had even reached the centre.

I was surprised by the numbers of these dramatic healings. Some could be put down to the patient's positive expectations, but this explanation fails to convince me. In particular it cannot explain successful outcomes in patients with strongly held beliefs that healing was all nonsense.

Consider the following case. Harry was asked to treat a man dying from terminal lung cancer. The man did not believe in healing so his wife asked Harry to try absent healing without his knowledge. This was done as requested. Next day there was a marked improvement and from then on the patient went from strength to strength, living for many years and going back to his old occupation of making hand-made violins.[11] Of course, Harry was an exceptional healer and few healers achieve results of this level. It requires great dedication to become a good healer and just like other therapists, some will be more talented than others.

Dr Norman Shealy documented more than 100 medical records where miraculous healing had taken place and confirmed them to be true. Osted Parvarandeh cured metastatic cancers and sarcomas, macular degeneration and paralysis following spinal surgery.[9] These were verified from medical records. Another gifted healer, John Sewell, had considerable success treating cancers and found many would dissolve after four days, although once chemotherapy had been used, he found, like Bill Bengston, that treatment was often not possible, presumably because of its negative effect on the immune system.

I was surprised by the sheer volume of solid data and research which exists on healing. The data on the exquisite correlation between the timing of brain changes in both the healer and the patient are compelling. All that is lacking is an explanation of how healing works.

I think healing leaves us with a dilemma. Here we have a mode of treatment with enormous potential and an outstanding track record, even with the most serious of illnesses. The reality though is that its impact may vary with the skill of the healer and this is not easy to assess and unfortunately fraudulent healers do exist.

A further difficulty is that even highly gifted healers have been known to lose their way. In the 1920s, the well known healer Annie Semple Mcpherson lost her abilities after she disappeared following an affair. Many other healers have shone brightly only for their star to fade, sometimes after they have been tempted by money, sex and power; many have died young. The best healers appear to have their lives centred on spiritual values and are involved in regular spiritual practice. They typically take no credit for the healing and instead attribute it to the divine. Harry Edwards felt that spirit doctors were working through him and his job was simply to attune to them. I think the best policy is to find the best healer you can and one you can trust.

Not everyone will want to use healing but it seems to me that there are few downsides. Absent healing, where healing is done from a distance, requires no contact with the healer, requires nothing from the patient and seems to me to be like a situation where there is nothing to lose and everything to gain. It is often possible to put your name down on lists for absent healing at healing centres.

2. Life force energy

Most systems of medicine assume that a vital force flows through the body. They recognise that the free flow of this force promotes health whereas blocks and stagnation cause disease. This contrasts sharply with modern medicine where no such understanding exists. However, if you have a major illness could this knowledge be important? Could we use this knowledge to enhance health or even cure major diseases? Let's first look at these mysterious energy channels, so well known to the ancients, which include meridians, chakras and auras.

Meridians

The meridians are thought to consist of 12 energy channels which run in lines through the body, supplying organs and tissues with this vital force.

Evidence for meridians

The lack of concrete proof for the existence of meridians has proved a stumbling block for mainstream medicine. North Korean surgeon and scientist, Professor Bong Han Kim, at the National Medical Research Institute, US, found minute tubular structures were present at the site of meridians. These took up the radioisotope P32. When they were severed in the ducts to the liver in frogs, the livers of those frogs became swollen and congested and, within three days, the frogs started to die.

Nevertheless, this ground-breaking work remained obscure until further confirmation came in 1985, when Dr Claude Darras and Pierre de Vernejoul injected radioactive technetium into human acupuncture points and found the tracers followed the pathways of the meridians for 30 cm over the next four to six minutes. To confirm that this was a genuine effect, they also injected the technetium into sham acupuncture points which produced a different, more random pattern in which the tracer diffused outwards in a circular fashion.

The meridians have since been found to contain larger quantities of DNA granules and to emit photons. It has been speculated that these channels allow photons to be easily emitted, in turn allowing rapid transmission of light energy through the meridian system.[13]

Slowly science is catching up with the physicians of ancient China. This has added credence to methods of healing which are based on the existence of the meridians, whether it be by acupuncture, *qigong* or *t'ai-chi* or the energy psychology techniques (discussed later).

Auras and chakras

Not only can 'sensitives' see energy flow within the body but they can also see an aura which surrounds it. In the 1950s, Semyon Kirlian made this visible to all when he developed a type of photography using high-frequency electrical fields known as Kirlian photography.[14] This showed beautiful multicoloured light which sparkled, with flares, and surrounded the bodies of plants, animals and people. Kirlian started using still photos and later developed moving pictures.

What made this discovery intriguing was this energy field disappeared on death and changed with disease. What impressed Kirlian most was the fact that changes in the energy field preceded disease. He called this field surrounding the body the 'biological plasma body'. He noticed it changed from moment to moment, altered with breathing and with different emotions. It was stronger after exercise. It changed in healers before, during and after healing. However, exactly what it is that is seen during Kirlian photography and whether this is the same as the aura has remained controversial.

Harry Oldfield, a scientist with a longstanding interest in Kirlian photography, developed a more sophisticated version of it called poly-contrast interference photography (PIP) scanning. This produced changing colour images of the body's energy field. He noticed disc-like areas of increased energy down the centre of the body. At the time he knew nothing about *chakras*, but later realised this was what he was seeing. The PIP scan proved to have considerable potential in the diagnosis of many diseases, including cancer. Cancer typically showed areas of chaotic increased energy. Even a PIP scan of the fingertips in a cancer patient showed an altered energy pattern.

At one time Harry worked full time in cancer research. However, he became concerned about the effects of some of the treatments. For instance, he noticed radiation would diminish or collapse the energy field. Eventually, he left cancer research. He then made a further fascinating discovery. He discovered that wholefoods and living foods had strong energy fields around them, but in contrast the energy field around processed foods was virtually zero.[15] Harry went on to develop a form of therapy which enhanced and balanced the chakras called 'electro-crystal therapy'.

We can sum up all this work on energy fields by stating that science is little by little uncovering evidence that the energy fields, in and around the body, which were postulated so long ago, do exist. We also now understand much more about what causes changes in this energy field. Kirlian noted how changes in both emotion and breathing altered it.[16] Harry Oldfield confirmed these facts but also found that processed food and radioactivity lowered the energy field whereas living foods and wholefoods raised it.[17]

The energy field, it turns out, was telling us something crucial about health, something we might have already guessed. It was telling us that we can boost our energy quite easily with good nutrition, positive emotions, exercise and deep breathing.

We know that a person is more likely to develop a disease when their energy is low. Logically it follows that if we want to recover from a disease we need to raise our energy and raise it to a high enough level to heal the disease.

Manipulating energy

Micheal Gearin-Tosh, in his recovery from myeloma, a cancer which is usually fatal, used nutrition in the form of the Gerson therapy (see page 33) and a Chinese 'bone-breathing' exercise he learned from a book by Jan de Vries called *Cancer and Leukaemia*.[16]

The author recommends cancer patients should do this exercise three times daily. It involves breathing slowly and imagining the breath coming up through the bones and then returning on the outbreath. This is done in a specific sequence. Gearin-Tosh felt 'deliciously warm and so airy he could float' after doing the breathing exercise. It is impossible to know how important this exercise was to his recovery but the technique has similarities with other Chinese exercises and breathing methods, such as those used in *qigong*.

From the perspective of Chinese medicine, when we breath in a certain way we are not just inhaling oxygen but we are also drawing energy into the body's energetic field and increasing our *qi*.

Indian traditions have advocated breathing exercises as a way of increasing *prana* in the body for centuries. Kirlian photography confirms breathing does indeed have a positive effect on the body's energy field.

Michael Gearin-Tosh used two methods in his recovery: high quality nutrition and breathing. Both are known to expand the energy field.

Shivani Goodman (see page 118) used a method she called the 'five-minute cancer cure', which she learned from a meditation teacher. She had previously experimented with this method and successfully cleared two fibroid tumours from her body. After she developed cancer she used it to help herself, and later others, recover from cancer.

It involves breathing in silvery light or sunlight through the solar plexus (whichever is easier to visualise) and then, during exhalation, directing it to different parts of the body in turn: each leg, the abdomen, the chest, each arm, the neck, the head, the aura and next the area with disease (she recommended trying to increase it by 100-fold).

An inspired idea was to direct healing energy to the diseased part whilst at the same time imaging it as perfectly normal. Then she saw the body as whole and perfect. Initially she repeated it three times a day.

Here we have simple and easily available methods which can enhance any healing programme.

Donna Eden

The Chinese have no monopoly when it comes to energy medicine. Some people possess the ability to see or sense energy in others. One such person was Donna Eden and her story is truly remarkable.

She had ongoing problems with her health from an early age, having been diagnosed with multiple sclerosis at the age of 16, and then having a mild heart attack in her 20s. She later developed severe allergies and asthma and then a breast tumour in her 30s. She became seriously ill after being bitten by a poisonous insect and went into a coma, coming close to death.

Her path back to health was unusual. When her doctors could do no more for her she turned to the local shamans in Fiji. For two days she was buried up to the neck in the sands for hours at a time, apparently to relieve the toxins. Her health recovered. She continued to improve on a diet of fresh organic food, daily swimming in the Pacific Ocean and living at the slow, easy pace of life in Fiji. Little by little she was able to say goodbye to all her illnesses.[17]

Later she returned to the USA. Here, her ability to see and feel energy combined with her success in curing herself led her to a highly successful career treating thousands of people, many of whom had failed to respond to conventional treatment. This in turn led her to develop and teach many new methods of healing. She called this 'energy medicine'.

Many people have heard of *chakras*, meridians and auras, but Donna could actually see them. They corresponded to those mapped out by Chinese physicians thousands of years before. She became aware of other, even more obscure, energy channels and, significantly, she could perceive when these channels were malfunctioning. This ability to see energy allowed her to use her own and other people's bodies almost like a laboratory, discovering exercises that corrected the abnormal energy flows.

Qigong

Does this knowledge of energy flow make a difference? The answer is yes as seen in the remarkable stories of Feng Jian and Guo Lin who recovered from cancers using *qigong* (also spelt *chi-gung*).

Qigong has a long history of use in China. It was in existence over 4000 years ago and a classic text *On Causes and Symptoms of Disease* from the seventh century AD outlined 260 *qigong* exercises for over 100 different diseases. *Qigong* has been studied in great detail by the Chinese and over 800 scientific articles have been published on it during the last 25 years and presented at eight international conferences.[18]

It can work in two ways. One is by performing *qigong* exercises to build up beneficial *qi* or life force energy in oneself. This was the method of healing used by Feng Jian and Guo Lin. In the second, it can be used to heal others.

Qigong masters have developed the ability to heal and transmit *qi* to an extraordinary degree. A dramatic example is recounted in Chapter 4 (page 135). The book *Qigong: Miracle Healing from China* gives many examples of healing by *qigong* masters and describes astonishing recoveries from metastatic cancer, multiple sclerosis, Parkinson's disease, strokes and cerebral palsy. An example from the book is an elderly man who recovered from lung cancer after 21 days of *qigong* treatment. This was confirmed when his x-rays returned to normal.[19]

Besides these anecdotal accounts there are scientific studies demonstrating *qigong* can improve heart and lung function and reduce blood pressure. In the laboratory, emitted *qi* has been shown to kill bacteria and cell cultures from a variety of cancers. It has been demonstrated to improve survival, quality of life and immunity in cancer patients, and reduce fatigue and inflammation. *Qigong* masters themselves have been studied and their hands have been found to emit microwaves, Raman and ultraviolet spectra and low frequency infrasonic emissions. This latter information is of some importance as there are cases in China of fraudulent healers claiming to be *qigong* masters. However, not all masters produce detectable emissions.

T'ai-chi can also be used for healing and a number of diseases have shown a positive response. These include rheumatoid arthritis, type 2 diabetes, multiple sclerosis, hypertension, fibromyalgia and osteoarthritis.

How then can we use this knowledge? It seems to me highly likely that whenever the total energy of the body reaches a critical level, and becomes greater than the energy of the disease, then healing will occur. Using *qi* is one of many ways to raise energy. It is not the only way and it may not be enough on its own. However, I believe when we add methods that increase energy, then healing becomes far more likely. This is why understanding energy makes total sense.

How do we do this? It is far from difficult. We can increase our intake of high-quality foods, we can breathe deeply and we can generate positive emotions. Donna Eden has created many techniques to improve our energy and advocates a five-minute routine to be used daily which improves and balances the body's energy. (This is easy to use and is demonstrated in the DVD contained in her *Energy Medicine Kit*.[20]) But there is more. A fascinating new group of therapies has emerged in recent years. They have a growing body of research behind them. These are the energy psychology therapies.

Energy psychology
Gill Edwards describes two cases of metastatic cancer that responded dramatically to intense treatment using a therapy

many have never heard of.[21] It was called the Emotional Freedom Technique (EFT) and it is one of a number of energy psychology therapies. But what are they and how did they develop?

The first of the energy psychologies was Thought Field Therapy (TFT) developed by Roger Callaghan. Working as a psychologist in 1980 he attempted, unsuccessfully, to treat a client named Mary who had the most severe water phobia he had ever known. She was unable to take a bath, wash her children or even look at the ocean. He had been treating her for over a year, using a variety of methods, with minimal success. At the time she was able to dangle her legs over the shallow end of his pool but still had a feeling of terror whenever she looked at the water. At one point she became agitated and told him she felt the fear in her stomach.

It was at this moment that Callaghan had a eureka moment. It was this that changed the direction of psychological treatments from that time on. Having some knowledge of Chinese medicine he suggested tapping on the stomach acupuncture point, situated under her eyes. After tapping for a while she stopped and said 'It's gone', ran towards the pool, sat down and splashed water onto her face stating she wasn't afraid any more. Later that night, even though she couldn't swim, she went to the ocean, immersing herself in water up to the waist. Mary was cured.

Callaghan experimented with this tapping treatment on other patients but frustratingly found successes like this were few and far between. However, when they did occur, they were dramatically effective. He finally worked out that he needed to use different tapping sequences for different conditions and this developed into TFT.[22]

This therapy was a huge step forward but somewhat complex. The next breakthrough came through Gary Craig. He simplified the approach by developing a single protocol which could be used for all conditions. This was the Emotional Freedom Techniques (EFT), the best known of the energy psychologies. Around this time other therapies appeared, including Eye Movement

Desensitisation and Reprocessing (EMDR), Tapas Acupressure Technique (TAT), Wholistic Hybrid and the Havening technique.

Research published in *Psychotherapy* in 2008 reviewed research on energy psychologies and found they dramatically improved a whole range of psychological problems, including depression, anxiety, phobias and post-traumatic stress.[23] A study of patients with generalised anxiety, treated with energy psychology treatments, documented changes in both EEG readings and brain scans after treatment.[24] Similar changes were recorded after cognitive behaviour therapy (CBT) but not with medication.

A remarkable feature of these therapies was the speed with which they worked. They have been notably successful in treating post-traumatic stress, a condition usually resistant to standard psychotherapy.

However, energy psychology is far from being just a treatment for psychological problems and our interest here is in the treatment of major physical illnesses. Gary Craig has produced a DVD for therapists on *Using EFT for Serious Diseases* where he is shown treating a range of major illnesses, such as cancer, multiple sclerosis, Parkinson's disease and many other conditions, with success (see www.emofree.com).

How can these methods work in physical conditions? The idea is that each treatment releases an energy block. (This is similar to the idea of acupuncture relieving an energy block with a meridian). The correction is typically permanent. It is like peeling an onion. My understanding is that when enough blocks to healing have disappeared, then healing can occur.

When it comes to using energy techniques to heal serious illnesses, we are still at an experimental stage. However, these tools do exist and I expect, in time, that more and more people will use them as an adjunct to standard treatments. Their advantage is that they are quick, simple, user-friendly and in a sense there is nothing to lose by trying them. The anecdotal cases are out there but, as always, it will take time for science to catch up.

3. Electromagnetic energy

All creatures produce electromagnetic fields and one, the shark, hunts by detecting these in other creatures. Electrical impulses make our hearts beat, our muscles move and our brains function. Movement of the bones and other structures generate piezo-electricity. Electricity controls another vital function: the movement of water and nutrients across the membrane of every cell.

After death, the chemicals in the body remain largely unchanged but electrical activity stops. Suffice it to say that the body cannot survive without electricity.

Research into the magnetic fields around the body has revealed an unexpected finding. Although these magnetic fields are small (being about a billion times less than that of the earth) they are intimately linked with, and change with, the magnetic cycles of the earth. The body is constantly being affected by and in rhythm with the earth.

The earth can be thought of as a giant battery. It has a negative charge on its surface. The circadian rhythms of all species tested have been found to coordinate with the earth's magnetic field. These are complex, including daily, weekly, biweekly and annual cycles. They include pulse, temperature, blood pressure and blood clotting; these wax and wane with the earth's magnetic field.

However, the earth's magnetic field is not static but changes with the movement of the sun, moon, solar flares and the sun's magnetic field. We could think of our bodies as being tiny magnets standing on top of a very large magnet, the earth, which in turn changes with another large moving magnet, the moon, and a gigantic magnet, the sun, and the massive magnetic storms created by it. We know rates of heart attacks go up with changes in solar flares as do psychiatric admissions and suicides.[25]

All this data is complex but confirms that our biological cycles, our hormone output, our overall health and probably our recovery from disease are intimately connected with the earth and its changing magnetic fields. In other words, our health and our connection to the earth are intimately connected.

Connecting to the earth

Clint Ober, a retired telecommunications engineer, was one of the first to wonder if our connection to the earth was important for health. He made the astute observation that most people are insulated from the earth either because they are indoors, with their feet on insulated floors, or outdoors wearing plastic or rubber soled shoes. He wondered what the consequences of this could be.

He performed an inspired experiment on himself, measuring his own electrical charge using a voltmeter. What he found was that the charge varied with each room he entered and depending on how close he was to electrical appliances. The charge was highest in his bedroom. He wondered what would happen if he earthed himself. So, whilst lying in his bedroom, he connected himself with a wire to a rod inserted into the ground outside his house. On connection, his voltmeter dropped to zero and the next thing he knew it was morning. After years of poor sleep he had one of the best nights he could remember. He repeated the process with a number of friends and found that grounding (as he called this connection) consistently produced beneficial effects, including improved sleep, reduced pain and more energy.[26]

More discoveries followed. Roger Applewhite published a study in 2005 showing that electrons move from the earth to the body with grounding and keep the body at the same negative charge as the earth. He found grounding also reduced the effect of electromagnetic fields (EMFs) on the body by a factor of 70.[27] Later studies noted quicker healing, increased energy, decreased inflammation and reduced pain with grounding.

The body acts like an electron sponge when in contact with the earth, absorbing and becoming saturated with electrons.

Grounding reduces viscosity, sometimes known as thickening of the blood, which is associated with heart and cerebrovascular disease.

Many diseases, notably autoimmune conditions, are characterised by excess inflammation. Could the absence of a connection to the earth, with its ready supply of beneficial electrons, be a factor? There is anecdotal evidence to support this. Ober witnessed improvements in a variety of inflammatory and autoimmune conditions with earthing, including fibromyalgia, rheumatoid arthritis, multiple sclerosis and lupus.

The Chinese have long recommended doing healing exercises outdoors on grass; they often combine this with imagining roots going down deep into the earth. Some Native Americans have a tradition of putting their sick into pits in the earth to help them to heal (as with Donna Eden) and vets have noted animals that live out of doors heal better than those kept indoors.

It will be some time before the full significance of grounding can be evaluated. Modern medicine has typically treated discoveries in the electromagnetic field with little enthusiasm. Survivors see things differently and typically act on hunches long before medical proof finally arrives.

Grounding is an intriguing discovery and may be a hunch worth testing in any chronic inflammatory condition. Fortunately, it is easy to test. As little as 15 minutes contact with the earth with bare feet will restore the necessary electrons. There are also devices available to create earthing connections in specific situations, such as during sleep.

The earth has other hidden treasures. Visiting forests exposes us to essential oils known as phytoncides which increase the activity of natural killer cells in our bodies. This positive effect on natural killer cells after a weekend in the forest can last for one month.[28] A 30-minute visit to a forest lowered cortisol and blood pressure, reduced depression and enhanced parasympathetic activity in one study.[29]

There seems to be a pattern here. Many of the factors that affect our health most positively are simple, natural and readily available. They include sunshine, exercise, high quality food, relaxation and happy thoughts. Typically they cost nothing. Grounding seems to fit into this pattern and suggests our disconnection from the natural world could be costing us dear in terms of our health.

Geopathic stress
However, not all earth energies are benign. One of the central tenets of this book is that the body has the ability to recover from most diseases once blocks to healing are removed. One little-known block is geopathic stress.

Geopathic stress refers to noxious energies arising from the earth, often from underground water. In the past doctors knew that certain buildings and locations could be associated with illnesses. The Chinese, in times gone by, used dowsing to decide whether a particular site was suitable for building houses on. However, these ideas have long since been lost and few doctors today would consider that illness could be connected to a particular location.

An exception was Dr Patrick Kingsley, a doctor who had an astonishingly successful record of treating 'no-hopers' with cancer and multiple sclerosis. He considered geopathic stress to be an important factor in many of his patients, and the evidence supports him.

Gustav Freiherr von Pohl mapped out the distribution of subterranean water currents in the town of Vilsbiburg using dowsing between 1928 and 1929. Independently, the health authority plotted the locations of all 54 patients who had died of cancer. There was a strong correlation with the location of the cancer patient's beds and underground water, as von Pohl had predicted.[30] His results were treated with scepticism so he repeated his investigation in another town, Garfenau, replicating his findings.

An interesting point about his work is that the zones of disturbance were plotted before the location of the cancer beds was known. Later work by the Scientific Association of Medical Doctors studied the location of 5000 people who had died of cancer in the German town of Stettin with the aid of a dowser. In all cases, their homes were in areas of geopathic stress.

Different workers have done the same work with the same results: Dr Hartmann investigated the beds of cancer patients in Eberbach using a high frequency detector. All registered a strong reaction. Russian geologist Dr Eugen Melnikov investigated geopathic stress in St Petersburg between 1989 and 1992 in a different way, testing with a geomagnetometer. He found the cancer incidence was three times higher in areas of geopathic stress.[31]

But what do we mean by 'geopathic stress' and what causes it? Subterranean water flowing under houses appears to be the most important cause. This can be from streams but also from drains and sewers. However, this is not the only cause. Other researchers have found currents of electromagnetic energy coming from the earth: these include the Hartmann grid and Curry lines, which are naturally-occurring grids of electrically charged lines that run diagonally to the poles.

Some of the most detailed work ever done on geopathic stress was conducted by Austrian dowser, Kathe Bachler, who examined several thousand houses and apartments.[32] She used strict scientific methods: she always worked blind, dowsing to detect harmful zones first before finding what was wrong with the people living there. She catalogued information on large numbers of diseases and spoke at many medical and scientific meetings at Salzburg and Vienna where geopathic stress is more accepted as a cause of illness than in the UK. She kept meticulous records of all her cases and many of these are recorded in her book *Earth Radiation*. Her ability to detect geopathic stress by dowsing has been confirmed using other scientific instruments.

She investigated 500 cases of cancer using dowsing and she

never found a case where geopathic disturbance was not present. And this was not all. In three cases, children became seriously unwell after sleeping in the beds used by relatives who had previously died from cancer. She also noted several cases where the person sleeping directly above or below the ill patient became unwell. (Geopathic stress typically affects everyone living directly above the stress lines no matter what floor they live on). She once treated a patient with severe pains who had seen eight specialists without benefit. The pain responded instantaneously once the bed was moved to a site free of geopathic stress.

Her book contains many short case histories of people who recovered after moving their beds to areas free of geopathic stress. She believes geopathic stress contributes to the vast majority cases of serious chronic illness and that there are people in every city and every country where it is causing major illnesses.

I believe most doctors in the UK would be highly sceptical of these ideas, partly because of their unfamiliarity with the concept and partly because the diagnosis is usually made by dowsing. Dowsing is certainly an unusual way to collect information but, before dismissing it, it is worth noting that some oil fields, including the one at Zisterdorf, were discovered by dowsing. Even more intriguing was the use of dowsing in bomb disposal units during World War II. Colonel Kenneth Merrylees used dowsing to find unexploded bombs, notably locating a 500-pounder under the swimming pool at Buckingham Palace.

In spite of these reservations and its inherent strangeness, I think there are several reasons why geopathic stress should be taken seriously. The first is the good correlation between the location of disease and the location of geopathic stress. This is especially convincing as lines of geopathic stress tend to be quite narrow. Bachler again and again noted the lines crossed at sites where cancer had been found; this included cases of abdominal and ovarian cancers. This, itself, is convincing, especially as she worked blind.

A second reason to take geopathic stress seriously is the tendency for illness to recur in different occupants of the same bed. She cited the case of three nuns who occupied the same room and bed at different times. All became seriously ill, with two contracting cancer.[33] Another reason to take geopathic stress seriously is that treatment is often simple, cheap and effective – just moving the bed. (Sometimes the geopathic stress zone is below a favourite chair or desk and this also needs to be moved).

A further reason is that there are some patients where every treatment tried has failed to work and it is here that geopathic stress needs to be considered. To illustrate this point, Bachler was asked by a Dr Kolitscher in Salzburg to investigate 107 patients who had failed to respond to standard treatments. She found geopathic stress was contributing in every case and the majority responded well to her recommendations, which usually involved moving the bed.

When should we suspect geopathic stress? The symptoms unfortunately are non-specific but the biggest clue is sleep disturbance and feeling run down in the morning or unrefreshed following sleep. Other symptoms include dizziness, pallor, aches and pains, coldness in bed, frequent illnesses, poor healing, headaches, loss of appetite, and, in children, poor school performance. Sometimes there is other supporting evidence such as the person sleeping directly above or below them becoming ill, cracks in the ceiling or paintwork above the bed and a tendency for mould to build up in these areas.

Animals provide another clue. Dogs avoid areas of geopathic stress whereas cats, ants and bees are attracted to them. If anyone becomes ill after moving to a particular bed, then be suspicious. Bear in mind that it can take months or even years before illness develops. A further clue is improvement in symptoms and better sleep after moving to another bed. Symptoms which abate whilst on holiday or living at a new location are a further clue. Improvement is sometimes instantaneous but can take a week or more. Sometimes there is an initial worsening after moving the bed as the body readjusts.

All this leaves most people with a dilemma. How do they know if they are affected by geopathic stress? Their doctor will not be familiar with it and will anyway be unable to test for it. However, there are clues. Are you better sleeping in a different bed? Is your cat or dog, if you have one, attracted to your bed? Try moving the bed or sleeping in a different room. Dr Kingsley often recommended the book *Are You Sleeping in a Safe Place* by Rolf Gordon to his patients.[33] It describes a simple method of home dowsing using two wire coat hangers adapted for the purpose. (The body is far more sensitive to energy than we often realise. We know this as we often talk about picking up the vibes of another person. Bachler suggests moving very slowly to different parts in the bedroom with eyes closed and sensing the energy at these points.) Finally, you could enlist the help of an experienced dowser. Some instruments are thought to be able to detect geopathic stress, such as an electromagnetic meter, available from Coghill Research Laboratories; however, there is little scientific data on these at present.

Other electromagnetic treatments
Various pioneers have used electromagnetic energy in novel ways to heal. One was Georges Lakhovsky. In 1924 he suggested that all living organisms emit light. He felt that twisted filaments in the cell act like oscillating circuits. Later research was to confirm some of his ideas. It has since been discovered that all organisms do indeed emit photons and that DNA is one of the major sources of this light emission (see page 310).

He believed that cells had their own oscillations and that life forms could be harmed by competing oscillations, including those from other organisms. He surmised that anything that increased the amplitude of the organism's oscillation would strengthen the organism and anything that gave a different competing oscillation could weaken it. It was an inspired idea. But was it true?

He put it to an ingenious test. He inoculated geraniums with a plant tumour. He then exposed some of these plant cancers to a device designed to strengthen the oscillation leaving other geraniums as controls. The result was dramatic: in less than three days the tumours fell off the treated geraniums and the plants remained in good health. All untreated plants died. He published his theory and results in a book *The Secret of Life* (of which various free downloads are available). He then turned his attention to people.

In France he is known to have treated cancer patients but fled to the USA during the war. He developed a machine called the 'multiple wave oscillator' which was used in a New York Hospital in 1941. He achieved good results in treating conditions like arthritis and ulcers. Recorded cases include a 25-year-old woman with a sarcoma of the hand who relapsed after two operations but was healed within two months of starting his treatment. Unfortunately, he died the following year and his treatment fell into disuse. But is there anything to support Lakhovsky's idea that we can transmit and receive oscillations?

Popp, who we will meet later, found that healthy seedlings can have a positive effect on the growth of unhealthy seedlings. This infers a non-local effect, as if healthy vibrations can be transmitted like a radio signal.

Disease can be transmitted too. A clever experiment done by Russian biologist S P Schurin in 1972 gave a clue.[15] He put two tissue cultures in air-tight vessels side by side. In one experiment these two cultures were separated by glass and in another by a quartz crystal. In both experiments he inoculated one of the two cultures with a lethal virus. As expected, this killed the cells in the inoculated cultures, but in the adjacent culture there was no effect when the vessels were separated by glass. However, in the cultures separated by quartz, something unexpected happened: the cells in the adjacent tissue culture also died though they had not been inoculated with the virus and were physically separate from the inoculated culture. Even so, the cells died as if they had been directly inoculated with the lethal virus. The only logical explanation was that the virus was giving off some form of toxic energy or radiation which was capable of killing the tissue cultures. Although this form of energy is, as yet undiscovered, we do know glass filters out ultraviolet radiation whereas crystals are good conductors of electromagnetic radiation.

This experiment changes our whole understanding of infection and toxicity. It implies that some sort of oscillation from the virus or the dying tissue culture produced a lethal effect on the second adjacent culture.

In another interesting experiment in 1965, Riviere was able to cause regression and sometimes cures of cancer in rats by using magnetic fields at a specific frequency in conjunction with microwaves.[15] This sounds similar to Lakhovsky's idea of strengthening the organism's oscillation. These findings suggest Lakhovsky was onto something of profound importance.

His ideas are not as far-fetched as they sound. We know that molecules and even intermolecular bonds emit specific frequencies. Biomolecules can act as semi-conductors and transmit electricity and resonate at particular frequencies. Can we use this knowledge practically?

A number of innovators have built frequency generators that can be tuned to the specific frequencies of viruses and bacteria. These frequencies, called 'mortal oscillatory rates' (MORs), kill the pathogens without causing harm to the body. There are also frequencies that help cell regeneration. The best known innovator was Royal Rife who developed equipment capable of killing bacteria and cancer cells. He was said to have treated cancer patients at the Pasadena County Hospital with 100% success in the early 20th century. However, his success did not go unnoticed. He was harassed, his laboratory was raided and his equipment was confiscated.

Another innovator who worked along the same lines was electrical engineer Antoine Priore. He developed a technology that emitted multiple electromagnetic signals. His work was initially funded by the French government in the 1960s. The machine he built proved highly effective in curing hundreds of laboratory animals with metastatic tumours and bacterial infections. His work was later suppressed. Again, success came at a price.[34]

Some machines have come on the market based on Rife's work but without the necessary electronic expertise. However, high quality machines of this type have produced remarkable results in diseases as diverse as rheumatoid arthritis, multiple sclerosis and autism. Where does that all this leave us? Lakhovsky's multiple wave oscillator and Rife's frequency generators appear to have enormous potential. What is frustrating is that these ideas have been simply left to rot without further investigation.

It seems tragic that gifted scientists with ground-breaking discoveries, highly relevant to the treatment of major diseases, have been forgotten, ignored or sabotaged. And not least, it has happened at a time when medicine is desperately short of new ideas and when trillions of dollars have been spent on cancer research with little to show for it. These are discoveries with the potential to transform the way we treat many of today's most serious illnesses. However, at the moment, frustratingly, they remain largely unused.

During this time mainstream medicine has embraced and, in fact, been transformed by electromagnetic and technological advances in diagnosis, such as the MRI scan and the endoscope.

Certainly electromagnetic treatments would need careful research as the body is extremely sensitive to very small currents and electromagnetic fields have dangers, but they also have huge potential and tested they should be. If I was a cancer researcher genuinely searching for new treatments, this would be one of the first areas I would want to explore. I have little doubt it would pay dividends.

In summary, we have postulated that if the energy of the body is higher than that of a disease then this will promote healing. These electromagnetic devices can help in two ways, by either increasing the energy of the organism or reducing the energy of the disease.

Conclusion

This chapter has explored some of the less well-known forms of energy. Many of these offer real hope to those with major illnesses. In the next chapter we will look at two other forms of energy: thought energy and organising fields and witness some more dramatic healings

Chapter 11

Energy within and around us

'How often have I said to you that when you have eliminated the impossible, whatever remains, however improbable, must be the truth.'

Sherlock Holmes by Sir Arthur Conan Doyle

Denise Linn, mentioned in Chapter 3 suffered a near fatal shooting at the age of 17. After this she had a near-death experience. During this experience she felt she was bathed in light and music, merging with that light and music. This was accompanied by a sense of unity with all life. Like so many who have been through these experiences, she was far from pleased to find herself back in a hospital bed on planet earth.

Her doctors didn't expect her to survive and told her that the best she could hope for was life as an invalid. However, her experience had given her a new and different perspective. She understood she was not her body; it was simply something she inhabited and because of this she knew she could heal. She recovered rapidly to the great surprise of her doctors. They considered it a miracle.[1]

My understanding of this is the reason she healed so rapidly was because of her certainty that she was really energy or spirit and anything was possible. It is an understanding that could benefit us all.

I would now like to look at the two other types of energy listed but not discussed in Chapter 10 – thought energy and organising fields.

Thought energy

It is said that energy follows thought. We know from Kirlian photography (page 284) that the energy fields surrounding our bodies do alter with our thoughts. Thoughts and emotions can create changes in our energy field in an instant. Emotions typically have the strongest impact.

Thinking creates changes within the body. Thinking about a particular part of the body activates the corresponding area in the brain.[2] This same brain activation occurs when that part of the body is touched and even on watching someone else having that part touched.[3]

However, the most intriguing fact about our thinking is that our consciousness, intention and expectations change the probability of any particular outcome. Quantum physics is quite clear about this. We can, in essence, mould the outcome of a disease with our thoughts and emotions. And we have been sitting on this knowledge for nearly a century. Perhaps it is time to act on it.

Does this mean we can heal illnesses with our thoughts? This is a huge question and the answer is that we do have this potential. But does this mean that a major disease, one which has perhaps developed over a long time, is going to reverse easily, with an occasional visualisation or a few positive thoughts? The answer here is clearly no.

The reason is that keeping our thoughts consistently positive in this situation is next to impossible and could be perceived as an added pressure. Faced with a major illness, such as cancer, most people initially will be able to think of little else but the illness, the treatment and the likely progression. An added problem is that the symptoms themselves act as a constant reminder.

Creating a strong belief that you will get better against the odds is no simple feat when there is nothing in medicine to support you. Survivors have often needed great determination, self-belief and perseverance to maintain this attitude. Some have had an attitude of defiance.

However, we can't get away from a simple fact: the mind does influence healing. Perhaps the most striking example of this is people who have died after having been wrongly being diagnosed with cancer. They have literally died from their mistaken belief.[4] In addition, wrong diagnoses are not uncommon.[5, 6] How do we use this knowledge, because use it we must? But to change your whole way of thinking all at one time is not realistic.

I think it is more useful to think in terms of altering the balance of our thoughts than to think in terms of positive and negative. No one with a major disease can be expected to keep their thoughts positive all the time. What is possible is to change the proportion of useful thoughts.

Imagine this hypothetical scenario in someone who is suffering from cancer. The forces of disease are pitted against the body's healing mechanisms. At that moment they are finely matched. The outcome is in the balance and could go either way. Imagine then that this patient decides to influence the immune cells by visualisations or affirmations, and this leads to an increase in the number and strength of the immune cells. This one act could be just what was needed to tip the balance. And if it could be tipped far enough and often enough, it is easy to see how healing would become much more likely.

A little positivity goes a surprisingly long way. At the HeartMath Institute in Boulder Creek, California, they measured the amount of immunoglobulin A (s-IgA) in the saliva. This is a marker of the strength of the immune system. After subjects held positive thoughts of care and compassion for five minutes in the morning, it was found that s-IgA swung upwards. The levels slowly dropped in the afternoon but stayed elevated all day.[7] Those who harboured thoughts of anger and frustration for five minutes had a depression of their s-IgA for five hours, which remained low for the rest of the day.

What strikes me about this is how little time was spent in either a positive or negative emotion and how prolonged the response was. This is surely knowledge that we can use. Starting the day with five minutes of positive thought is far from impossible.

One of the greatest gifts some cancer survivors have given us is to draw our attention to the value of focused thought and intention. Specifically they have shown us that by focusing on health rather than disease, we can influence the progression of a disease. Survivors have experimented with many methods, but the bottom line is that they have been able, eventually, to shift their focus away from their disease towards a belief that they could heal.

There is another aspect of all this that I think is important. It is how a disease is perceived and about steering energy in the direction of healing. Once a diagnosis has been made, people often assume the disease has become a part of them or, more likely with a cancer, resembles an alien growing inside them. So much of the fear produced by cancer is caused not so much by the disease itself but by the anticipation of a relentless downhill progression. In reality, the situation is more complex. Any disease is in a constant state of change.

A more useful and accurate way to think about disease is to see it in a state of flux, something that the body is always trying to heal, sometimes succeeding, sometimes not. Perhaps more importantly, it is something that we can deliberately modify.

Gill Edwards has suggested using the disease as a verb.[8] In other words, if someone has cancer and is worrying about it, thinking about it or talking endlessly about it, then she would describe this as 'cancering'. In energy terms it would be like adding fuel to the fire. Being in a relaxed or distracted state would be like pouring water on the fire. We have explored many ways to do this in previous chapters.

Although keeping the emotions positive and relaxed is beneficial, several authors have emphasised the value of not being attached to the outcome – in other words, not being attached to the need for a cure, perhaps aiming for being at peace. An intense need for a cure creates resistance which is counterproductive. Better to just observe this need, let it be and release it.

To conclude, we possess the ability to augment healing at any time by simply changing our thoughts and emotions. Research studies confirm this. Survivors, as ever, have been ahead of the game and quick to understand the crucial role of the mind. Norman Cousins has described this as 'our beliefs become our biology'. There are three main points here:

1. Focusing on health as opposed to illness assists healing.
2. Intention and expectation influence healing.
3. Disease is not constant and the body can go into healing mode at any time.

Organising fields

How the body regulates itself has long puzzled scientists as I first discussed in Chapter 9. The complexity of a system capable of running the body is mind-boggling. There are an estimated 30-trillion cells, undergoing 100,000 chemical reactions a second, and these need to be co-ordinated perfectly. All parts of the body are interconnected and each part has to be aware of what other parts are doing at that time. This requires a system of extraordinary sophistication which is able to process information at lightning speed.

The reality is we know virtually nothing about how it is done. Neither the nervous system (which is estimated to produce signalling at 10-100 metres per second) nor our biochemical processes are remotely fast enough to coordinate the multitude of processes. We need to look further.

One candidate is electron transmission. When we plug in an electrical device we get power instantly. There is good evidence that the body works in a similar way. Proteins in connective tissue are aligned as semi-conductors in a way that seems designed to promote rapid electron transmission through the body.[9] Cells contain microtubules which are ideal for high speed wave movement of electrons and photons. Water is perfect for the communication of these signals. It can store, carry and amplify the frequencies of charged particles and molecular signalling cannot occur without it.[10, 11]

In other words, the body is probably using an electronic system rather than a chemical pathway. This is like the difference between the internet and a landline, using information in the form of waves and frequency rather than chemicals. Physicists know that wave patterns can store vast amounts of data and this is why so much information can be accessed using mobile phones and wifi.

Fritz-Albert Popp, a German biophysicist (introduced in Chapter 10, page 300), suggested photon emission is the likely mechanism for orchestrating the body's complex communication and processes (this works in the same way as electron emissions). Photons are tiny particles of light which have no mass but carry electromagnetic energy.

Popp made the pioneering discovery that all species emit light in the form of photons. And DNA is a major source of these photon emissions. Higher species typically emit fewer photons and these emissions are more coherent. This means they resonate together, acting like one big wave rather than many small ones – more like a laser and less like ordinary light. This level of coherence is rare in the world and only occurs in specialised substances such as superconductors.

The work of physicist, Herbert Frohlich, has demonstrated

that at a certain level of energy, vibration of molecules can produce coherence allowing wave communication and hence action at a distance.[12] These ideas are remarkably similar to those of Lakhovsky.

There are practical implications. Photon emission is increased by stress whereas better health is associated with fewer emissions and more coherence. Popp noted that free-range eggs showed a more coherent pattern than battery-produced eggs and went on to find that the healthiest food had the most coherence and the lowest level of light. Photon emission in a healthy person is also cyclical, following rhythms of day and night[13] coupled with more complex rhythms and they also mirror solar activity. In cancer this rhythm disappears. Perhaps this is the reason why maintaining contact with the earth's electromagnetic fields benefits us (see page 293).

Popp also made another fascinating discovery. This was the difference between carcinogenic chemicals and other chemicals: carcinogens absorb the frequency of light necessary for photo-repair of cells and DNA and re-emit it at a different frequency. The danger of these chemicals lies in their ability to block DNA repair.

I think the main point here is that with any disease there is distortion of energy. When we produce healthy coherent energy fields it helps correct this. And this could be one of the key reasons why eating healthy food and having positive thoughts benefit us so much. Carcinogenic chemicals, stress and poor quality food block our ability to transmit these coherent frequencies and hence impair our ability to heal. A further point is that transmission of these signals is partly dependent on water and this may explain why getting enough water is important for our wellbeing.

Making it easier for others
Could one person's breakthrough with a major illness unwittingly help others with a similar illness, even if they know

nothing about this breakthrough? It sounds improbable, perhaps preposterous, but let's explore this further.

Rupert Sheldrake developed the theory of 'morphic resonance'. He wondered how it was that an egg becomes a chicken. He hypothesised that there was an energetic blueprint that contained all the information needed. He also postulated that these blueprints could be modified by information learned from previous generations of the species, allowing the species to evolve.[14] For this to happen there would need to be a mechanism that allows members of the species to communicate with each other, both at a distance and at an unconscious level. This stretches the imagination, but keep in mind that Bell's theorem formulated over 50 years ago, maintains that the reality of the universe is non-local. And consider these two examples.

In a cruel experiment by the Russians in 1956, baby rabbits were separated from their mother and put in a submarine and one was killed off every hour. A submarine was used as it was thought impossible to transmit any sort of electromagnetic information whilst under water. Each time a baby rabbit was killed the mother rabbit responded with a detectable change measured in electrodes implanted in her brain. Though we have no idea of the mechanism, this experiment confirmed the existence of non-local effects.[15]

Even more surprising are the experiments done by the US army which involved taking DNA samples from subjects and moving them to a distant location. After this, the subjects were exposed to films with strong emotional content, with sexual and violent imagery. At the time they were watching the films their DNA, now in another place, also responded with strong electrical discharges at exactly the same moment, demonstrating the same non-local effect.[16]

We also know many people have described responding to pain at just the moment a close friend or family member has been injured. In an intriguing experiment, researchers were given two different puzzles with hidden visual pictures within them. They were then sent to remote parts of the world and were shown to hundreds of people. Later the hidden figure on one but not the other was shown on a British TV programme. It was postulated that once it was shown on TV the solutions would become easier to solve for everyone.

Researchers then went back to the remote areas to retest the puzzle. Remarkably, people proved to be much better at locating the figure shown on the TV programme (even though there was no chance they could have seen it) but no better at finding the other figure. The implication was that as one group solve a problem it makes it easier for everyone to do the same, as suggested by Sheldrake. It is easy to see how biologically useful this could be, making a species more adaptable.

The effect has also been demonstrated in animals. Researchers in Melbourne put rats in a situation where they had to negotiate an underwater maze. The task was difficult and it took a long time for the rats to solve it. Successive generations did the task progressively faster. After 50 generations of rats trained to do this, they *and* other rats of different stock, with no training in the maze, were all able to navigate the maze in the same rapid way. Eventually all rats of this species developed this unique and strange ability.[17]

Is there evidence that this happens in the context of healing disease? Certainly some diseases seem to disappear. A trivial example is car sickness, common in the early days of the motor car, but now less common. It suggests the whole species has adapted.

Although it is still conjecture, it implies that one person's successful battle against a serious disease is not just a personal triumph, but may enhance everybody's ability to fight that same disease. It means these healings have a significance way beyond the individual who achieves them.

Quantum healing

Ultimately, as Einstein told us, everything is energy and we too are made up of patterns of energy. If so how should we regard diseases? Surely as disturbed patterns of energy, and perhaps more importantly, patterns with the potential to be transformed? So let's look at disease through the eyes of a physicist rather than through the eyes of a doctor.

Consider the composition of the human body? At one level we could say it is made from tissues and organs, or perhaps cells; at another level, molecules of proteins, fats and similar substances. This is where the standard medical understanding of the body stops.

But molecules are made from atoms which can be subdivided further into neutrons, protons and electrons and subdivided yet again into even smaller particles such as quarks and neutrinos. Here things start to get interesting as some of these sub-atomic particles have bizarre properties. They can change from particles to waves; they can come in and out of existence; and they can even be in two places at once. In other words, at this level the dividing line between energy and matter starts to become blurred.

If we shrink ourselves down to this dimension we would see tiny particles or units of energy surrounded by vast amounts of nothingness. The solid matter would start to disappear. This might sound academic but when it comes to healing, it is not. The reason is that our thoughts and emotions are also energy and interact with other parts of the energy field. Heisenberg's Uncertainty principle tells us we cannot observe a system without entering into it and changing it. So our observations and beliefs about a disease need to be factored in as they will alter and modify the outcome.

Put another way, the building blocks of our bodies are tiny sub-atomic waves and particles that change their behaviour as we change our perspective and expectations. Think of them as millions of tiny coloured dots that are continually changing colour as our thoughts and beliefs change. The implications are huge. It means that our bodies are far more pliable and changeable than we give them credit for.

This insight also begins to explain things that have long since puzzled doctors. For instance, why do some patients sometimes get better when they have no right to do so? How can some illnesses spontaneously disappear? Why do some patients die after being wrongly diagnosed? How is it possible that *qigong* healers in China can consistently make tumours disappear within minutes using only their energy and thoughts? And how can visualisation sometimes reverse a major disease?

Understanding illness from this perspective means the numerous studies and larger numbers of anecdotal cases cataloguing unexpected cures make more sense. But how can we use this extraordinary knowledge? Is there anyone using these ideas today? To some extent visualising a disease disappearing or visualising optimum health is applying this knowledge. The common belief amongst survivors that they will find a way to get better when nothing in the world supports their view, is another example. They say: 'I will get better, no matter what'. This could literally be true.

Some have used ideas based to some degree on quantum science. Matrix energetics, developed by Richard Bartlett, is perhaps the closest match. This system presupposes that we can transform our energy and produce extraordinary healings. Bartlett believes that we are made up of patterns of light and information. He is open to the possibility of instantaneous and miraculous change. He considers the biggest barrier to healing is our low expectation of what is possible.

His cases border on the miraculous. After a bizarre healing of a child with eye problems, he found his own energy changed markedly. After this, whenever he touched someone with a feeling of positive intent he was able to produce dramatic healings, for instance making chronic pain disappear and bones realign. He described breaking his leg on stage in front of hundreds of people, feeling a pop followed by severe white-hot pain, worse with any movement. Many unpleasant thoughts crossed his mind, including the urgent need to get to a hospital. However, he decided to practise what he preached. He was able to shift into a different state of reality where he didn't have a broken leg or pain and continued lecturing, with some difficulty. He followed this the next day by a group healing. He went on to make a full recovery.[16]

He describes cases of scoliosis of the spine and frozen shoulders recovering in moments. He believes we can manipulate time and describes healing his son's chickenpox within an hour by taking the illness back in time to before it started. From the current medical perspective these feats are impossible but from the perspective of quantum science they are not.

How does Bartlett achieve these extraordinary results? He says that he sees himself, the patient and the space between them as an ever-changing field of interlocking energy. He believes that the waves can disassemble and reassemble in a new, more useful form. His method involves using a focused positive healing intent and a strong belief that changes for the better will take place. He then lets go, feels an expanded state and trusts that this change will take place.[17] The last part, the trusting, is not an easy mind set to achieve; it involves a belief that change will occur almost miraculously (although I anticipate that Bartlett would say not being able to trust is a limiting belief).

He considers he is simply allowing energy to re-organise itself in the best possible way and has no idea what will happen next. He avoids being hooked into the idea of a disease or a cure. He notes a disease like cancer has a huge field of negative energy and fear associated with it. It would be unwise to tackle such a large negative field directly; it is better to focus on changing energy and to be open to what develops. Sometimes he sees the disease as simply not there. His says his aim is transformation not healing, and he does not specify what the positive outcome should be. The therapy seems quite intuitive as he responds to and can change images which appear spontaneously in his mind about what is happening. It appears he is manipulating fields of quantum reality.

As there are no controlled studies on his work it is difficult to judge the long-term results, but they certainly look dramatic. There are parallels with the Chinese *qigong* healers. They visualise the patient as whole and healthy during healing.

At the moment I think these types of healing are so astonishing that they are outside the belief systems of most people, but let's simply note that they exist and are with us today. Bartlett, with his extraordinary and innovative ideas, has shown everyone that the ideas behind quantum physics are not just abstract theory but can produce results in the real world. Rapid and miraculous healing is always a possibility, even if a remote one, and, as Bartlett points out, one predicted by quantum science. I expect to see more of these types of therapy appearing in the future as people change their mindsets about what is possible.

The more the better

Mark Hansen tells the story of Amy Graham in the book *Chicken Soup for the Soul*. Amy, a 17-year-old girl with terminal leukaemia, had been given days to live. Mark Hansen, a motivational speaker, was addressing an audience of over 1000 people. He was aware that Amy was amongst them and that she wished to attend one of his seminars before she died. This gave Mark an idea. He asked the audience to learn how to heal, suggesting to them that this is an ability that we all innately have. He further suggested that about 5% of us have this to such a degree that they could become healers. First, he asked them to work in pairs and attempt to heal each other. He next asked a very frail Amy to come on stage with him. Finally, he asked the audience to send their healing energy to Amy, all at once. This they did enthusiastically. Then they all gave her a standing ovation.

Two weeks later she was discharged after a total remission of her leukaemia. Two years later she called Mark to say she was married.[20] Mark's comment was that he has learned never to underestimate our own healing ability, a remark I have come across many times whilst researching this book.

This story made quite a big impression on me. Of course, it is a remarkable tale of healing in its own right, but there was something else. I sensed that there was something immensely important going on here. The question I asked myself was whether healing of this type was reproducible, and, if so, could others, with a variety of serious illnesses, be healed in a similar fashion.

What makes this more likely is that it is not unique. In the Chinese Zhi Neng Qigong Hospital hundreds of people practise *qigong* together. The director at the hospital is Dr Pang Hemiong. He asks patients with cancer to stay in the middle of the group and has noticed that the cancers often shrink or even disappear after this experience. And, of course, as we saw in Chapter 4 (page 135), the Chinese healers in the medicineless hospital in Beijing, acting in unison, were able to heal cancer as a group.

Richard, in the *Heart of Healing*, describes how he was diagnosed with serious heart disease. His angiogram showed up major blockages in his arteries and he was scheduled for bypass surgery. However, the day before surgery he felt much better and a further angiogram showed these blockages had completely disappeared. It seemed like a miracle had taken place, but how? Only later did he discover why. His friend, a Native American medicine man, had held a healing ceremony for him, leading a group in songs, prayers and movement. He was in excellent health 15 years later.[21]

Lynne McTaggart, founder and co-editor of the magazine *What Doctors Don't Tell You* (now renamed *Get Well Magazine*) ran workshops on intention around the world. Participants were put in groups of eight and given the intention of healing one member of the group who had a physical or mental problem. The groups were shown how to send healing thoughts, in unison, for 10 minutes while holding hands and forming a circle around the person selected. She later asked the people receiving the healing what had happened. She received hundreds, perhaps thousands, of accounts of incredible and immediate healings, including remissions from arthritis, multiple sclerosis, insomnia, cataract, depression and chronic fatigue.[22]

Looking at all these many varied group healings, there is a pattern. It implies that groups with an intention to heal can have a powerful impact and that numbers do count. Could it possibly, one day, become an accepted mode of healing? As an aside I believe many people would love to take part as healers working as a group and that it would be a wonderful collective experience to participate in. Lynne McTaggart noted those doing the healing often noticed remarkable positive shifts in their own lives too. It would be a win-win situation.

The intention of the group is key. Where people gather together, with the same condition, such as can happen with support and rehabilitation groups, there can be a tendency to dwell on negative aspects of the illness, to talk and obsess over problems and to become too comfortable with the disease. This is not to say these groups aren't useful, but when the focus is on the disease rather than healing the outcome is likely to be different.

These are early days and we are yet to test the full power of focused healing intention in group settings. My guess is that it will depend partly on the innate healing abilities of some of the individuals within the group but also on the sheer numbers involved. Although talented individuals like Richard Bartlett, and small groups of highly trained individuals, like the Chinese *qigong* healers, may be able to produce near miraculous results, I suspect that using larger groups could be an easier way of achieving the same result. With Amy there were over a thousand people acting in unison. Might the energy here be so powerful that it could heal almost any disease under the sun? I would love to know the answer.

Summary of the three chapters on energy

How can a person use energy to help recover from a major illness? Some of the data are straightforward:

1. Just about any illness will be helped by consistent, regular exercise. If this is not possible then visualising exercise can help.
2. Most illnesses will be helped by exposure to the sun (but avoid sunburn or prolonged exposure at the hottest time of the day). The benefits of regular exposure to morning and evening sunshine, ideally enough to cause tanning, have given dramatic benefits in some diseases. Sunlight through the eyes also appears to be beneficial so beware of glasses and contact lenses blocking this.
3. Changes in the body's energy precede disease and also precede healing. A positive change in energy is a useful indicator of improvement.
4. Healing, including distant healing, has been intensively investigated. Results have varied with different healers but there is solid evidence for its validity and results can sometimes be extraordinary. Consider adding this to any healing regime as there are no known downsides.
5. The body has energy channels. These have long been recognised in Chinese medicine. These energy channels can be seen by 'sensitives'. New technologies have also demonstrated their presence. Boosting the flow of the body's energy (*qi*) is not difficult. It can be enhanced by

exercises developed long ago such as *qigong*, by new methods developed by Donna Eden and by the various energy psychology techniques. One of the simplest methods of increasing *qi* is through breathing exercises.

6. The body is an electromagnetic organism affected by both natural electromagnetic fields such as the earth, sun and moon, and by artificial electromagnetic fields. Enhancing exposure to natural rhythms and reducing exposure to artificial electromagnetic fields benefits health. Geopathic stress, usually from sleeping over lines of negative energy, can be a rarely recognised but important block to healing.

7. Thoughts are energy; they create physiological changes within the body, altering its biochemistry, neurotransmitters, gene expression and immunity. Keeping the focus on health rather than disease enhances health. Our thoughts, our intentions and our expectations all impact on our well-being. We can deliberately put ourselves into healing mode by entering a positive state, such as in the relaxation response.

8. Quantum science predicts any outcome is possible, including the healing of diseases thought to be incurable. We know that dramatic healings have happened with most, if not all, major diseases. Restructuring the energy of the body should restructure matter. Some methods such as matrix energetics are attempting to do this. This is probably what happened with the Chinese healers who reversed cancer within minutes. These methods are in their infancy but I expect to see more of therapies of this type in the future. At the very least it is worth having an attitude that anything is possible.

9. Groups with an intention to heal have produced powerful and dramatic healings. There is little research

on this at present but I believe this is an area with enormous potential.

Finally I would like to look at energy again from the perspective of Georges Lakhovsky. I believe his ideas were ahead of his time and his observations are central to understanding energy and health. I would add that it is difficult to understand health without understanding energy.

My understanding of this is that healing will be enhanced whenever the body's innate energy or vibrations are increased and will be reduced whenever harmful energies are present. It is rare to find a single cause or a single cure for most of today's major diseases. What is much more realistic is to tilt the scales in the direction of health. This is a useful model for healing.

Another key observation is that energetic changes precede disease. Similarly we would expect energetic changes to precede healing. So if we want healing to occur then it logically follows that we must first change our energy.

One strategy is to enhance anything that boosts energy. We know that high quality foods help heal many diseases: this may be because of their nutritional content but, equally, could be due to the transmission of coherent energy fields throughout the body. In Lakhovsky's terms this would be strengthening the body's fundamental oscillation.

Food, however, is not the only way of amplifying energy. Positive thinking, meditation, exercise, healing, sunlight, connection to the earth and boosting *qi* would all be ways to strengthen the body's innate vibration. The more methods we have to increase our energy, the better chance we have of modifying an illness. And it is reassuring to know that most of these are easy to do. We can often sense this change in our own energy once we use them. For those dealing with a serious disease, an increase in energy is an important sign, pointing to the fact that healing is taking place.

Equally important is reducing harmful energies. Popp discovered that carcinogenic chemicals are not just poisonous but also prevent DNA repair. Reducing our exposure to harmful chemicals, geopathic stress, electro-pollution, poor quality food and negative emotions allows the innate healthy frequencies to gain the upper hand.

Whether a disease gets better or worse most likely depends on the balance between the competing energies of health and disease. The crucial message here is that most of these factors, both positive and negative, are under our control and if we can increase the healthy ones and reduce the unhealthy ones, long enough and often enough, then we can reach a tipping effect where healing can occur.

Part V

Combine what works for you

Chapter 12

Putting it all together

You can't do the same thing in the same way and expect to get a different result.

Albert Einstein

What happens following the diagnosis of a major illness? The first step for most people is speaking to their doctor. Naturally they will be told what treatments are currently available. The next step many then take is to look elsewhere, maybe speak to friends and family and look in books or on the internet. However, once the initial drama subsides, other questions arise.

'Is there anything else I need to do that could make a difference?' 'Are there other useful methods of treatment that I don't know about?' 'Are there treatments that my doctor has not considered or perhaps is not even aware of? If so, what are they?'

These questions are especially crucial if the disease is one without an effective treatment. One of the aims of this book is to help answer these questions.

The answer to most of these questions is usually yes. There are almost always other ways to move the illness in the direction of healing.

To give one example: there is now solid and wide-ranging evidence that good nutrition alters the outcome not only with cancer but with virtually every serious disease. This

327

evidence comes from a multitude of sources: population and epidemiological studies, research on the anti-carcinogenic properties of foods, animal research and case studies of individuals using nutrition as the mainstay of their treatment.

However, doctors are often unfamiliar with this. They are not taught it. They may ignore it, or worse, deny it. As the saying goes, 'If you're not up on it, you're down on it'. But facts are facts, and to treat a major disease without good nutrition is like treating it with one hand tied behind your back.

There are other ways forward. We have discussed the influence of the mind, but again doctors are likely to be unfamiliar with this. Yet it could affect the outcome.

Spontaneous remission

Even without treatment we know that some cancers simply disappear. Accounts of spontaneous remission date back to the beginning of the 20th century. The Spontaneous Remission Project, which researches these unexpected events, contains thousands of references on these remissions (mostly from cancer) from hundreds of different medical journals. Spontaneous remission seems rare but one study in a small area in Holland in the 1980s uncovered as many as seven cases of spontaneous remission in 18 months, suggesting that these events are commoner than previously thought.[1]

But even this may still be a serious underestimate. A study of breast cancer in Norway revealed some unexpected and surprising findings. The study investigated the incidence of this cancer in two groups of randomly selected Norwegian women aged between 50 and 64. Some had had breast screening and some had not. They compared one group who had received two-yearly screening (under the national screening programme between 1996 and 2001) with another group (who would have been screened if the national screening programme had been in place between 1992 and 1997). The unscreened group were invited to have a single mammogram and then compared with the screened group.

If breast cancer was a disease which inevitably progressed then the incidence of breast cancer should have been the same in the two groups. However, this was not what the data showed. In the screened group the incidence of breast cancer was 22% higher.[2]

Why was this? These figures imply something surprising: that breast cancer may have been resolving spontaneously in about one in five cases (in the unscreened group). The only other explanation would be a large increase in the incidence of breast cancer during this time period but, although breast cancer has risen, a difference of this magnitude is highly unlikely.

This figure of one in five breast cancers resolving spontaneously appears high but support comes from an unlikely source: autopsy studies of women dying from unrelated causes. These women, not known to have breast cancer during life, were found to have breast cancer growths in surprisingly large numbers. This included both invasive cancer (around 1% with a range of 0% to 1.8%), carcinoma-in-situ (usually 9% with a range of 0% to 14.7%) and atypical hyperplasia (around 10%).[3] A few studies found higher rates of malignant change.[4, 5] Rates of breast cancer were higher in those over 40 but in one study even younger women, with an average age of 39 years, had cancerous or precancerous lesions in 18% of cases.[6]

Admittedly, most of these cases were cancers in the very early stages, but the studies suggest that cancer could be far commoner than we suppose and that between one in five and one in 10 women experience spontaneous remission of breast cancer on an almost routine basis – remissions from cancers that they never knew they had.

Suffice it to say, spontaneous remission of cancer does happen and may be much commoner than we suppose. What do we make of this? It means that the body is always attempting to heal us from any condition we suffer from. It often succeeds and who knows how many of us have had a cancer that has healed without us knowing.

Our remarkable ability to heal ourselves

With any disease there is always the possibility of recovery and the bottom line is that there is no disease from which someone, somewhere, has not recovered. I think it is a useful assumption, with almost any illness, that the body knows how to heal itself. However, the persistence of any illness may indicate some block to healing or the absence of a key healing factor.

Evidence that the body has hidden powers of healing comes from an unlikely source: the humble placebo. In Chapter 3 (page 101), I covered the story of Mr Wright and his remarkable response to Krebiozen. What was extraordinary was that his body already had the capacity to heal his cancer, and in this case, to do it at speed. But is this innate ability unique to Mr Wright? I very much doubt it.

Deepak Chopra recounts the story of a woman in her 50s who, during an operation for suspected gallstones, was found to have widespread cancer that had metastasised to the liver. The case was thought hopeless so no further surgery was attempted. Her daughter begged him to tell her mother that she was okay so he simply informed her that the gallstones had been successfully removed.

Eight months later, to his surprise, she returned to the clinic in good health. After another year of good health he started to become curious for he guessed that something remarkable had taken place. The patient admitted to him that she had suspected cancer all along. However, once she had been told that it was only gallstones she was so pleased she vowed never to be sick again.[7] Her body responded to her vow and cleared the cancer.

Although the two stories are different, the effect was identical: the immune system mobilised its enormous powers and removed the cancer. Somehow it knew how to do it. However, this leaves us with a dilemma. Short of being tricked into remission by being given the perfect placebo by the most persuasive doctor on the planet, how else can we switch on this remarkable healing power?

Remission by design

Our main interest here, however, is not spontaneous remission or finding the perfect placebo; it is therapeutic remission, and we can gain an insight into this by observing those pioneering individuals who have reversed cancers and other major illnesses. What do these accounts tell us? And how can we use this information to increase our chances of healing?

Let's think of a disease as an event or series of events that have overwhelmed the body's healing mechanisms. Assuming this to be so, it makes perfect sense to strengthen the body as much as we can and to remove anything that reduces the body's power to heal. This is a key theme in this book. We need to strengthen the body enough and reduce negative influences enough that the immune system can overcome the disease, but how do we achieve this?

I propose that the first step is a decision. It is a decision made by the person deciding that they are now going to get better. It doesn't matter if they have no idea how to achieve this; answers can come later. It is the belief that it is possible that matters. This is the mindset seen over and over again with survivors. It attracts solutions. It orchestrates a chain of events in the outside world which facilitates healing. Often survivors intuitively sense what will work.

The first ingredients needed are hope and belief. Next comes a determination to recover. This is essential as recovery is rarely straightforward and set-backs are the rule. The fourth is the knowledge of how to do it. This is where other people's experiences come in, and there is always more than one way to heal a disease. The best starting points are nutrition and the mind. These are strategies with a track record of success. There is substantial evidence behind both. Let's start with the well-known saying that you are what you eat and you are what you think. If this is true, and I think the evidence speaks for itself, then it makes logical sense to change your diet and to change your mind-set.

As we have seen throughout this book, there are many stories of survivors who have cured themselves using nutrition. These include William Kelly, Dr Eva Hill, Jane Plant, Michael Gearin-Tosh (all from cancer, including metastatic cancer). Others have reversed their tumours predominantly by changing their thoughts and beliefs (Louise Hay, Shivani Goodman and Brandon Bays).

However, putting these methods into practice is not easy. Survivors have needed patience, determination and consistency to achieve their goals. It is not for the faint-hearted. I know from my experience as a doctor that it is only a minority of patients, even when confronted with a life-threatening illness, who are prepared to make major lifestyle changes.

Committing to a strict diet means changing habits, eating differently from friends and relatives, and perhaps missing out on social events. Additionally, for some people, the work involved in preparing healthy foods and juices can be a source of stress. The flip side is that you cannot heal your body if you don't eat healing foods. On the positive side, these diets are typically energising, boosting health and well-being, and sometimes taking the person to a level of health they have never experienced before.

Keep in mind that the number of people who have reversed major diseases in these ways is still small but what is more important is that they have done it at all; they have shown what is possible. They have shown that the body does have its own healing mechanism.

In the past, few people had access to the necessary information and resources to put healing diets into practice, but numbers are now increasing. People are becoming more and more aware that this is a real option and they are learning from those who have already travelled this path.

When it comes to using mental strategies the data are less clear cut. However, even here, we are in a better position than a decade or two ago, thanks to trail-blazers such as the Simontons, Louise Hay, Bernie Siegel and Shivani Goodman, and researchers like Dean Ornish. We have a better understanding of which mental strategies make a difference. However, as we have seen, diet and mind techniques are not the only means to heal a serious disease. Reducing toxicity and healing and energy techniques all have a part to play.

There is, however, another piece of the jigsaw and I think it is fundamental. Typically in medical research, one method of treatment is tested in isolation. This approach can be useful but may, in the long run, prove short-sighted, for the evidence strongly suggests that more is better. This evidence comes from the pioneering research of Dr Dean Ornish. What he discovered is that 'lifestyle' treatments work better when combined rather than in isolation.[8] This fits in well with the idea of using as many methods as possible to boost the body's innate powers and at the same time dealing with any blocks to cure.

More is better

Dr Ornish did research on the effects of lifestyle changes on patients with early prostate cancer. The patients in this study had elected to undergo active surveillance before a decision was made about further treatment. This is an accepted strategy in prostate cancer. Unlike the majority of cancers, the course of prostate cancer can be followed with a blood test, the prostate specific antigen (PSA) which monitors the activity of the disease.

Ornish compared an experimental group who used lifestyle changes with a control group. Those in the experimental group used a combination of exercise (walking for half an hour a day, six days a week), vegetarian diet, vitamins and supplements (vitamins E, C, selenium and omega 3 fats), stress management techniques (mental imagery, relaxation, breathing exercises and yoga) and weekly participation in a support group. The control group used none of these.

Today it may be hard to believe how radical this research was. Most of the methods were considered controversial or of dubious benefit. However, the results were unambiguous. After one year the two groups were performing quite differently. Six out of 49 in the control group developed deterioration of their cancer and went on to have surgery, radiotherapy and chemotherapy. None of the experimental group needed such treatments. The PSA increased by an average of 6% in the control group with much higher levels in those requiring further treatment. By contrast, the PSA in the experimental group decreased, on average, by 4% and this was accompanied by a sevenfold increase in the ability of their blood to inhibit cancer growth.

However, the most fascinating finding was not just that these lifestyle methods made a difference. It was that the more of these methods were used, the stronger the effect and the greater the inhibition of cancer cells. Those with high adherence to the programme had blood that inhibited cancer cell growth by 72% whilst those with low adherence had blood that inhibited growth by 7%.

Thirty of the intervention group had prostate biopsies before and after the study and gene expression was assessed. The results showed an alteration in genes in a direction which favoured tumour inhibition.[9] There was an up-regulation of 48 genes and a down-regulation of 453.

Telomeres (described earlier in Chapter 4) are structures that protect the chromosomes. A fascinating property is that they get shorter as we age, usually going down by 1% per year. They also shorten with illness and give a unique insight into overall health. In this study, there was a 3% decrease in telomere length in the control group but an astonishing 10% increase in the experimental lifestyle group.[10]

These studies were truly ground-breaking. They demonstrated not only that lifestyle changes work, but, more importantly, that they work best when combined.

Many of the lifestyle methods used in this study have been discussed in previous chapters. These are not, however, the only choices available. I personally believe the methods used here, though excellent in themselves, could be enhanced and made even more powerful.

Personalising a strategy

However, the question anyone with a serious illness is likely to ask is 'will these methods work for me?' or 'are results guaranteed?' Unfortunately, it is not possible to say. The reason is that, for each person, the causes of their disease will vary and the most appropriate methods of treatment will vary too. A diet that produces wonderful results in one person may fall short in another person who might need to make changes more in the mental arena. Although this sounds a bit vague and woolly, I think we all have some idea of what makes us healthy and happy and, more crucially, what we need to change in order to become as healthy as we can. Let me explain further.

Doctor and author, Lissa Rankin, gives a fascinating insight into this conundrum. In her holistic practice in California she found she could get most patients to recover from a variety of ailments, using a combination of healthy diets, exercise and supplements. However, some patients stubbornly refused to get better, even when doing all the right things. She wondered why.

Puzzled by this failure of some patients to improve whilst outwardly living very healthy lives, she started to ask deeper questions. She enquired: 'What do you think is at the root of your illness?' and 'What does your body need to heal?' Surprisingly, many of them already knew the answers. They told her 'I hate my job'; 'I need to end my marriage'; 'I need more time to myself'; 'I need to find my life's purpose'.

One simply told her she needed to move to Santa Fe (her symptoms disappeared when in Santa Fe). Although this patient took lots of exercise, practised yoga, avoided alcohol and cigarettes and had an excellent diet she had a list of chronic health problems as long as your arm. In the end, she did move to Santa Fe, she made major changes in her life, sold her company, took up art, divorced her husband and went on to make a complete recovery.[11] For her it was changing her whole life, not her diet, that ultimately turned her health around.

I realise that completely changing our whole life is often not an option, but it is does tell us something fundamental. It tells us that the factors which influence health vary greatly from person to person. It also goes some way to explaining why not every person with cancer responds to an excellent diet or to a supposedly healthy lifestyle. For that person, removing the major stresses in their life may be more crucial.

It can also work the other way round: some people have a very positive mindset and a life that they love but continue to smoke, take little or no exercise or eat junk food. Not surprisingly, it eventually takes a toll on their health.

What approach should we use?

The approach to healing disease advocated in this book is best suited to those diseases where mainstream medicine has no effective treatment. This applies to some cancers but also to many chronic diseases.

Some cancers, such as breast and testicular cancer, do well with mainstream treatment, and when this is the case it makes absolute sense to go down this route. Modern medicine can make a real difference when early diagnosis is combined with early surgical treatment. But what about people diagnosed with cancers not in this category?

For many cancers, such as cancers of the pancreas, lung and stomach, the results with mainstream treatment remain poor. In addition, mainstream medicine has almost nothing to offer in metastatic cancer. If the results are poor then it is logical to consider other options. When it comes to cancer treatment, you cannot afford to be an uneducated consumer. You need to know what else is available. If the treatment doesn't feel right, it probably isn't.

It is a little-known fact that some nutritional treatments have proved superior to mainstream treatment. For example, JP Carter compared treatment using a macrobiotic diet with standard treatment in pancreatic cancer. Those on standard treatment had a 9% one-year survival whereas those on a macrobiotic diet for three months or longer had a 52% one-year survival.[12]

This is only a single study but the results don't surprise me. Many years ago I came across the story of Dr Hugh Faulkner, a retired GP, who developed pancreatic cancer at the age of 74. He was given three months to live. He put himself on a macrobiotic diet and after a few weeks was feeling better than he had felt for years. Eight months after diagnosis, his scan confirmed that his tumour had shrunk. He went on to live another seven years.[13]

So understanding the success and failure rates of mainstream cancer treatments is an essential first step. In many other diseases, like multiple sclerosis (MS) and chronic fatigue syndrome (CFS/ME), where standard treatments have limited effectiveness, using the methods advocated here is a sensible option.

Many survivors seem to intuitively know what will work best for them and what would not. Sometimes survivors have used alternative methods as their sole treatment. I believe this is generally unwise without thoroughly researching the pros and cons of conventional treatment first.

Michael Gearin-Tosh, mentioned in Chapter 10, is an excellent model here. After being diagnosed with myeloma, he consulted numerous doctors, many of whom were experts in the field. After doing his research, he realised that the results achieved by mainstream medical treatment were poor and, taking this into account, he opted for a very different method (Gerson diet and healing exercises).[14] The outcome was remarkable and far better than could have been expected with conventional treatment. He died nine years later from an unrelated condition.

Unfortunately, patients with cancer are often rushed into treatments before they have a chance to fully assess the advantages and disadvantages of conventional therapy and with a haste that is rarely necessary. There is nearly always time to research the best way forward.

Let's summarise what we need for healing:
1. Strengthen the body.
2. Remove any obstacles to health.
3. Combine effective treatments where possible.

Also:
- Don't be rushed into a treatment before you have had time to research its benefits and downsides.
- Don't be an uneducated consumer.

Understanding healing

Let's go back to the idea that we are what we eat and we are what we think. Could these work through a common mechanism? Biologist, Bruce Lipton, performed a fascinating set of experiments exposing stem cells to different environments.[15] Stem cells have the unique ability to differentiate into more specialised cells, such as those of a particular organ, under the right conditions. He found the environments not only influenced which cells the stem cells turned into, as expected, but they also determined whether the cells stayed healthy or not. Crucially, he found that once unhealthy cells were put back into a healthy environment, in this case surrounded by healthy extracellular fluid, they became healthy again.

This was a ground-breaking observation. In cancer research, scientists have spent huge amounts of time and energy studying abnormal cells, looking for a way to treat them, but have largely ignored the extracellular fluid surrounding the cells. Yet this experiment suggests that if we could create a healthy environment surrounding the cells, then abnormalities within the cells would revert to normal. But how do we create a healthy extracellular fluid?

We already know that healing is enhanced once the body becomes more alkaline. One experiment involved injecting turpentine into the legs of rabbits whilst their bodies were kept in either an acidic or an alkaline state. Would it make a difference? In fact the difference was profound. Those in an alkaline state had minimal damage whilst the same injection, done in an acidic state, caused sloughing of tissues, inflammation and death. A study on mice with metastatic breast cancer found that those given sodium bicarbonate (an alkalinising salt) had inhibition of tumour formation and inhibition of spontaneous metastases. It reduced liver metastases and lymph node involvement.[16] But how can we make the body more alkaline?

The most obvious way is by changing our diet. Fruit and vegetables have an alkalinising effect whilst sugar, starch and meat are acid-forming. It is also possible to use alkalising substances to achieve an ideal pH. This is outside the scope of this book but involves monitoring the pH of the urine (see *Cancer: The Complete Recovery Guide* by Jonathon Chamberlain for more details).

It is not just diet, however, that influences the extracellular fluid. So too does the mind. In response to our thoughts and emotions we produce hormones, peptides and neurotransmitters which are pumped into the bloodstream and extracellular fluids on a moment by moment basis. These changes are then picked up by receptors on cell walls. Stress hormones create a negative environment in contrast to the relaxation response which releases hormones, peptides and neurotransmitters which are healing, activating the parasympathetic system.

The way I imagine this is that the cells of someone on a standard western diet, packed with sugar and chemicals, would be surrounded by thick, stagnant fluid whereas the cells of someone from a long-lived culture or on a healing diet would be surrounded by a clean, flowing, nutrient-rich liquid. I would see negative emotions producing dark, pungent secretions and positive ones as having a cleansing, revitalising effect.

Here we have a mechanism whereby both food and mental factors interact, altering the fluid surrounding the cells. This in turn either enhances or impairs healing within the cells. From this perspective it is easy to see why both diet and mental influences are central to health and healing.

More on nutrition

As mentioned, fruit and vegetables are alkaline or, in the case of citrus fruits, have an alkalinising effect on the body. Note, however, that although fruit and vegetables are alkaline when still fresh, they become acidic within a few days of being picked. Animal produce, starch, sugar, cereals, legumes and nuts make the body more acidic. The typical western diet is 20% alkaline and 80% acid, while the ideal ratio for the body is probably 80% alkaline and 20% acidic. The Gerson diet and the diets of long-lived cultures are much closer to the ideal healing ratio. (However, note there may be exceptions and Kelley found a few tumours, especially lymphomas and leukaemia, needed a more acidic diet).

Clearly it makes total sense, when faced with almost any serious disease, to go on the healthiest diet possible. My hope is that this vitally important knowledge becomes accepted by the medical profession, and patients could be supported when they wish to do so.

The full Gerson diet, which involves drinking large volumes of fresh juices, may prove too difficult, too time-consuming and perhaps too stressful for many people. However, it is a truism that the more serious the illness, the more radical the dietary changes need to be. I think with cancer or serious chronic illness, a good starting point is to have raw fruit and vegetables for the first month. This is a very healing diet. Usually a one-month trial with a diet will let you know which way things are going. However, sometimes this needs to be built up gradually as too much change can create stress.

Patrick Kingsley's recommendation for cancer (page 366), of avoiding animal milks and their products, avoiding beef, sugar and all refined carbohydrates, and all caffeine, alcohol and chemical additives, is a good compromise. In autoimmune and many other chronic diseases the 'paleo' diet is often the best diet to start on.

Combining this with juicing, which is equivalent to giving the body an infusion of nutrients, is not hard to do. This should rapidly boost immunity, improve well-being and make the diet more alkaline. Nearly everyone will feel better on this. There are many books which have useful tips on diet for cancer (see Appendix I). For most cancers, especially hormonal cancers (breast, prostate, ovary), avoiding milk with its mix of growth factors and hormones is an essential change to make. Removing sugar is important with virtually every disease, notably cancer. Using key supplements can also be very beneficial (see Appendix III).

More on the mind

We also know the mind powerfully affects health, but where does someone start when faced with a life-threatening illness? This is a time when the mind is already in turmoil and it is far from the easiest moment to switch on a new, more positive way of thinking. This dilemma may explain some of the mixed results seen in mind-body medicine. Nevertheless, we do have some hard data to guide us.

Dean Ornish's regime of stress management included relaxation, imagery, breathing exercises and support groups. It showed a positive effect in early prostate cancer, with an enhanced ability to inhibit cancer.[10]

As I have said, a key facet of healing seems to be a belief that recovery is possible. Survivors typically have had this belief and a feeling that they would somehow find a way to recover. Although they haven't universally succeeded, this belief has typically propelled them forward.

We also know that the relaxation response and meditation create a positive mix of chemicals and push gene expression in the direction of health. However, these are not the only methods used by survivors. Visualisation is the mental technique most strongly associated in the mind of the public with fighting cancer. Although this method won't appeal to everyone, it is relatively easy to use. There are many accounts of people who have reversed cancer using visualisation. Unfortunately, it doesn't work consistently, perhaps because some find it easier to use than others.

There are excellent guides to visualisation, including the Simontons *Getting Well Again* (page 368) and David Hamilton's *How your Mind Heals your Body* (page 369). Shivani Goodman's methods, using a combination of visualisation and related ideas, represent a fairly comprehensive, and in her case successful, attempt to reverse cancer, and this approach is again fairly easy to use (page 368).

Some survivors have considered illness to be a feedback mechanism. They have speculated that their life was off course and out of balance. They felt they needed to follow their bliss, take up their passion and change the direction of their life. I suspect the changes people need to make will vary from person to person. Asking what these changes are and trusting your intuition has proved valuable strategy for many.

In summary, there are plenty of mental strategies which have proved effective. We will never get proof or double-blind studies confirming these as they are so individual. It is a matter of going with your instincts and your intuition. Synchronistic events are another clue that you're on the right track.

However, sometimes the main cause is physical not mental. To take an extreme example, occupational medicine has found that some synthetic dyes, such as aromatic amines, cause cancer in virtually everyone who works with them after about 20 years.

Energy, toxicity and balance

When it comes to strengthening the body, energy medicine has much to offer. Plenty of good research shows that exercise, sunlight and healing can powerfully enhance health. Techniques to increase qi, the Chinese concept of body energy, are easy to use and will reinforce the body's innate healing capacity.

Detoxification is the other pillar of healing, and strategies to enhance this have been discussed. Fasting is one and has an excellent track record for healing a wide range of illnesses.

The dangers from mobile phones (particularly the advanced ones carrying the most information) deserve a special mention. We now know that they block DNA repair and create oxidative stress. For anyone trying to heal a major disease such as cancer, this is a potential block to healing that it would be dangerous to overlook.

If you can identify and remove the underlying cause of a

disease, whether it be a toxic exposure, a specific food or a key allergen (as in Patrick Kingsley's case of MS – see page 366 – with allergy to flowers), then recovery is much more likely.

For the Chinese good health was all about balance. Other systems of medicine such as ayurdevic medicine also stress the importance of balance.

Good health is not that complicated. There have been many societies where it has been the norm. Eating natural, unadulterated food, getting fresh air, sunlight, clean water and plenty of exercise and being happy are some of the key factors needed for health. Break with these principles and disease is an inevitable result.

These cultures contrast hugely with our society with its massive burden of chronic disease combined with its immense health costs. The message we are being given, in no uncertain terms, is that our whole civilisation is out of balance. Survivors have often returned to the ways of healthier societies, with perhaps a few modern tweaks thrown in.

Clearly there are many ways to heal, but keep in mind Gill Edward's sage advice (see page 289) that if you do so many things that you have no time for living and just being happy then it could prove counterproductive. Just enjoying life is healing in itself. However, using a combination of methods is a successful strategy and is typical of the majority of survivors. Dean Ornish's research testifies to its effectiveness.[10] Again it is about finding the right balance.

Putting it together

So let's assume you've been diagnosed with a serious disease and you have carefully weighed up the pros and cons of using conventional treatment and are considering using an approach such as outlined in this book. Let's recap on the basic principles outlined thus far:

Diet

The principle here is to reduce or cut out the foods that are detrimental to health and increase those that stimulate healing. Some survivors stated they would only eat food that healed them. Foster's group (of spontaneous remission from cancer) used 'foods that heal' almost exclusively.

FOODS THAT HARM	FOODS THAT HEAL
Sugar	Fruit and vegetables
Refined carbohydrates	Seeds and nuts
Modified starches	Oily fish (from unpolluted
(These three food groups	sources)
make up 50% of the modern	
diet)	Foods high in antioxidants
	(fruit and vegetables but
	especially herbs and spices)
Milk	
Hydrogenated fats	Foods high in phytonutrients
Colouring and additives	(multi-coloured fruit and
Processed food	vegetables)

Some foods have especially powerful healing properties as noted below:

HEALING FOODS
Raw food
Fruit and vegetable juices
(if freshly made and organic)
Sprouting seeds
Bone broth

Another principle is to make the diet more alkaline.

The Mind

Key principles

1) Putting the body in relaxation mode switches on healing (stress does the opposite)
2) The Mind is creative (affirmations, visualisation and the placebo response use this ability)

Other considerations

Believe healing is possible
Ask for help and trust the Universe. Assistance may come in the form of strong intuitions and synchronicities
Release negative emotions, especially resentment
Use intuition to decide the best treatment for you
Find your sense of purpose

Detoxification

REDUCE TOXICITY

Reduce toxicity in water (filter), in food (fewer chemicals and pesticides, less processed food, using organic), in the home (using natural products), in the air (filters, avoiding sprays and chemicals) and on the skin (use natural products)

Reduce dental toxicity

Reduce exposure to mobiles, wifi, phone masts and DECT phones

---

AID DETOXIFICATION

Fasting
Increase sweating (exercise, saunas)

Add foods and nutrients that assist detoxification
Use soluble fibre

ENERGY ENHANCERS	ENERGY DRAINS
Exercise	Poor quality foods
Sunlight	Drugs and radiation
Sleep	Toxicity
High quality foods	Electromagnetic pollution
Positive thoughts, positive states, positive people	Negative thoughts, negative states, negative people
Healing	Geopathic stress
Qi (e.g. qigung, breathing)	

Of all these categories, energy may yet prove to be the most important. The energy within the body needs to be powerful enough to overcome the disease. I believe this will allow the immune system to function at full throttle and do the healing. Certainly, an improvement in energy levels is an early sign and important clue that healing is taking place

Notice that foods act on several levels: they improve nutrition, they enhance detoxification; they also have energetic properties. This may explain why they are often so crucial to healing.

A final point is that with many natural methods of healing symptoms can get worse before they get better, although typically energy remains positive. This is known as a healing crisis. There is an example in Appendix III (on using supplements – see page 384).

Never underestimate the body's capacity to heal

I hope I have given enough examples of different successful healing methods and that these will help others with serious illnesses. A message that comes through over and over again from survivors is that we underestimate our body's innate capacity to heal, once it has been given the right conditions.

The all-important immune system

One way of assessing the value of a treatment is to consider its overall effect on the body. We particularly want to know whether it strengthens the body, especially the immune system, and whether it removes blocks to healing. Remember that in most major diseases the immune system is already in trouble. At present no treatments used by mainstream medicine are known to enhance immunity.

For the majority of illnesses the methods covered here combine well with conventional medical treatments. However, I believe there is an exception and it is an important one. The exception is where a treatment damages the immune system. Here the philosophies of the two types of treatment depart. Using a treatment that damages the immune system should, in my opinion, never be undertaken lightly. It may permanently reduce your chance of recovery.

It is useful to think of the immune system as a sleeping giant. There have been several recorded cases of patients developing cancer following organ transplants. This arises when undetected cancer cells are transplanted from the donor organ. The cancer then starts to spread. When this takes place there is only one course of action left and this is to stop the immune suppressants given to protect the donor organ. Once these are stopped, the immune system rapidly goes into action, ridding the body of cancer. Sadly the donor organ is also lost in the process. This demonstrates the innate power of the immune system and its ability to rapidly remove cancer under normal circumstances. Anything which damages this capacity (in this case, immune suppressants) is a block to healing.

Whatever treatment is used, it is the immune system which must ultimately clear the cancer or any other disease. Even if antibiotics are taken for a simple infection it is still the immune system that finishes the job. The approach of this book is to preserve, and wherever possible enhance, the immune system.

Many of today's treatments have a negative effect on immunity. Antibiotics (especially if repeated), steroids, anti-inflammatory drugs, acid-blocking drugs and the contraceptive pill all damage immunity, principally due to their negative effect on the microbiome which is thought to be responsible for 70 to 80% of our immunity (see Appendix II).

I would always recommend working with your doctor but would also suggest researching the methods of treatment being recommended, and be very wary of any treatment that damages immunity.

Chemotherapy

As mentioned, cancer often responds well to early surgery and most patients understand this (but ideally build up your nutrition before having the surgery). However, in my experience many have concerns about chemotherapy. I think they are right to have these concerns because chemotherapy has the capacity to seriously and irreversibly damage the immune system.

The idea behind chemotherapy is to cause more damage to the cancer than to the host and thereby remove the cancer. This has always been a high-risk strategy.

About 5% of cancers do respond well to chemotherapy. These include some leukaemias (especially in children), some lymphomas, including Hodgkin's lymphoma, ovarian, penile and testicular cancers and retinoblastomas. Even when successful, chemotherapy comes at a cost. Childhood chemotherapy creates a 15-fold higher incidence of further tumours and 40% of those who have it develop serious health problems in later years. The higher incidence of cancer in chemotherapy nurses tells its own story.

Although chemotherapy can be useful in selected cases and is now generally less toxic than in the past, treating cancer with carcinogens has always struck me as illogical. I am particularly worried by the fact that chemotherapy has repeatedly been shown to increase the incidence of metastases.[16, 17, 18, 19, 20, 21, 22, 23, 24] in animal studies.

However, what concerns me most is that chemotherapy is being given for 75% of all cancers. This means 70% of the time it is being given for cancers that respond poorly to chemotherapy and where the chances of success are small and where its use is inappropriate. A meta-analysis of all major trials in the USA and Australia between 1990 and 2004 reported that the contribution of chemotherapy to overall survival in common cancers (breast, colon, lung) was 2.1% in the USA and 2.3% in Australia.[24] In other words, the benefits were miniscule.

Against this questionable benefit, the downsides of chemotherapy are significant: adverse effects occur in 80% and in 64%, these are severe. So why is it being used in these types of cancers? The reason is because initially treatment with chemotherapy can be quite promising and typically will reduce tumour size and tumour markers. This is encouraging for both patient and doctor. Oncologists call this a response.

But there are two snags to this strategy and they are major ones.

First, this 'response' to chemotherapy is only temporary and does not kill the cancer stem cells which means the cancer will sooner or later return.

Secondly, during chemotherapy some of the cancer cells inevitably become resistant. These cells remain, multiply, become stronger and return with a vengeance. This resistance is a well recognised phenomenon and it is the reason why several chemotherapy drugs are often used together. The resistant cancer cells typically become more aggressive and, by definition, drug-resistant. The eventual outcome is further relapse and, by this time, the chemotherapy will prove ineffective. When this scenario happens, the body's final defence, the immune system, may have been irretrievably weakened.

Chemotherapy is a complex subject which changes year by year. Because of its complexity doctors will leave decisions to oncologists, who have expertise in this field. The oncologist advises the patient who understandably is likely to take this expert advice. What is less well known is that oncologists are not so ready to use chemotherapy on themselves. One study from the McGill Medical Center in Montreal in 1986 asked oncologists if they would treat themselves with chemotherapy if they had cancer: 58 out of 79 said they would decline. This would make me very cautious.[25]

I believe good information is essential before agreeing to chemotherapy. Good questions to ask oncologists are whether the specific chemotherapy they are recommending will usefully extend life (not just shrink the tumour) and whether they would use this treatment on themselves. The answer will usually be no to both these questions and, more often than not, oncologists only use chemotherapy because they have no other strategy left to treat the disease. I would also look at independent sources of information, free from commercial bias, such as the charity CANCERactive.

In my experience, it is rarely made clear to patients that the aim of chemotherapy, in the majority of cases, is palliation rather than cure. One study found that 80% of patients with metastatic lung and colon cancer, who had been given chemotherapy, thought they were being given the treatment to cure their cancer although this was never the intended aim.[26]

This palliative approach might still be acceptable for the majority of people, but if the patient's real aim is cure, however poor the odds, then using chemotherapy in this way would be counterproductive. Certainly, chemotherapy has a place in the treatment of a few less common cancers, but its destructive effect on the immune system is a major downside. Shrinking tumours is an entirely different thing to curing cancers.

Chemotherapy is a treatment where it is unwise to assume that the doctor knows best. Sometimes doctors say 'We will give it as insurance so we get all the cancer cells', but this simply isn't true. A tumour the size of a pin head has a million cells and a 2-cm tumour (just visible on a scan) has 10 billion cancer cells. There is no way in the world that these can all be removed. The only protection is a strong immune system.

The basic principles underlying medicine are using the safest methods of treatment first, doing no harm and strengthening the body wherever possible. These remain as true today as ever. We should veer away from these sensible principles with great caution. So the pros and cons of chemotherapy need weighing up very carefully. Be very wary of being carried down this course if your intuition is telling you otherwise.

Pros and cons of treatments

There is another aspect to treating a major disease like cancer. Clearly there are numerous approaches, but before embarking on any new method of treatment it is prudent to look at the possible downside. Anyone with a life-threatening illness needs to consider how they would feel if they followed a particular path, especially one not recommended by the medical profession, and later found out it didn't work. After all, there is never a guarantee of success. Survivors typically, let go of their attachment to getting better. They do all they can and leave the rest in the lap of the gods.

This attitude is important because without it you could end up feeling like a failure, perhaps blaming yourself for not trying hard enough or making the wrong choice. With many treatments we are in uncharted territory.

And sometimes a person's time is up for reasons we can't fathom. There may be good reasons why this is so, but these are probably beyond our understanding. Some schools of thought believe that illness can allow us to grow in unexpected ways, perhaps allowing us to be vulnerable and allowing others to care for us. Perhaps a serious illness pushes us to examine our lifestyle. Usually we simply don't know. There is now much interest in dying well and making this as good an experience as possible. Some have felt a sense of serenity at this time that they have never felt before. Surrendering and being at peace with the outcome, whatever it turns out to be, is the ideal mindset and paradoxically this also helps the healing process.

Those that didn't make it

Some of the authors who have written books about how they got better have eventually succumbed. I think this deserves comment.

Anne Frahm has described her recovery from a metastatic breast cancer that had infiltrated her bones, including her spine. She relapsed after intensive treatment, including surgery, radiotherapy, chemotherapy and a bone marrow transplant. At this point the medical profession told her that there was nothing more they could do.

Normally when someone has cancer this serious and this extensive, death follows within weeks, certainly within months. However, this didn't happen. She initiated a programme of nutritional treatment with regular juicing and began to recover.[27] She went on to live another nine years. This in itself was remarkable, given the severity of the cancer and the aggressiveness of her treatment. Eventually she did die, although the exact cause of her death remains unclear. Whatever the cause, her story still remains an amazing testament to the healing powers of the human body when all seems lost.

A recovery for nearly a decade with metastatic cancer is something that most doctors have never seen and would find inexplicable. Something very unusual had taken place. The fact

that she ultimately died suggests to me that, although she was on
the right track, there were still things to learn; still pieces of the
jigsaw missing. Importantly her story is not unique and this type
of healing has been used by many others, as noted previously.
In spite of her death, I believe her story will have helped many
people with cancer. She was a pioneer in new territory, providing
much needed maps.

Shivani Goodman's illness was similar but the healing path
she took was different. She also developed metastatic breast
cancer, starting first in the left breast and later recurring on the
right. She also had surgery and chemotherapy. After her third
relapse she decided to treat herself.[28] She decided against a
dietary approach as she hated the thought of not being able to
eat normally. As a psychotherapist she had successfully treated
many people with psychosomatic disorders. In spite of the pleas
from her family to continue with conventional treatment, she
declined and gave herself three months to treat herself using
her own methods. (Louise Hay also persuaded her doctors to
give her three months to heal (see page 369). There were other
parallels; she had also helped others to heal using mind-body
techniques and she also went on to make a full recovery.)

During this period her tumour shrank by half and, after
16 months, it had finally disappeared. What was going on?
Shivani didn't regard cancer just as an illness but as feedback
on her lifestyle. She felt there were psychological and spiritual
issues which she needed to address. So, she listened to her body
wisdom and got a message back that she needed to live a life of
joy. Her body told her it would check out on her if she didn't do
this. With some difficulty she stopped working (she considered
herself a workaholic). She divorced her husband and moved
location, making this seem like an exciting adventure.

She developed many healing exercises and practised them for
an hour, three times a day. One included an exercise to create
a feeling of certainty that she would recover. She developed

exercises for pain, anxiety and dealing with the frightened part of herself. It was basically a mental and spiritual approach to disease. What was fascinating, and may give encouragement to others, is that she was initially plagued with doubts about her ability to succeed and felt fearful exploring new ideas as she still had reservations about them. It is tough to road-test a new psychological treatment on yourself, knowing that if you fail you will die.

Some of her observations were intriguing; she accurately observed the negative impact on her well-being when she heard stories of other people dying of cancer and after listening to her relatives' fears about her doing her own programme.

She died about 10 years later, although it is not clear why. Some have suggested her death negates her work. I do not accept this. Her recovery was still astonishing, given the severity of her disease, and it was clear that she had a great desire to bring this knowledge to the world at large. Not only did she reverse her own disease, she also successfully helped others to heal from AIDs and cancer and even successfully treated a dog with cancer (by creating certainty in the owner that her dog would recover).

I think a clue to her thinking is in one of her affirmations: 'I choose to live in perfect health until an age when I have completed my life on earth with fulfilment and satisfaction'. She died soon after her book was published. Hers was an outstanding achievement and a new and original approach to healing. I think she pushed the psychological treatment of cancer an important step forward and many will benefit from her insights.

Completing a work is a powerful reason to survive. David McFall, the Scottish sculptor was commissioned to produce a large statue of Christ outside Canterbury Cathedral. At the time he had been diagnosed with inoperable cancer, had lost several stone in weight and had stopped working. However, the challenge of producing his final great work spurred him on, even though the hard manual work proved exhausting. He successfully completed his work and died soon after.

Dr David Servan-Schreiber developed a brain tumour at the age of 31. The statistics gave him a life expectancy of less than six months, even with the best treatment available. As it turned out, his life was far from over. He researched the literature on cancer, looking for a fresh approach. He went on to make an incredible recovery. One result was the wonderful book *Anti-cancer: a new way of life*, which gives his vision of how to reverse cancer, using methods such as optimising diet, developing mental harmony and reducing toxicity,[29] based on extensive research. He died almost 20 years later.

As his health deteriorated, he agonised over whether his relapse undermined the credibility of his methods – the methods he had recommended to so many patients in his best-selling book. His answer, after much soul-searching, was the ideas were as valid as ever. He had lived an exceptionally long time for someone with an aggressive brain tumour of this type and he felt that the measures he had taken had dramatically improved both the quality and quantity of his life.

He admitted that, rather than keeping to his own recommendations, he had thrown himself into an exhausting, over-loaded work schedule which included speaking all over the world during the last two years of his life.[30] The work was so absorbing and rewarding that he ignored his own health. In his own words, he forgot to look after himself, thinking himself invincible.

In retrospect, he felt that he had been unable to maintain his sense of inner calm. He compared himself with a woman he knew who had the same illness. She had maintained a prolonged remission for over a decade. She kept her sense of peace by taking daily walks in nature. At the end he had no regrets and was happy to have taken the path he had, which ultimately may have helped to change the way cancer treatment is perceived world-wide, even though it was at some cost to himself.

All of these patients died, although only David Servan-Schreiber is known to have died from cancer. None had any right to live as long as they did. The strategies they used were all different and proved effective for long periods of time. Mainstream medicine uses a one-size-fits-all approach to treatment, but these stories show how patients can not only recover but tailor treatments to their own needs and individuality. They were all true pioneers and have given us new, valuable and much needed maps of how to tackle cancer.

Lessons from survivors

What survivors have given us is a much better knowledge of the key factors involved in healing. We live in exciting times and we have more ideas about healing now than at any time in history. Many have travelled down this road and acted as guides. At the very least, their methods enhance the chance of conventional methods succeeding. Sometimes they do far more.

At one time, anyone who took their own initiative in the treatment of a disease as serious as cancer would have been ridiculed as an oddball and thought to be a little crazy. Cancer was a disease left to the professionals. But times have changed and there are good reasons for this.

Firstly, the search for a cure for cancer has been the single most unsuccessful and expensive quest in medical history. The treatments that do exist are harsh, some would say medieval, and the results frequently disappointing. Secondly, the evidence that other methods can work has been steadily mounting and the science behind them accumulating.

In 2012 the conservative American Cancer Society reported that there is overwhelming evidence that complementary therapies, including diet, exercise and weight control, can increase cancer survival and prevent recurrence.

Where does this leave the ordinary person diagnosed with

cancer or another major illness? This book is certainly not suggesting anyone ignores medical advice. What it is advocating is knowledge and choice. The more informed you are, the better are your chances. The days are gone where oncologists could insist that there is no evidence that diet or mental strategies make a difference. Such a view has long since been proved untrue and is now untenable.

In 100 years' time, nearly all of the drugs in current use will be obsolete and medicine will have changed beyond recognition, but some things won't change. Diet will still be as fundamental to good health as it was at the time of Hippocrates. Exercise and sunlight will continue to have the same health-sustaining properties that they always had. The way we use our minds when faced with a serious illness will be as important as it ever was and it will, no doubt, have been studied in even greater detail. Reducing toxicity will be a recognised as an essential part of healing, and patients will be routinely checked for toxicity. I predict energy medicine will have moved forward in leaps and bounds and will be widely used. In the medicine of the future whatever is fundamental to health will remain.

Hopes for the future

It is my hope that treatment of cancer will start to include many of the methods of healing that have been used successfully by survivors. My wish is that people who have been diagnosed with cancer will not be rushed into treatments they have doubts about, and will be advised on all the available options and not pushed into treatments that intuitively feel wrong to them. I would like to see a move towards cancer centres incorporating methods known to make a difference, such as high-quality nutrition and nutrient infusions. At the very least I would like to see hospital food that encompasses the best nutritional knowledge available.

I hope doctors will do everything possible to enhance the

body's health and remove obstacles to healing. I would hope doctors keep to the principle advocated by Hippocrates: first of all do no harm and use the least toxic therapies first. I realise we are a long way from this ideal but I believe more and more people would like to be treated this way. These strategies would have a useful by-product: they would save millions of pounds for these treatments are far, far cheaper.

I would like to see a systematic and thorough investigation of patients who get better using non-conventional treatment. This would allow both patients and doctors to learn from them and benefit from them. Then treatments would inevitably improve. I believe this would speed up progress in cancer care more than any other single factor. This is not rocket science; it is simply learning from success.

I would also like to see the same principles used in the treatment of other serious illnesses.

And finally...

This chapter sums up what I have learned from survivors. My hope is that this book has given an insight into the many different therapies available that can help to heal a life-threatening illness. If you have a major illness, my hope is that it has given you new ideas and strategies, perhaps ones you had never realised existed. I have included Appendices on supplements which can help in serious disease and some related topics.

I believe survivors have much to tell us and some of this knowledge goes beyond surviving a serious disease. They are canaries telling us about the damage we are doing to ourselves by poisoning our world and adulterating our food. They have shown us how crucial our mindset is to our health and how we can all benefit from this knowledge and live richer lives. They have taken our knowledge about disease and living healthily to a new level.

My hope is you too can emulate the success of these survivors. If so I would love to hear from you and perhaps add your story to the ever-growing band of pioneers who have beaten the odds. Maybe others will benefit from *your* story and be inspired in turn.

Appendices

**I: Useful books on health
and healing
II: More on food and health
III: The use of supplements**

Appendix I

Useful books on health and healing

Anti-cancer: a new way of life

By Dr David Servan-Schreiber

Penguin Books: 2017

This book combines the story of the author's own battle with an aggressive brain tumour, diagnosed whilst he was a young doctor, with up-to-date scientific information. He was given months to live but wrote this book 14 years later. The book contains fascinating information on the influence of food, the mind, toxicity and exercise on cancer and an insider's insight into understanding the benefits and limitations of current medical treatments. There is an excellent colour-pullout at the end of the book on the influence of specific foods on specific cancers.

Everything You Need to Know to Help You Beat Cancer, 5th edition

By Chris Woollams

Health Issues: 2015

In my view this is one of the best books on cancer. Chris Woollam's daughter died after developing a brain tumour. He was unhappy about the quality of her care and resolved to learn more. His book is packed with useful information. This could make a real difference to anyone faced with cancer. The research on nutrients and herbs is especially good. The sections on chemotherapy and radiotherapy and how to minimise side effects are also excellent. There are good sections on specific cancers and their treatments. Chris Woollams runs the excellent website, CANCERactive, which is full of up-to-date information on everything about cancer. Another of his books, *The Rainbow Diet*, expands on the theme of food and cancer.

Radical Remissions: Surviving Cancer Against All Odds

By Kelly A Turner

Bravo Ltd: 2015

This is an excellent book about people who survived cancer against the odds and how they did it. It looks at case histories of cancer survivors submitted to her website. She identified 75 healing factors but nine factors came up most frequently. Two were physical: diet and supplements; the other seven factors were psychological or spiritual. There are chapters on each of these. This is a terrific book for people with cancer or any other serious disease and will give lots of new and positive ideas about healing.

Your Life in Your Hands

By Jane Plant

Virgin Publishing: 2007

Professor Jane Plant describes her recovery from terminal breast cancer. She was given three months to live after all conventional treatments had failed. She tells the fascinating story of her search for a cure and her light-bulb moment when she realised that milk products could be the major factor maintaining her cancer. After stopping milk products she went on to live for nearly three decades. It could be one of the most important discoveries in medicine. It includes other dietary recommendations and accounts of people who turned breast cancer around using her methods. This is also a good book for hormonal cancers, including ovarian or prostate cancer, and much of the advice can be applied to other cancers. (She has also written a book on prostate cancer along the same lines: *Prostate Cancer: Understand, Prevent & Overcome Prostate Cancer*).

The Wahls Protocol
By Dr Terry Wahls
Avery: 2015

This book describes the author's gradual deterioration with multiple sclerosis which continued despite having access to the best treatments currently available. It goes on to describe how she experimented with diet and other therapies and eventually found a successful formula which reversed her MS. The therapy is based on the 'paleo' diet but has important modifications. There are many case histories which include not only MS but other autoimmune diseases which responded to the same treatment. I believe this a ground-breaking book which will give much hope to those with MS and other autoimmune diseases.

Do You Want to Know What We Did to Beat Cancer?
By Sue and Robert Olifent
Active Cancer Therapy Support: 2017

This is a small book which could be read in an evening. However, it is full of useful information. It describes the experience of Sue Olifent, who was diagnosed with a large (two and a half inch) liver tumour, with smaller tumours in her pancreas. No treatment was offered as it was considered inoperable and incurable. Her husband had become interested in nutritional treatments after his parents had died from cancer. She started on nutritional treatment. A scan done six weeks after this was started found only scar tissue where the cancer had been. Three years later she was in good health. The book describes the methods they used.

Cancer: The Complete Recovery Guide
By Jonathon Chamberlain
Long Island Press Ltd: 2008
This is a comprehensive review of the many alternative therapies that have proven useful in cancer with some inspiring histories of people who got better against the odds and how they did it. There is also a useful section on the pros and cons of conventional treatment. The author has also written a smaller book, *The Cancer Recovery Guide: 15 Alternative and Complementary Strategies for Restoring Health*.

The Choice
By Bernadette Bohan
Ted Smart: 2005
Bernadette Bohan suffered from lymphatic cancer and later developed breast cancer. Two thirds of the book is about her own inspiring story. She decided to learn all she could about treating cancer and made a full recovery. Eventually she went on to advising others on simple methods that make a big difference with an emphasis on high quality nutrition. The last three chapters describe her approach to cancer. Her follow-up book *The Choice – the Programme* looks at her methods in more detail (half of this book is about her methods and the other half is recipes). These are books to get you started.

The New Medicine
By Dr Patrick Kingsley
SureScreen Life Sciences: 2013
The late Dr Kingsley had a worldwide reputation for dealing with 'no-hopers' with cancer and multiple sclerosis. He achieved extraordinary results. This book describes his methods. Some of the tests and methods he used, such as intravenous infusions of nutrients, are not easy to access but the book gives an insight into his methods.

A Living Miracle
By Pat Reeves
Pathfinder: 2008
This details her journey of recovery from both a brain tumour and an osteosarcoma using a raw food diet, fasting and exercises. Available through her website www.foodalive.org

Living Proof
By Michael Gearin-Tosh
Simon & Schuster: 2008
The author was diagnosed with myeloma, a cancer which still has a very poor prognosis. He describes the methods he used to recover after thoughtfully examining the pros and cons of the available conventional treatments. He used a version of the Gerson (juice) diet (see page 33) and breathing exercises.

Love, Medicine and Miracles and Peace, Love and Healing: the path to self-healing
By Bernie Siegel
Rider: 1999
Bernie Siegel, an American surgeon, was one of the first doctors to investigate patients who recovered from terminal cancers against the odds, after forming a group of exceptional patients. These best-selling books contain many inspiring stories and ideas which could assist recovery.

Foods to Fight Cancer: what to eat to reduce your risk
By Richard Beliveau and Denis Gingras
DK: 2017
This small book by the world's leading expert, Professor Beliveau, on the effect of common foods on cancer, is easy to read. He gives details of his research, showing how many common foods have powerful effects on cancer.

Metaphysical and mind-body approaches

9 Steps to Reversing or Preventing Cancer and Other Diseases: learn to heal from within
By Shivani Goodman
New Page Books: 2004
This book describes how the author developed her own successful regime to treat her breast cancer. She had conventional treatment for a cancer of the left breast but the cancer recurred in the right breast a year later and spread to her lymph glands.

After the third recurrence she decided to use her own methods, partly derived from her work as a psychotherapist using psychological and spiritual principles. She gave herself three months to test her methods. During this time the cancer halved in size; it later disappeared. She continued to live in good health for nine years. She also describes how her method helped others, including a sceptical doctor who rapidly dissolved a colon cancer. Her book gives a daily healing routine and many other techniques. She has also produced CDs which allow people to put her visualisations into practice.

Getting Well Again: a step-by-step guide to overcoming cancer for patients and their families
By Carl Simonton and Stephanie Matthews-Simonton
JP Tarcher: 1978
This is a classic book about the work of the Fort Worth Center where patients diagnosed with incurable cancer were treated, mainly using a mind-body approach. They achieved remarkable results as described in the book. This is often thought to be a book about visualisation, but it is far more than this. Exercise was also a mainstay of treatment. The book is full of useful insights.

How Your Mind Can Heal Your Body
By David R Hamilton
Hay House UK: 2018
This is a book about visualisation, a technique which has been used by many cancer sufferers with success. The book gives up-to-date scientific evidence on studies supporting its use. There is a chapter on cancer with inspiring stories and information on specific visualisations which can be used. The book is easy to read, and perhaps the most useful section is an appendix which give specific visualisations for a variety of diseases.

You Can Heal Your Life
By Louise L Hay
Hay House: 1984
Louise Hay used the methods outlined in her book to cure herself of cervical cancer and describes her beliefs. It includes a comprehensive section describing what she understands to be the message behind different illnesses and appropriate affirmations for these illnesses.

The Dynamic Laws of Healing
By Catherine Ponder
DeVorss & Company: 1999
This is a metaphysical approach to disease with many stories of healing and how people have used psycho-spiritual techniques and affirmations to heal themselves. It is strong on affirmations.

Appendix II

More on food and health

Neither gut bacteria nor food intolerance have been covered in the food chapters yet both have a far-reaching impact on health. Despite the good science behind them, these areas have been largely ignored by mainstream medicine so it is important to include them here.

Gut bacteria

One of the fastest-growing areas of knowledge in medicine concerns the microbes in our gut, with over 20,000 studies in the last 10 years. One of the fascinating discoveries of the American Microbiome Project was that most illness starts in the gut and we do not fully recover until our microbiome has recovered.[1]

The microbiome is the collection of bacteria living in our gut. It is responsible for 85% of our immunity and 38% of the molecules circulating in our bloodstream at any one time. For a healthy microbiome we need to have both a high number and a high diversity of beneficial bacteria. These normally keep any harmful bacteria or fungi under control.

The major proportion of the microbiome is made up of families of bacteria called bacteroidetes and firmicutes; these represent 90% of the total. The ratio is critical and, the higher the ratio of bacteroidetes to firmicutes, the better it is for our health. Firmicutes are characteristically higher in people who are obese.[2]

We know that the microbiome of those living on a western diet differs significantly from the microbiome of rural Africans with the western microbiome having less diversity of bacteria and, in particular, more firmicutes.

Unfortunately, many of today's medicines damage the microbiome: these include antibiotics, acid-blocking drugs, the contraceptive pill, vaccinations, steroids, anti-inflammatory drugs and chemotherapy drugs. Other factors that are harmful to the microbiome include a diet high in sugar and gluten and one low in vegetables and fermented foods. Caesarian sections, bottle-feeding, chlorinated water and pesticide residues add to the problem. The bottom line is that if we want good health we have to look after our microbiome. It is fundamental to good health.

Why should these microbes be so important, though? Firstly, there are a lot of them (about 100 trillion), compromising 10,000 species. Our own cells are greatly outnumbered by microbial cells and our DNA is greatly outnumbered by bacterial DNA. This complex collection of microbes acts like an organ within our body. If the balance within the microbiome is good, we stay healthy; if not, we will likely develop disease.

These microbes are chemical factories and can act like a friend or a foe. In an optimum state they produce useful vitamins, like vitamin K which protects against heart disease, valuable neurotransmitters, like serotonin which protects against depression, and short-chain fatty acids like butyric acid, which protect against colon cancer. The microbiome can also aid digestion, regulate the immune system and detoxify chemicals, taking the strain off our over-taxed livers.

Conversely, when the microbiome is out of balance it can produce highly inflammatory substances, including cytokines and lipopolysaccharides (LPS), and dangerous short-chain fatty acids, like proprionic acid, known to be toxic to the brain.

The fact that a change of microbiome can change our health

was demonstrated dramatically in a landmark study by Dr Nieuwdorp and colleagues from the University of Amsterdam.[3] He was able to reverse many of the markers of diabetes in 250 diabetic patients by using microbial faecal transplants from donors without diabetes. Now this is an entirely new way to treat chronic illness, and it is still very early days, but clearly our bacterial flora have a profound influence on us, one that goes far beyond anything that we previously imagined.

How then do we promote a healthy microbiome? A good way is through diet. A low-carbohydrate diet, with a high proportion of vegetables, is ideal. The fibre from vegetables that we can't digest acts as food for beneficial microbes. Onions, garlic, artichokes, leeks and asparagus are particularly useful. Fermented foods, such as sauerkraut and kefir, add beneficial microbes to our gut flora.

In the past, we humans ingested small amounts of useful bacteria from the soil and from eating freshly-picked and unwashed food.

Fasting also supports a healthy microbiome while fascinatingly, exercise increases bacteroidetes and reduces firmicutes.[4]

We can also add probiotics (combinations of beneficial bacteria are now widely available at health-food stores and supermarkets), but be aware that many of the live-yoghurt products are high in unhealthy sugars and processed milk derivatives. Probiotics are useful in the short term but, unless you eat foods to support the bacteria they contain, they will ultimately be a waste of money. Ideally, probiotics should be rotated so we develop more diversity in the microbiome.

Dr David Perlmutter in the *Brain Maker* has found that using high quantities of probiotics through an enema has been one of the most powerful interventions he has used in 30 years of practice.[5]

Sometimes gut bacteria can damage health in unexpected ways. There has been a profusion of publications in the last 10 years linking harmful organisms with arthritic conditions. This is thought to be caused by molecular mimicry. An example is the immune system creating antibodies against the bacterium *Klebsiella*, which then cross-react with the antigen HLA B27, damaging spinal ligaments and triggering ankylosing spondylitis. Other examples include rheumatoid arthritis being linked with the protozoa (parasitic amoeba), *Naegleria*,[6] and with the bacterium *Proteus mirabilis*;[7] reactive arthritis being linked with *Yersinia*,[8] *Shigella*,[8] *Chlamydia*,[8] and *Campylobacter*[8] and polyarthritis being linked with *Strongyloides stercoralis*.[9] It may take specialised testing to reveal these.

Some conditions such as autism are almost always accompanied by a highly abnormal gut flora and marked gut symptoms. It is now well understood that toxins released from harmful microbes damage the brain and this is thought to be a likely mechanism in autism. Typically, autistic children can handle protein, fats, most fruit and non-starchy vegetables but are made markedly worse, in terms of gut symptoms and autistic behaviour, by sugar and complex carbohydrates. Gluten and milk can also trigger symptoms. These foods are not broken down normally and act as building blocks for inflammatory chemicals.[10]

The 'specific carbohydrate' diet (also used for ulcerative colitis) and the 'gut and psychology' (GAPs) diet, which remove these from the diet, are effective but complex treatments for healing the microbiome in autism. It typically takes two years for them to be effective. The GAPs diet (a refinement of the specific carbohydrate diet) was developed by Dr Natasha Campbell-McBride, a neurologist and author of many books, after her son developed autism. He made a complete recovery as have many others who have used this regime. It is a classic survivor story of having to find a new way to treat an illness that has no satisfactory treatment.[11]

Many other childhood brain conditions, such as attention

deficit disorder (ADHD),[12] and adult disorders such as schizophrenia, have been linked to abnormal gut flora.[13]

As we can see, and as Hippocrates wisely commented so many years ago, most diseases start in the gut. The microbiome project has now confirmed his observations. Certainly, the gut is central to the healing of many diseases.

Food intolerance

Even healthy foods can cause illness if we become intolerant to them. Pioneers in this field have often achieved results far exceeding those from standard treatments. The reason is that recovery from some illnesses will only occur after the offending foods have been removed from the diet. These illnesses include some cases of eczema, irritable bowel syndrome, Crohn's disease, ulcerative colitis, rheumatoid arthritis (RA) and migraine. Conversely, in any chronic illness, if the causative foods continue to be eaten then the illness will remain in place. Finding food intolerances can therefore make a profound difference.

Rheumatoid arthritis serves as an example. A trial published in the *Lancet* in 1986 found 75% of patients with the condition experienced major improvements or became totally well after eliminating foods they were intolerant of.[14] Another major trial, done in three environmental control units in the USA, produced similar results: 80% had fair to excellent responses after removal of foods they were intolerant of. The remaining 20% of non-responders were those who had received prolonged steroid treatment.[15, 16] Wheat, corn and animal proteins were the foods which most often triggered arthritis.

Two later studies of food intolerance in RA were negative but these were seriously flawed as they did not eliminate grains, known to be the most potent trigger for the condition.[17] A further study from the University of Oslo compared those on an exclusion diet with controls. Those on the diet had highly significant improvements in joint swelling and pain and in blood test results.[18]

These results, taken as a whole, are impressive, confirming RA responds well to the detection and elimination of food intolerances. It is surprising and disappointing that such an effective treatment remains hidden away in medical archives, virtually unused by conventional medicine.

Sometimes food exclusion can produce spectacular results. Tom Warren was diagnosed as having Alzheimer's disease in 1983. Even when your mind is sharp it is difficult enough to arrest a major disease, but to do so when your mind is failing is even more challenging. There was much to learn and many lifestyle changes for him to negotiate.

He read voraciously but forgot most of what he read within a short space of time. However, one thing made an impression on him. Dr Bernard Zussman described a patient with a hole in his skull following an operation. This patient observed that when he ate foods he was allergic to his brain would swell, expanding out through the hole in his skull. Warren wondered if this could apply to him. He experimented and discovered he was intolerant to sugar, wheat flour, coffee, fruit juices, colourings and monosodium glutamate (MSG). Like many survivors, he found there were several factors contributing to his illness and he knew that he needed to tackle all of them: toxicity from his mercury fillings, food intolerances, and poor nutrition (his absorption was impaired due to low stomach acid). He initially dealt with the mercury toxicity using chelation, but when this failed, he had his amalgams removed. Of course, not everyone with Alzheimer's has food intolerances or mercury toxicity, but if this is the cause then that is what must be dealt with. After 18 months he was substantially improved and after four years his CAT scan indicated his disease had gone into remission.[19]

Food intolerance is almost never considered as a treatment by mainstream medicine despite the fact that detailed and well-referenced works on the subject exist.[20] Suffice it to say that many patients are not doing nearly as well as they should, partly due to the medical profession's lack of understanding of food intolerance. Although this subject is beyond the scope of this book, it does illustrate what could be achieved if we used currently-existing knowledge and relied less on a narrow pharmaceutical approach.

Appendix III

The use of supplements

We all know that eating fruit and vegetables is good for us yet the amount we eat is declining. With supplements the story is different; we are using more and more of them. For good health it might be better if it was the other way around. Ideally, we should not need supplements. Long-lived and healthy populations don't use them. Food should give us all the nutrients we need. Combination of nutrients found in foods work synergistically unlike those in supplements. Supplements can never give us all the benefits of good food.

In addition, supplements have many potentially toxic ingredients such as excipients (inactive substances added to pills). These include binders and fillers. Supplements can be heated, crushed, irradiated and fumigated. Generally speaking, capsules, liquids and powders are preferable to tablets and the more natural the supplement the better. Recent work shows that food from plants has energetic properties thought to augment healing. These again are absent from supplements. However, many survivors, especially those with cancer, have used supplements extensively so we must explore this important area.

In today's world, supplements are needed. Almost everybody has nutritional deficiencies. Studies have found 85% of the population is deficient in at least one mineral. The National

Health and Nutrition Examination Survey (NHANES)[1] between 2007 and 2010 showed high levels of nutritional deficiencies in the US population. For instance, 94% of people surveyed were deficient in vitamin D, 88.5% in vitamin E, 67% in vitamin K, 52% in magnesium, 44% in calcium deficient and 43% in vitamin A. In the UK, the National Diet and Nutrition Survey[2] also found micronutrient deficiencies were common.

There are several reasons for this. The soil has become increasingly deficient in minerals and these, in turn, lead to deficiencies in our food. Storage of foods causes further vitamin and mineral loss. This is happening at a time when the body requires more nutrients than ever before, not least to detoxify pollutants present in the environment and food. In practice it has become nearly impossible to obtain all the minerals we need from today's food. Let's look at examples of some nutrients which have potentially life-changing benefits.

Vitamin C

One of the most controversial areas in cancer care has been the use of intravenous infusions of nutrients by alternative practitioners, particularly vitamin C. Even though there have been international conferences on the use of vitamin C in cancer, this topic is still hotly debated.

The perfect cancer treatment would kill cancer cells and leave healthy cells unharmed (or perhaps healthier). Vitamin C comes close to achieving this.

Vitamin C was first noted to kill cancer cells as long ago as 1969.[3] More importantly, it *selectively* kills cancer cells. Cancer cells are thought to absorb the vitamin C, causing them to release hydrogen peroxide which then destroys them.[4] Mice with cancer given vitamin C or a raw vegetable diet lived 20 times longer than controls.[5] Vitamin C also enhances cell-mediated immunity and increases synthesis of interferon (an antiviral signalling protein). Cancer patients are typically deficient in vitamin C so it seems extremely plausible that it should help.

Ewan Cameron, a consultant surgeon at the Vale of Leven Hospital in Scotland and a Fellow of the Royal College of Surgeons, became interested in vitamin C in the 1970s whilst searching for something to help his incurable cancer patients. He experimented with a combination of intravenous and oral vitamin C. Some of his patients responded dramatically. Here was another great observation by an astute doctor. These are the type of observations that have the potential to change medicine.

He followed his initial findings up by conducting two trials on terminal cancer patients, working with two-time Nobel prize winner, Linus Pauling. Pauling knew that most animals produced their own vitamin C but humans had lost this ability. He also knew that they increased production of this vitamin when ill or under stress. A goat normally produces about 1 gram of vitamin C daily, but increases this to 10 grams per day during illness. He reasoned we would do the same if we had the capacity.

The first trial matched 100 terminal cancer patients given 10 grams of intravenous vitamin C with 1000 control patients, also with terminal cancer, given routine treatment. The results were significant: those in the vitamin C group lived, on average, 4.2 times longer. A small number of the terminal patients given vitamin C survived long-term; none in the control group did so.[6] A second trial compared 296 incurable cancer patients given vitamin C with 1532 matched controls who had similar cancers. Again, survival time was much greater in the vitamin C group and the results were highly significant.[7]

However, controversy was soon to follow. Dr Moertel, a vitamin C sceptic, did his own trial which seemingly showed no benefit. It soon became apparent, however, that his trial had major flaws. Many patients did not receive the full amount of vitamin C, others received it for too short a time or had the treatment stopped when symptoms appeared (see below). Linus

Pauling suspected foul play, famously declaring 'the war against cancer is largely a fraud'.

But what struck Ewan Cameron about vitamin C treatment was not so much the prolonged survival but the sense of wellbeing and enhanced quality of life that followed. Others have noted the same.

Cameron was not the only one to find that vitamin C helped in cancer. Dr Hugh Riordan, an American doctor, started using intravenous vitamin C for cancer after a patient with metastatic renal cancer, having heard about Cameron's work, approached him for treatment with vitamin C. Fifteen months later this patient had no signs of cancer. Impressed, Riordan went on to treat others this way and described seven cases of metastatic cancer treated with intravenous vitamin C: five recovered, one died (from pancreatic cancer) with a greatly extended survival and another died from an unrelated condition.[8] Other studies followed: Hoffer and Pauling reviewed 134 patients who had received 12 grams of oral vitamin C daily or placebo. The vitamin C group lived 21 times longer.[9] The same authors then looked at cancer patients given vitamin C combined with other nutrients and found even better survival times with 50% of the vitamin C group surviving over five years.[9]

Abram Hoffer was a psychiatrist, with an interest in nutrition. He originally used vitamin C combined with other nutrients to treat several of his psychiatric patients who had developed inoperable cancer. Some cases were dramatic. A 16-year-old girl with Ewing's sarcoma was due to have her arm amputated to remove her tumour. Hoffer gave her 3 grams of vitamin C and 3 grams of niacinamide (vitamin B3) daily. She recovered and never did have the amputation. This patient received a surprisingly low dose of vitamin C. Hoffer more commonly gave 12 to 40 grams daily. He gave this orally, combined with other nutrients.

Word got around and he was soon inundated with cancer

patients requesting treatment, mostly people with advanced cancer. Eventually he went on to treat over 1000 cancer patients. His survival rates were between 72% and 77 % at one year and between 23% and 46% at five years. Standard treatments gave survival rates between 24% and 28% at one year and between 5% and 11% at five years.[9]

Dr Murata treated 99 terminal cancer patients with vitamin C in two hospitals in Japan between 1973 and 1977 (oral, supplemented by intravenous) and found they had an average life expectancy of 246 days compared with 43 days in controls.[10] Case-control studies had also observed that high-dose vitamin C causes regression of tumours.[11, 12]

Consider the following case. Philip was a 60-year-old industrial designer who developed cancer in his neck. Surgery and radiotherapy failed to stem the cancer and left him, in his own words, a physical wreck. Hearing of the work of Cameron, he persuaded his doctors (he lived in Switzerland) to give him intravenous vitamin C. On the fifth day of treatment he began to feel much better. By the 10th day he switched to oral vitamin C. Six week later, a dramatic event occurred. His whole neck swelled up and he naturally assumed his cancer had returned, but, oddly, this change was accompanied by a feeling of wellbeing. The swelling then started to diminish. After two months the swelling had disappeared and later, he was confirmed to be cancer-free.[13]

Three things strike me about this controversy. Firstly, the amount of vitamin C used by Ewan Cameron was conservative (10 grams daily). Many alternative practitioners use 10 times this amount; some have gone up to 250 grams daily. I suspect the higher doses would work better, lead to more cures and a better prolongation of life. Adverse effects are extremely rare, even at these high doses, but testing for glucose-6-phoshate deficiency is necessary. The latter is rare but haemolysis can occur with large doses of intravenous vitamin C in patients with this condition, so it needs to be considered.

Secondly, what is remarkable about these infusions is the feeling of wellbeing that follows; this is so different to chemotherapy. Another feature is marked pain relief. Surely these features alone would justify its use? It is so much more humane than current cancer treatments.

Thirdly, the healing crisis experienced by Philip was fascinating; this is typical of what occurs when the body's immune system gets the upper hand. The symptoms get temporarily worse but the patient feels better. Yet in the Moertel trial, treatment was stopped as soon as symptoms occurred, at the very point when it should have been continued. We can learn so much by observing individual cases.

So where does this leave someone with cancer? Vitamin C is one of the most promising treatments available but infusions are not readily available. The jury is out about whether infusions are superior to oral treatment. Some think sustained oral treatment may be better than short doses of intravenous treatment and that once levels of vitamin C drop, then resistance of cancer cells is possible. However, Hoffer used oral treatment only.

As a GP with cancer sufferers among my patients, I think treatment by mouth has many advantages: it is readily available, cheap and relatively easy to use. It should be used up to bowel tolerance – this is the dose that gives mild diarrhoea – and then it should be slightly reduced. The aim is to get the maximum daily dose possible: ideally 10 to 30 grams per day. As levels of vitamin C drop 50% in two hours, the ideal is to give many doses spaced out over the day.

Most doctors working in this field would not recommend vitamin C alone and have found it works better when combined with other nutrients. Hoffer, for example, used 10-40 grams of vitamin C daily combined with vitamin B3 (300-3000 mg), vitamin B6 (2-300 mg), folic acid (1-30 mg), co-enzyme Q10 (300-600 mg), selenium (200-1000 mcg), zinc (25-100 mg), mixed carotenoids (as carrot juice), a multivitamin/multimineral and a calcium/

magnesium supplement. He also stopped junk food in the diet.

Chemosensitivity testing also supports the use of vitamin C. This blood test, though expensive, can be useful in cancer. It allows the cancer to be tested against a variety of chemotherapy agents but also against nutrients. Using this method, 95% of cancers have been found to respond to vitamin C. To sum up, there is now compelling evidence that vitamin C should become part of the treatment of the great majority of patients with cancer.

Vitamin C has other uses too. In the 1940s, Dr Fred Klenner discovered it to be an effective agent against a wide range of viruses, including influenza, herpes, hepatitis, tetanus and polio. This was confirmed by Japanese researchers in the 1970s; they found vitamin C could inactivate most viruses in the test tube.[14] When used intravenously it hastens recovery in chronic hepatitis.[15]

In 2016, researchers at the Eastern Virginia Medical School compared the effect of different approaches on patients treated for sepsis at their intensive care unit. Of these patients, 47 patients were given standard treatment and 47 were given intravenous vitamin C together with thiamine and hydrocortisone. They found 4.5% of the vitamin C patients died compared with 40.4% of those given standard treatment, a reduction in death rate of 500%.[16]

Here we have a treatment of immense value, especially for viruses. At the moment there is virtually nothing in modern medicine's arsenal available to treat viruses. Vitamin C could do for viral infections what antibiotics did for bacterial infections. Despite this, it is almost never used in these situations.

I remember a patient of mine, a man in his early 30s, who was admitted to hospital with a serious viral infection. There was no effective treatment and he subsequently died. I often wondered what would have happened if he had been given a simple, cheap vitamin C infusion. The scientific knowledge that could have saved his life already existed, but doctors were unaware of it.

Sadly the situation is no better today. Certainly, it would have been worth a try.

You can watch youtube: *Vitamin C: The Miracle Swine Flu Cure.* It describes a New Zealand farmer who developed swine flu and was given up for dead. However, the family insisted the doctors try vitamin C before switching off his life support. The story documents how he improved each time he was given vitamin C, the difficulties he had in receiving this inexpensive and effective treatment, the deterioration when doctors forbade the treatment and his eventual recovery. As ever with medicine, it is not that we don't have the answers, it is bias and ignorance that prevent their use.

However, there is an even more remarkable story about vitamin C that needs to be told. On 11th March 2011 a major earthquake hit Japan. This earthquake was so severe that it seriously damaged the Fukushima nuclear power plant and released dangerously large amounts of radioactive caesium into the atmosphere (168 times more than released from the Hiroshima bomb). Even today, nine years later, the area is out of bounds and access is prohibited within 20 km of the plant. Doctors were concerned about protecting emergency workers, who were still going into the plant, and also the local population. In the meantime, the government issued bland reassurances. In reality they predicted that the radioactive discharge would lead to an excess of 25,000 cancers.

Doctors led by Dr Atsuo Yanagishawa started to look for answers. At this point they didn't know what to do. However, they came across a key piece of research. It was a study on mice exposed to radiation. As we shall see, it was truly ground-breaking. In this study, the mice in one group were given a large dose of radiation. They all died, succumbing to lethal gastrointestinal syndrome. A second group of mice were given the same dose of radiation but only after they had received 150 grams per kilogram of body weight of vitamin C for three days.

Of these, 60% survived two weeks, and the 42% who survived 24 days all survived long-term. This study concluded that vitamin C gave significant and often life-saving protection from radiation.[17]

This is in keeping with what we know about the effects of radiation: only 20% of the damage caused by radiation is from its direct impact; 80% occurs later. This secondary damage is due to reactive oxygen created by the radiation which in turn produces massive damage to genes and cell membranes. Vitamin C can prevent this secondary damage if given at an equivalent dose in humans (about 8 to 10 grams daily). The authors of the study realised how crucial this information could be, if there was ever to be a nuclear incident in the future. No other treatment exists that could help.

Dr Yanagishawa and his colleagues sent out press releases; they expected it would provoke intense media interest. However, there was silence; no one wanted to know. Nevertheless, they gave preventative doses of vitamin C to the emergency workers. They went on to conduct tests on them. Despite the treatment, five out of 16 emergency workers developed pre-cancerous genetic changes. In response to this, the Japanese doctors treated them with intravenous vitamin C and other antioxidants, such as selenium and alpha-lipoic acid. In every case, the genetic changes reverted to normal within two months. In stark contrast to what happened at Chernobyl, all the emergency workers survived and remained well. It was a first for science.[18]

This incident proved that vitamin C and other anti-oxidants can not only prevent radiation damage but can reverse genetic damage brought about by radiation.

Alpha-lipoic acid

Alpha-lipoic acid was one of the antioxidants used by the Japanese doctors; it has an impressive record itself and deserves a mention. People who ingest the amanita group of mushrooms (the commonest being the 'deathcap') normally die rapidly or need a liver transplant. Forty years ago, American physician, Dr Burt Berkson, developed a protocol for treating these patients with intravenous alpha-lipoic acid. He researched this method between 1974 and 1978 and this led to 67 full recoveries and eight patients dying.[19] The time lapse between the mushroom poisoning and giving the intravenous alpha-lipoic acid proved critical to recovery.

Sadly, this highly successful treatment has been ignored by medicine ever since, even though in this case it was undoubtedly life-saving. Dr Berkson also used intravenous alpha-lipoic acid in acute hepatic necrosis on a variety of occasions, with equally dramatic results, saving these patients from liver transplantation. He also used it successfully in chronic hepatitis C infections.

Glutathione

Glutathione infusions have been found to be remarkably effective in Parkinson's disease. A study of patients given twice daily intravenous glutathione for 30 days found it reduced disability by 42%, and after these infusions the benefit lasted for two to four months.[20] Dr David Perlmutter, an American neurologist who uses this treatment, describes it as nothing short of miraculous. It has no reported side effects. Many patients improved rapidly in as little as 15 minutes. As with vitamin C, the treatment is accompanied by a general feeling of wellbeing. He has seen patients who no longer need to use their wheelchairs after receiving this treatment.

Normally Parkinson's disease is extremely difficult to treat. Like vitamin C, glutathione infusions are rarely used, principally because of the prevailing bias against nutritional treatments rather for any reason connected to good science. Of course, nutritional remedies cannot be patented and there is little financial gain in promoting their use; cynics believe this is the reason behind the bias. However, I think lack of familiarity and teaching also play a part.

Macular degeneration

Macular degeneration, another disease which is extremely difficult to treat conventionally, has been found to respond well to nutrient infusions (particularly those containing zinc, selenium and taurine). Practitioners who use these methods report that over half the patients given these infusions, together with oral supplements, have sustained improvements in visual acuity, usually starting after four to six weeks. Those taking just oral supplements have not fared as well.[21]

The problem as ever, in medicine, is not so much finding successful treatments but making this knowledge more widely known and available.

Conclusion

This is a brief look at a big topic. Determining which supplements are best for any disease is beyond the scope of this book. What we can say is that fighting cancer without supplements or high-quality foods is like fighting a disease with one hand tied behind your back.

References

Introduction

1. Foster HD. Lifestyle changes and the "Spontaneous" Regression of Cancer: An Initial Computer Analysis. *Int J Biosocial Res* 1988; 10(1): 17-33

2. Price W. *Nutrition and Physical Degeneration*. La Mesa, California, USA: Price-Pottenger Nutrition Foundation; 1939.

3. Visintainer MA, Volpicelli JR, Seligman ME. Tumour rejection in rats after inescapable and escapable shock. *Science* 1982; 216(4544): 437-439.

4. Boik J. *Natural Compounds in Cancer Therapy*. Oregon, USA: Oregon Medical Press; 2001.

5. Bredesen D, *The End of Alzheimers*. London, UK: Vermillion; 2017.

6. Nussbaum E. *Recovery from Cancer*. New York, USA: Square One Publishers; 2004.

7. Pleshette J. *Cures that Work*. London, UK: Arrow Books Limited; 1986.

8. Hill N, Stone WC. Success through a positive mental attitude. (CDs/audio) UK: Thorsons; USA: Nightingale Conant, 1997.

9. Steward F, Wibberley G. Drug Innovation: What's slowing it down? *Nature* 1980; 284: 118-120.

10. Sattar N, Preiss D, Murray HM, et al. Statins and risk of incident diabetes: a collaborative meta-analysis of randomised statin trials. *Lancet* 2010; 375(9716): 735-742.

11. Fabian CJ, Kimler BF, Hursting SD. Omega 3 fatty acids for breast cancer prevention. *Breast Cancer Research* 2015; 17: 62.

12. Hin-Peng L. Diet and Breast Cancer: An epidemiological

perspective. *Critic Rev Oncol Haematol* 1998; 28(2): 115-119.

13. Atoum M, Alzoughool F. Vitamin D and Breast Cancer: Latest Evidence and Future Steps. *Breast Cancer* 2017; 11: 1-8. doi: 13.1177/1178223417749816

14. Wu K, Helzisouer KJ, Comnstock GW, et al. A Prospective study on folate, B12 and pyridoxal-5-phosphate (B6) and breast cancer. *Cancer Epidemiology, Biomarkers and Prev* 1999; 8(3): 209-217.

15. Self-reported chemicals exposure, beliefs about disease causation, and risk of breast cancer in the Cape Cod Breast Cancer Study: a case-control study. *Environ Health* 2010; 9(4): 40.

16. Lopez-Carillo L, Hernandez-Ramirez RU, Calafat AM, et al. Exposure to phthalates and breast cancer risk in northern Mexico. *Environ Health Perspect* 2010; 118: 539-544.

17. Crouse DC, Goldberg MS, Ross NA. Postmenopausal breast cancer is associated with exposure to traffic-related air pollution in Montreal, Canada: a case-control study. *Environ Health Perspect* 2010; 118: 1578-1583.

18. Colditz GA, Hankinson SE, Hunter DJ, et al. The use of estrogens and progestins and risk of breast cancer in postmenopausal women. *N Eng J Med* 1995; 332: 1589-1593.

19. Langman L, Burr HS. Electromagnetic studies in women with malignancy of cervix uteri. *Obstetric and Gynaecology Survey* 1947; 2(5): 714-721.

Chapter 1: Using food to cure

1. Wahls T. *The Wahls Protocol*. New York, USA: Penguin Group; 2014.
2. Foster HD. Lifestyle changes and the "Spontaneous" Regression of Cancer: An Initial Computer Analysis. *Int J Biosocial Res* 1988; 10(1): 17-33.
3. Nussbaum E. *Recovery from Cancer*. New York, USA: Square One Publishers; 2004.
4. Bohan B. *The Choice*. London, UK: Element; 2005.
5. Price W. *Nutrition and Physical Degeneration*. La Mesa, California, USA: Price-Pottenger Nutrition Foundation; 1939.
6. McCarrison R. *Nutrition and Health*. London, UK. The McCarrison Society; 1936.
7. Kenton L, Kenton S. *Raw Energy: eat your way to radient health*. UK: Arrow Books Ltd; 1986.
8. Plant J. *Your Life in Your Hands*. London, UK: Virgin Books Ltd; 2003.

References

9. Rowlands MA, Gunnell D, Harris R, et al. Circulating insulin-like growth factor peptides and prostate cancer risk: a systematic review and meta-analysis. *Int J Cancer* 2009; 124 (10): 2416-2429.

10. Gonzalez N. The Enzyme Therapy of Cancer. Conference at the Royal Society of Medicine. 18 April 2009.

11. Somers S. *Knockout*. New York, USA: Harmony Books; 2009: Chapter 8 – Dr Nicholas Gonzalez.

12. Cohen JH, Kristal AR, Stanford JL, et al. Fruit and Vegetable Intakes and Prostate Cancer Risk. *J Natl Cancer Inst* 2000; 92(1): 61-68.

13. Zhang SM, Hunter DJ, Rosner BA, et al. Intakes of Fruits, Vegetables and related Nutrients and the Risk of Non-Hodgkin's lymphoma Among Women. *Cancer Epidemiol Biomarker Prev* 2000; 9: 477-485.

14. Giovannucci E, Michels KB, et al. Fruit, Vegetables, Dietary Fibre and Risk of Colorectal Cancer. *J Natl Cancer Inst* 2001; 93(7): 525-533.

15. Zhang M, Huang J, Xie X, et al. Dietary intakes of mushrooms and green tea combine to reduce the risk of breast cancer in Chinese women. *Int J Cancer* 2009; 124(6): 1404-1408.

16. Eliassen AH, Liao X, Rosner BA, et al. Plasma carotenoids and the risk of breast cancer over 20 year of follow-up. *Am J Nutr* 2015; 101(6): 1197-1205.

17. Farvid MS, Chen WY, Rosner BA, et al. Fruit and vegetable consumption and breast cancer incidence: Repeated measures over 30 years of follow-up. *Int J Cancer* 2019; 144(7): 1496-1510.

18. Desai G, Schelske-Santos M, Nazario CM, et al. Onion and Garlic and Breast Cancer, a Case-control Study in Puerto Rico. *Nutr Cancer* 2019; 12: 1-10. doi:10.1080/01635581.2019.1651349

19. Lowcock EC, Cotterchio M, Boucher BA. Consumption of flaxseed, a rich source of lignans, is associated with reduced breast cancer risk. *Cancer Causes Control* 2013; 24(4): 813-816.

20. Brasky TM, Lampe JW, Patter JD, et al. Speciality supplements and breast cancer risk in the VITamins and Lifestyle (VITAL) Cohort. *Cancer Epidemiol Biomarkers Prev* 2017; 19(7): 1696-1708.

21. Lof M, Sandin S, Lagiou P, et al. Fruit and vegetable intake and risk of cancer in the Swedish women's lifestyle and health cohort. *Cancer Causes Control* 2011; 22(2): 283-289.

22. Boivin D, Lamy S, Lord-Dufour S, et al. Antiproliferative and antioxidant effect of common vegetables: a comparative study. *Food Chem* 2009; 112: 374-380.

23. Zhang NQ, Ho SC, Mo XF, at al. Glucosinolate and isothiocyanate intakes are inversely associated with breast cancer risk: a case-control study in China. *Br J Nutr* 2018; 119(8): 957-964.

24. Kolonel LN, Hankin JH, Whittemore AS, et al. Vegetables, Fruits, Legumes and Prostate Cancer: A Multi-ethnic Case-Control Study. *Cancer Epidemiol Biomarkers Prev* 2000; 9: 795-804.

25. Brown LM, Gridley G, Pattern LM, et al. Diet and Nutrition as Risk Factors for Multiple Myeloma Among Black and Whites in the United States. *Cancer Causes Control* 2001; 12: 117-125.

26. Budhathoki S, Hidaki A, Yamaji T, et al. Plasma 25-hydroxyvitamin D concentration and subsequent risk of total and site-specific cancers in Japanese population: large case-cohort study within Japan Public Health Center-based Prospective Study cohort. *Br Med J* 2018; 360: k671.

27. Buijsse B, Feskens EJ, Schlettwein-Gsell D, et al. Plasma carotene and alpha-tocopherol in relationship to 10 yr all-cause and cause-specific mortality in European elderly: The survey in Europe on Nutrition and the Elderly, a Concerted Action (SENECA). *Am J Clin Nutr* 2005; 82(4): 876-886.

28. Khadge S, Thiele GM, Sharp JG, et al. Long-chain omega 3 polyunsaturated fatty acids decrease mammary tumour growth, multi-organ metastasis and enhance survival. *Clinic Exp Metastasis* 2018; 35(8): 797-818.

29 Benade L, Howard T, Burk D. Synergistic killing of Ehrich Ascites Carcinoma Cells by Ascorbic Acid and 3-Amino-1,2,4-triazole. *Oncology* 1969; 23: 33-43.

30. Doskey CM, Buranasudja V, Wagner BA, et al. Tumour cells have decreased ability to metabolize H2O2: Implications for pharmacological ascorbate in cancer therapy. *Redox Biol* 2016; 10: 274-284.

31. Rock CL, Natarajan L, Pu M, et al. *Longitudinal biological exposure to carotenoids is associated with breast cancer-free survival in the Women's Healthy Eating and Living Study*; and, Braakhus AJ, Campion P, Bishop KS. Reducing Breast Cancer recurrence: The role of dietary Polyphenolics *Cancer Epidemiol Biomarkers Prev* 2009; 18(2):486-494. doi: 10.1158/1055-9965.EPI-08-0809.

32. Chatenoud L, La Vecchia C, Franceschi S, et al. Refined-Cereal Intake and Risk of Selected Cancers in Italy. *Am J Clinic Nutr* 1999; 70: 1107-1110.

33. Bakker N. Adipose Fatty Acids and Cancers of the Breast, Prostate and Colon: An Ecological Study. *In J Cancer* 1997; 72: 587-591.
34. Johnson K. Dairy Products linked to Ovarian Cancer Risk. *Family Practice News* 2000; 8: 34619.
35. Nguyen T, Duran RV. Glutamine metabolism in cancer therapy. *Cancer Drug Resist* 2018; 1: 126-138.
36. Henslet CT, Wasti AT, DeBerardinis RJ. Glutamine and Cancer: Cell Biology, Physiology and Clinical Opportunities. *J Clin Invest* 2013; 123: 3678-3684.
37. Nanba H. Maitake D Fraction: healing and preventative potential for Cancer. *J Orthomol Med* 1997; 12: 43-49.
38. Patel S, Goyal A. Recent developments in mushroom as anti-cancer therapeutics. *3 Biotec* 2012; 2(1): 1-15.
39. Yang P, Liang M, Zhang Y, et al. Clinical application of a combination of lentinon, multi-electrode RFA and TACE in HCC. *Adv Therap* 2008; 25: 787.
40. Bright S. Biobran and the fight to empower the immune system. JAFRA 2006.

Chapter 2: Food and health

1. GBD 2013 Rick Factors Collaborators. Global, regional and national comparative risk assessment of 79 behavioural, environmental and occupational and metabolic risks of clusters or risks in 188 countries, during 1990-2013: a systematic analysis for the Global Burden of Disease Study 2013. *The Lancet* 2015; 386: 2287-2323. doi: 10.1016/S0140-6736(15)00128-2.
2. Sanchez A, Reeser JA, Lau HS, et al. Role of sugars in human neutrophil phagocytosis. *Am J Clin Nutr* 1973; 26: 1180-1184.
3. Ringsdorf WM Jr, Cheraskin E, Ramsay RR Jr, et al. Sucrose, neutrophilic phagocytosis and resistance to disease. *Dent Surv* 1976; 52(12): 46-48.
4. Nalder BN, Mahoney AW, Ramakrishnan R, et al. Sensitivity of the immunological response to nutritional status in rats. *J Nutr* 1972; 102: 535-542.
5. Demetrokopoulos GE, Brennan MF. Tumoricidal Potential of Nutritional Manipulation. *Cancer Res* 1982; 42(Suppl): 756s-765s.
6. Stattin P, Bjor O, Ferrari P, et al. Prospective study of hyperglycaemia and cancer risk. *Diabetes Care* 2007; 30(3): 561-567.
7. Seeley S. Diet and breast cancer: the possible connection with sugar

consumption. *Med Hypothesis* 1983; 11(3): 319-327.

8. Saydah SH, Loria CM, Eberhardt MS et al. Abnormal glucose tolerance and the risk of cancer death in the United States. *Am J Epidemiol* 2003; 157: 1092-1100.

9. La Vecchia C, Negri E, Franceschi S, et al. A case-control study of diabetes and cancer risk. *Br J Cancer* 1994; 70: 950-953.

10. Chan JM, Stamfer MJ, Giovannucci E, et al. Plasma insulin-like growth factor-1 and prostate cancer risk: a prospective study. *Science* 1998; 279(5350): 563-566.

11. Goodwin PJ, Ennis M, Pritchard KI, et al. Fasting insulin and outcome in early-stage breast cancer: results of a prospective cohort study. *J Clinic Oncol* 2002; 20(1): 42-51.

12. Wolpin BM, Meyerhardt JA, Chan AT, et al. Insulin, insulin-like growth factor axis and mortality in patients with non-metastatic colorectal cancer. *J Clin Oncol* 2009; 27(2): 176-185.

13. Santisteban GA, Ely JT, Hamel EE, et al. Glycemic modulation of tumour tolerance in a mouse model of breast cancer. *Biochem Biophys Res Commun* 1985; 132(3): 1174-1179.

14. Pan J, Chen C, Yin Y, et al. Differential impact of structurally different anti-diabetic drugs on proliferation and chemosensitivity of acute lymphoblastic leukaemia cells. *Cell Cycle* 2012; 11(12): 2314-2326.

15. McGirt MJ, Chaichana KL, Gathinji M, et al. Persistent outpatient hyperglycaemia is independently associated with decreased survival after primary resection of malignant astrocytomas. *Neurosurgery* 2008; 63(2): 286-291.

16. Priebe A, Tan L, Wahl H, et al. Glucose deprivation activates AMPK and induces cell death through modulation of Akt in ovarian cancer cells. *Gynaec Oncol* 2011; 122: 389-395.

17. Shim H, Chun YS, Lewis BC, et al. A unique glucose-dependent apoptotic pathway induced by c-Myc. *Proc Natl Acad Sci USA* 1998; 95: 1511-1516.

18. Yang Q, Hang Z, Gregg EW. Added sugar intake and Cardiovascular Disease Mortality amongst US adults. *JAMA* 2014; 174(4): 516-524.

19. Levi F, Pasche C, Lucchini F, et al. Refined and whole grain cereals and the risk of oral, oesophageal and laryngeal cancer. *Eur J Clinic Nutr* 200; 54(6): 487-489.

20. Chatenoud L, La Vecchia C, Franceschi S, et al. Refined-cereal

intake and risk of selected cancers in Italy. *Amer J Clinic Nutr* 1999; 70(6): 1107-1110.

21. McRae MP. Health Benefits of Dietary Whole Grains: An Umbrella Review of Meta-analyses. *J Chiropr Med* 2017; 16(1): 10-18.

22. Ho VW, Leung K, Hsu A, et al. A low carbohydrate, high protein diet slows tumour growth and prevents cancer initiation. *Cancer Res* 2011; 71(13): 4484-4493.

23. Venkateswaran V, Haddad AQ, Fleshner NE, et al. Association of diet-induced hyperinsulinemia with accelerated growth of prostate cancer (LNCaP) xenografts. *J Natl Cancer Inst* 2007; 99(23): 1793-1800.

24. Shan Z, Rehm CD, Rogers G, et al. Trend in Dietary Carbohydrate, Protein and Fat Intake and Diet Quality Among US Adults, 1999-2016. *JAMA* 2019; 322(12): 1178-1187.

25. Hadjivassillou M, Grunewald RA, Davies-Jones GAB. Gluten sensitivity as a neurological illness. *J Neurol Neurosurg Psychiatry* 2002; 72(5): 560-563.

26. Stott-Miller ML, Stanford JL. Consumption of deep-fried food and risk of prostate cancer. *The Prostate* 2013; 73(9): 960-969. doi:10.1002/pros.22643

27. Aschero A, Willett WC. Health Effects of Trans Fats. *Am J Clinic Nutr* 1997; 66(Suppl): 1006S-1010S.

28. Mozaffarian D, Katan MB, Ascherio A. Trans Fatty Acids and cardiovascular disease. *N Eng J Med* 2006; 354: 1601-1613.

29. Dhaka V, Gulia N, Ahlawat KS, et al. Trans fats – sources, health risk and alternative approach. A review. *Food Sci Technol* 2011; 48(5): 534-541.

30. Chavarra JE, Minguez-Alarcon L, Mediola J, et al. Trans fatty acid intake is inversely related to total sperm count in young men. *Hum Reprod* 2012; 29(3): 429-440.

31. Hooper L, Martin W, Abdelhamid A. Cochrane Corner: What are the effects of reducing saturated fat intake on cardiovascular disease and mortality. *Heart* 2015; 101: 24. doi.org/10.10136/heartjnl-2015-308521

32. De Souza RJ, Mente A, Maroleanu A. Intake of saturated fatty acids and trans unsaturated fatty acids and risk of all-cause mortality, cardiovascular and type 2 diabetes: systematic review and meta-analysis of observational studies. *Br Med J* 2015; 351: h3978

33. Lawrence F. *Eat your Heart Out*. London, UK: Penguin Books; 2008: pp 223.
34. Deol P, Evans JR, Dhahbi J, et al. Soybean oil is more obesogenic and diabetogenic than coconut oil and fructose in mouse: Potential role for the liver. *Plos One* 2015; 10(7): e0132672.
35. Fiolet N, Srour B, Sellem L et al. Consumption of ultra-processed foods and cancer risk. *Br Med J* 2018; 360: 270-271.
36. Ershoff BH. Synergistic toxicity of food additives in rats fed a diet low in dietary fibre. *J Food Sci*1976; 41: 949-951.
37. McCann D, Barrett A, Cooper A, Crumpler D, Dalen L, Grimshaw K, et al. Food additives and hyperactive behaviour in 3-year-old and 8/9-year-old children in the community: a randomised, double-blinded, placebo-controlled trial. *The Lancet* 2007; 370: 1560-1567.
38. Pritchard C, Mayers A, Baldwin D. Changing pattern of neurological mortality in the 10 major developed countries 1979-2010. *Public Health* 2013; 127(4): 357-368.
39. Ahmed H, Abushouk A, Gabr H. Parkinson's disease and pesticides: a meta-analysis of disease connection and genetic alteration. *Biomed Pharamcother* 2017; 90: 638-649.
40. Bristow A. Organic processed food. *Which* 2002; April: 22-23.
41. Rohrmann S, Overvad K Bueno-de-Mesquita AB, et al. Meat consumption and mortality- results from the European Prospective Investigations into cancer and Nutrition. *BMC Med* 2013; 11: DOI: 63. 10.1186/1741-7015-11-63
42. Etamadi A, Sinha R, Ward MH, et al. Mortality from different causes associated with meat, heme iron, nitrates, and nitrites in the NIH-AARP Diet and Health Study: population based cohort study. *Br Med J* 2017; 357; j1957. DOI:10.1136/bmj.j1957
43. Thomas D. A Study of Mineral Depletion on the Foods available to us as a Nation over the period 1940-1991. *Nutr Health* 2003; 17(2): 85-115.
44. Key TJ, Appleby PN, Crowe FL, et al. Cancer in British vegetarians: updated analysis of 4998 incident cancers in a cohort of 32,491 meat eaters, 8612 fish eaters, 18,298 vegetarians and 2246 vegans. *Am J Clin Nutr* 2014; 100(suppl 1): 378S-385S.
45. Alfaia CPM, Alves SP, Martins SIV, et al. Effect of the feeding system on intramuscular fatty acids and conjugated linoleic acid isomers of beef cattle, with emphasis on their nutritional value

and discriminatory ability. *Food Chemistry* 2009; 114: 939-946.
46. Yang A, Lanari MC, Brewster M, et al. Lipid stability and meat colour of beef from pasture- and grain-fed cattle with or without vitamin E supplement. *Meat Science* 2002; 60: 41-50.
47. Insani EM, Eyherabide A, Grigioni G, et al. Oxidative stability and its relationship with natural antioxidants during refrigerated retail display of beef produced in Argentina. *Meat Science* 2008; 79: 444-452.
48. Yang A, Brewster MJ, Lanari MC, et al. Effect of vitamin E supplementation on a-tocopherol and ß-carotene concentrations from tissues of pasture- and grain-fed cattle. *Meat Science* 2002; 60: 35-40.
49. Daley CA, Abbott A, Doyle PS. Review of fatty acid profiles and antioxidant content in grass-fed and grain-fed beef. *Nutr J* 2010; 9(1): 10.
50. Lymbery P. *Dead Zone*. London, UK: Bloomsbury Publishing; 2017: chapter 5.
51. Ewald J. Chicken and obesity. *Life and Health Network* https://lifeandhealth.org/nutrition/chicken-and-obesity/093184.html (accessed 5 February 2020)
52. Wang Y, Lehane C, Ghebremeskel K, et al. Modern organic and broiler chickens sold for human consumption provide more energy from fat than protein. *Public Health Nutr* 2010; 13(3): 400-408.
53. Sirri F, Castellini C, Bianchi M, et al. Effects of fast-, medium- and slow-growing strains on meat quality of chickens reared under the organic farming method. *Animal* 2009; 5: 312-319.
54. Rohrmann S, Linseisen J, Nöthlings U, Overvad K. Meat and fish consumption and risk of pancreatic cancer: results from the European Prospective Investigation into Cancer and Nutrition. *Int J Cancer* 2013; 132(3): 617-624.
55. Rohrmann S, Linseisen J, Jakobsen MU. Consumption of meat and dairy and lymphoma risk in the European Prospective Investigation into Cancer and Nutrition. *Int J Cancer* 2011; 128(3): 623-634.
56. Johnson ES, Ndetan H, Lo KM. Cancer mortality in poultry slaughtering/processing plant workers belonging to a union pension fund. *Environ Res* 2010; 110(6): 588-594.
57. Lymbery P, Oakeshott I. *Farmaggedon*. London, UK: Bloomsbury Publishing Ltd; 2014: chapter 6.
58. Pickett H. Nutritional benefits of higher welfare products. 2012. www.compassioninfoodbusiness.com/media/5234769/

Nutritional-benefits-of-higher-welfare-animal-products-
June-2012.pdf (accessed 27 April 2020)

59. Snowdon DA. Animal product consumption and mortality because
    of all causes combined, coronary heart disease, strokes, diabetes,
    and cancer in Seventh-Day Adventists. *American Journal of Clinical
    Nutrition* 1988; 48(3): 739-748.

60. Tat D, Kenfield SA, Cowan JE,et al. Milk and other dairy foods in
    relation to prostate cancer recurrence: Data from the cancer of
    the prostate strategic urologic research endeavor (CaPSURE™).
    Prostate 2018 ; 78(1): 32-39.

61. Kroenke CH, Kwan ML, Sweeney C, et al. High- and Low-Fat Dairy
    Intake, Recurrence, and Mortality After Breast Cancer Diagnosis.
    JNCI J Natl Cancer Inst 2013; 105(9): 616-623. First published
    online: March 14, 2013.

62. Larsson SC, Bergkvist L, Wolk A. Milk and lactose intakes and
    ovarian cancer risk in the Swedish Mammography Cohort. *Am J
    Clin Nutr* 2004; 80(5): 1353-1357.

63. Jiang W, Ju C, Jiang H, et al. Dairy foods intake and the risk
    of Parkinson's disease: a dose-response meta-analysis of
    prospective cohort studies. *Eur J Epidemiol* 2014; 29(9): 613-619

64. Seely S. Diet and coronary disease: a survey of mortality and food
    consumption statistics of 24 countries. *Med Hypotheses* 1981; 7:
    907-918.

65. Grant WB. Milk and other dietary influences on coronary heart
    disease. *Alter Med Rev* 1998; 4: 281-294.

66. Potter JD. Your mother was right: eat your vegetables. *Asia Pacific J
    Clin Nutr* 2000; (9 Suppl): S10-S12.

67. Block G, Patterson B, Subar A. Fruit, vegetables, and cancer
    prevention: a review of the epidemiological evidence. *Nutr
    Cancer* 1992; 18: 1–29.

68. Oyebode O, Gordon-Dseagu V, Walker A, Mindell JS. Fruit and
    vegetable consumption and all-cause, cancer and CVD mortality:
    analysis of Health Survey for England data. *J Epidemiol Community
    Health* 2014; 68: 856-862. DOI:10.1136/jech-2013-203500

69. Thomas J, Sutcliffe K, Harden A, et al. EPPI Report: Children and
    Healthy Eating: A systematic review of barriers and facilitators.
    EPPI Centre, part of Social Science Research Unit, University of
    London; October 2003.

70. Beliveau R, Gingras D. *Foods to Fight Cancer*. London, UK: Dorling

Kindersley Limited; 2007.

71. Davis DR, Epp MD, Riordan HD. Changes is USDA food composition data for 43 garden crops, 1950 to 1999. *J Am Coll Nutr* 2004; 23(6): 669-682.

72. McManus T. *Bircher-Benner Nutrition Plan for Raw Food and Juices.* 1977. Jove/HBJ Book, New York, USA.

73. Collin LJ, Judd S, Safford M, et al. Association of Sugary Beverage Consumption with Mortality risk in US Adults. *JAMA Netw Open* 2019; 2(5): 193121.

74. Evers J. Diet therapy of Multiple Sclerosis: Case Report and Epicrisis of my First Multiple Sclerosis patient cured by Diet Therapy after an Observation of 20 years and Report on my other 9000 Dietetically Treated Multiple Sclerosis patients. *Med Welt* 1969; 31: 1700-1707.

75. Kollath W. *Der Vollwert der Nahrung und seine Bedeteutung fur Wachstum und Zellersatz.* [The Full Value of Nutrition and its Importance for Growth and Cell Replacement.] Germany; 1950.

76. Oldfield H, Coghill R. *The Dark Side of the Brain.* Shaftesbury, Dorset, UK: Element; 1988: pp 165.

77. Bao Y, Han J, Hu F, et al. Association of Nut Consumption with Total and Cause-Specific Mortality. *N Engl J Med* 2013; 369: 2001-2011.

78. van den Brant PA, Schouten LJ. Relationship of tree nut, peanut and peanut butter intake with total and cause-specific mortality: a cohort study and meta-analysis. *Int J Epidemiol* 2015; 44(3): 1038-1049.

79. Binzel P. *Alive and Well.* Westlake Village, California, USA: American Media; 1994.

80. Li Y, Korkaya H, Liu S, et al. Sulforaphane, a dietary component of broccoli/ broccoli sprouts, inhibits breast cancer stem cells. *Clinic Cancer Res* 2010; 16(9): 2580-2590.
DOI: 10.1158/1078-0432.CCR-09-2937

81. Ding Y, Paonessa JD, Randall KL, et al. Sulforaphane inhibits 4-aminobiphenyl-induced DNA damage in bladder cancer cells and tissues. *Carcinogenesis* 2010; 31(11): 1999-2003.
DOI: 10.1093/carcin/bgq183

82. Fernandez E, Chatenoud L, La Vecchia C, et al. Fish consumption and cancer risk. *Am J Clinic Nutr* 1999; 70(1): 85-90.

83. Hengeveld LM, Praagman J, Beulens JWJ, et al. Fish consumption

and risk of stroke, coronary heart disease, and cardiovascular mortality in a Dutch population with low fish intake. *Eur J Nutr* 2018; 72(7): 942-950.

84. Norrell SE, Ahlbom A, Feychting M, et al. Fish consumption and mortality from coronary heart disease. *Br Med J* 1986; 293(6544): 426.

85. Van Cauwenberghe L, Janssen C. Microplastics in bivalves cultured for human consumption. *Environmental Pollution* 2014; 193: 65-70.

86. Wallin A, Orsini N, Forouhi NG, et al Fish consumption in relation to myocardial infarction, stroke and mortality among women and men with type 2 diabetes: A prospective cohort study. *Clin Nutr* 2018; 37(2): 590-596.

87. Burr ML, Fehily AM, Gilbert JF et al. Effects of changes in fat, fish and fibre intakes on death and myocardial reinfarction: Diet and Reinfarction Trial (DART). *The Lancet* 1989; 8666; 757-761.

88. Pietinen P, Ascherio A, Korhonen P, et al. Intake of fatty acids and risk of coronary heart disease in a cohort of Finnish men: the Alpha-tocopherol, Beta-carotene Cancer Prevention study. *Am J Epidemiol* 1997; 145(10): 876-887.

89. Guallar E, Sanz-Gallardo MI, van't Veer P, et al. Mercury, Fish Oils and the Risk of Myocardial Infarction. *New Eng J Med* 2002; 347(22): 1747-1754.

90. Clover C. Radioactive waste found in supermarket salmon. *The Telegraph* 23 June 2003.

91. Zhang VW, Van Horn L, Cornelis MC, et al. Associations of Dietary Cholesterol or Egg Consumption with Incident Cardiovascular Disease and Mortality. *JAMA* 2019; 321(11): 1081-1095.

92. Qin C, Lu J, Guo Y, et al. Association of Egg Consumption with Cardiovascular Disease in a Cohort of 0.5 million Chinese adults. *Heart* 2018; 104: 1804-1805.

93. Alexander DD, Miller PE, Vargas AJ, et al. Meta-analysis of Egg Consumption and Risk of Coronary Heart Disease and Stroke. *J Am College Nutr* 2106; 35(8): 704-716. DOI.org/10.1080/08731524.2016.1152928

94. Richman EL, Kenfield SA, Stampfer MJ, et al. Egg, red meat and poultry intake and risk of lethal prostate cancer in prostate specific antigen-era: incidence and survival. *Cancer Prev Res* 2011; 4(12): 2110-2121.

95. Beare S. *The live-longer diet.* London, UK: Piatkus; 2003: pp 77-78.

96. McCarrison R. The Relation of Manure to the Nutritive and Vitamin

Value of Certain Grain. *Br Med J* 1924; 1(3300): 567–569.

97. United Nations Sustainable Development. United Nations Conference on Environment and Development, Rio de Janeirio, Brazil, 3-14th June, 1992.

98. Cai X, Wong C, Yu W, et al. Selenium Exposure and Cancer Risk: An updated Meta-analysis and Meta-Regression. *Sci Rep* 2016; 6: 19213.

99. Stahelin HB, Gey KF, Eichholzer E, et al. Betacarotene and Cancer Prevention: The Basel Study. *Am J Clin Nutr* 1991; 53(1 Suppl): 265S-695S.

100. Baudry J, Assman KE Touvier M, et al. Association of Frequency of Organic Food Consumption with Cancer Risk: Findings from the NutriNet-Sante Prospective Cohort Study. *JAMA Intern Med* 2018; 178(12): 1597-1606.

101. Baranski M, Srednicka-Tober D, Volakakis N, et al. Higher antioxidant and lower cadmium concentrations and lower pesticide residues in organically grown crops: a systematic literature review and meta-analyses. *Br J Nutr* 2014; 112(5): 794-811. DOI: 10.1017/S0007114514001366.

Chapter 3: Belief, expectation and purpose

1. G Klopfer B. Psychological variables in human cancer. *Journal of Projective Techniques* 1957; 12(4): 331-340.

2. Miller SD, Triggiano PJ. The psychophysiological investigation of multiple personality disorder: Review and update. *American Journal of Clinical Hypnosis* 1992; 35(1): 54. (Citing unpublished study by Shepard and Braun.)

3. Gramling R, Klein W, Roberts M, et al. Self-rated cardiovascular risk and 15 year cardiovascular mortality. *Annals of Family Medicine* 2008; 6(4): 302-306.

4. Hirshberg C, Barasch MI. *Remarkable Recovery*. London, UK: Headline Book Publishing, 1995.

5. Ouelette CP. *Miracle of Suggestion*. Virginia Beach, USA: Inner Vision Publishing Co; 1988.

6. Siegel B. *Love, Medicine and Miracles*. London, UK: Rider; 1986.

7. Canfield J, Hansen MV. *Chicken Soup for the Soul*. Florida, USA: Health Communications Inc; 1993.

8. Cui Z, Willingham MC, Alexander-Miller MA, et al. Spontaneous regression of advanced cancer: identification of a unique

genetically determined, age-dependent trait in mice. *Proc Nat Acad Science (USA)* 2003; 100: 6682-6687.

9. Simonton OC, Matthews-Simonton S, Creighton JL. *Getting Well Again*. New York, USA: Bantam Books; 1978.

10. Hastorf AH. Lewis Terman's Longitudinal Study of the Intellectually Gifted: Early Research, Recent Investigations and the Future. *Gifted & Talented International* 1997; 12(1): 3-7. https://doi.org/10.1080/15332276.1997.11672858 (The Terman study of gifted children started at Stanford University in 1921)

11. Rosenthal R, Jacobson L. Pygmalion in the classroom. *Urban Rev* 1968; 3: 16–20. DOI:10.1007/BF02322211

12. Alimujiang A, Wiensch A, Boss J, et al. Association between Life Purpose and Mortality Amongst US Adults Older than 50 years. *JAMA Netw Open* 2019; 2(5): e194270.

13. Dossey L. *Healing Beyond the Body*. London, UK: Piatkus; 2001.

14. O'Connor D. *The Healing Code*. Dublin, Ireland: Hodder Mobius; 2006.

15. Linn D. *The Soul Loves the Truth*. Carlsbad, California, USA: Hay House; 2006.

16. Goodman S. *Nine Steps for Reversing or Preventing Cancer and Other Diseases*. Franklin Lakes, New Jersey, USA: New Page Books; 2004.

17. Myss SN. *The Creation of Health*. New York, USA: Bantam Books; 1999.

18. Buettner D. *The Blue Zones*. Washington DC, USA: National Geographic; 2008.

19. Beck M. *Finding Your Own North Star*. London, UK: Piatkus; 2001.

Chapter 4: How the mind heals

1. Dispenza J. *Evolve your Brain: The Science of Changing Your Mind*. Deerfield Beech, Florida, USA: Health Communications Inc; 2007.

2. Segerstrom S, Miller GE. Psychological stress and the human immune system: a meta-analytical study of 30 years of enquiry. *Psychological Bulletin* 2004; 130(4): 601-630.

3. Segerstrom S, Miller GE. Psychological stress and the human immune system: a meta-analytical study of 30 years of enquiry. *Psychological Bulletin* 2004; 130(4): 601-630.

4. Thaker PH, Han LY, Kamat AA, et al. Chronic stress promotes tumour growth and angiogenesis in a mouse model of ovarian cancer. *Nature Medicine* 2006; 12(8): 939-944.

5. Locke SE, Kraus L, Leserman J, et al. Life change stress, psychiatric

symptoms and natural killer activity. *Psychosomatic Medicine* 1984; 46: 441-453.

6. Bennett MP, Zeller JM, Rosenberg L, McCann J. The effect of mirthful laughter on stress and natural killer cell activity. *Intern Ther Health Med* 2003; 9(2): 38-45.

7. Bhasin MK, Dusek JA, Chang B. Relaxation Response Induces Temporal Transcriptome Changes in Energy Metabolism, Insulin Secretion and Inflammatory Pathways. *PlosOne* 2013; 8: e62817.

8. Orme-Johnson DW, Herron RE. An innovative approach to reducing medical care utilization and expenditure. *American Journal of Managed Care* 1997; 3(1): 135-144.

9. Conkin QA, King BG, Zanesco AP, et al. Insight meditation and telomere biology: The effects of intensive retreat and the moderating role of personality. *Brain, Behavior and Immunity* 2018;. 70: 233-245.

10. Gawler I. *You can Conquer Cancer*. Melbourne, Australia: Thorsons; 1984.

11. Wallace RK, Dillbeck MC, Jacobe E. Effects of TM Meditation and TM-Sidhi program on the aging process. *Psychosomatic Medicine* 1997; 49: 493-507.

12. Simonton OC, Matthews-Simonton S, Creighton JL. *Getting Well Again*. 1978, Bantam Books, New York. (See also Chapter 3)

13. Achterberg J, Lawlis GF. *Bridges of the Bodymind: Behavioural approaches for Health Care*. Champaign, IL: Institute for Personality and Ability Testing Inc; 1980.

14. Schneider J, Smith W, Witcher S. The relationship of mental imagery to white blood cell (neutrophils) function in normal subjects. Paper presented at the 36th Annual Scientific Meeting of the International Society for Clinical and Experimental Hypnosis, San Antonio, Texas. 1984.

15. Goddard N. *The Neville Reader*. Camarillo, California, USA: DeVorss Publications; 2005.

16. Edwards G. *Conscious Medicine*. London, UK: Piatkus; 2010: pp28.

17. Braden G. *The Science of Miracles. The Quantum Language of Healing, Peace, Feeling and Belief*. DVD. Carlsbad, CA, USA: Hay House; 2009.

18. Chopra D. *Quantum Healing*. USA: Penguin Random House; 2015.

Chapter 5: More on the mind

1. Fawzy I, et al. Malignant melanoma: Effects of an early structured psychiatric intervention, coping, and affective state on recurrence and survival 6 years later. *Archives of General Psychiatry* 1993; 50(9): 681-689.

2. Ventegodt S, Morad M, Hyam E, et al. Clinical Holistic Medicine: Induction of Spontaneous Remission of Cancer by Recovery of the Human Character and the Purpose of Life (the Life Mission). *Scientific World Journal* 2004; 4: 362-377.

3. LeShan LL, Gassman ML. Some observations on psychotherapy with patients with neoplastic disease. *American Journal of Psychotherapy* 1958; 12: 723-744.

4. Bays B. *The Journey*. Northampton, UK: Thorsons; 1999.

5. Hay L. *You Can Heal Your Life*. London, UK: Hay House; 1984.

6. Ader R, Cohen N. Behaviourally conditioned immuno-suppression. *Psychosomatic Medicine* 1975; 37(4): 333-340.

7. Marchant J. *Cure: A Journey into the Science of Mind over Body*. Edinburgh, UK: Canongate Books; 2017.

8. The Placebo Experiment. *Horizon* BBC2 Oct 2018, with Michael Mosley.

9. Ghanta VK, Miura T, Hiranoto NS, et al. Augmentation of Natural Immunity and Regulation of Tumour Growth by Conditioning. *Annals of New York Sciences* 1988; 521: 29-42.

10. Gorczynski RM, Macrae S, Kennedy M. Conditioned immune response associated with allogeneic skin grafts in mice. *Journal of Immunology* 1982; 129: 704-709.

11. McCullough ME, et al. Religious involvement and Mortality: A Meta-analytic Review. *Health Psychology* 2000; 19(3): 211-222.

12. Strawbridge WJ, Cohen RD, Shema SJ, et al. Comparative strength of association between religious attendance and survival. *International Journal of Psychiatry in Medicine* 2000; 30(4): 299-308.

13. Pargament KI. The psychology of religion and spirituality?: Yes and No. *International Journal for the Psychology of Religion* 1999; 9(1): 3-16.

14. Dossey L. *Prayer is Good Medicine: How to reap the Healing Benefits of Prayer*. UK: Bravo Ltd; 1997.

15. Owen R. *Qualitative Research: The early years*. UK: Grayhaven Books; 1988.

16. Ironson G, Stuezle R, Fletcher MA, et al. View of God is associated with disease progression in HIV. Paper presented at the annual meeting of the Society of Behavioral Medicine; March 22–25, 2006; San Francisco, California; 2006: pp S074.

17. Gauds C. *The Energy Prescription*. New York, USA: Bantam Books; 2005.

18. Hirshberg C, Barasch MI. *Remarkable Recovery*. London, UK: Headline Book Publishing; 1995. (See also Chapter 3)

19. Peale NV. *Positive Imaging*. New Delhi, India: Orient Paperbacks; 2002.

20. Burk L. Dreams that warn of breast cancer. *Huffington Post* 13 October 2015, updated 6 December 2017. www.huffingtonpost. com/larry-burk-md/dreams-that-warn-of-breas_b_8167758.html.

21. Ingerman S. *Welcome Home: Life after Healing*. San Fancisco, CA, USA: Harper-San Francisco; USA. 1993.

22. Carson JW, Keefe FJ, Goli V, et al. Forgiveness and chronic low back pain: a preliminary study examining the relationship of forgiveness to pain, anger and psychological distress. *J Pain*, 2005; 6(2): 84-91

23. Pleshette J. *Cures that Work*. London, UK: Arrow Books Limited; 1986. (See also the Introduction)

24. Cunningham AJ, Phillips C, Stephen J, Edmonds C. Fighting for Life: a qualitative analysis of the process of psychotherapy-assisted self-help in patients with metastatic cancer. *Integr Cancer Ther* 2002; 1(2): 146-161.

Chapter 6: Toxicity and health

1. Green NS. *Poisoning Our Children*. Chicago, USA: Noble Books; 1991.

2. Davis D. *The Secret History of the War on Cancer*. New York, USA: Basic Books, 2007.

3. Carr BR, Griffin JE. Fertility control and its complications. In: Wilson JD, Foster DW (eds). *Textbook of Endocrinology*. 7th Edition. Philadelphia, USA: WB Saunders; 1985: pp 452-475.

4. Roth J, Grunfield C. Mechanisms of action of peptide hormones and catecholamines. In: Wilson JD, Foster DW (eds). *Textbook of Endocrinology*. 7th Edition. Philadelphia, USA: WB Saunders; 1985: pp 33-75.

5. Steingraber S. *Living Downstream*.London, UK: Virago Press; 1999.

6. Callahan MA, Moraski RV, Nauman CH. (Executive Summary) US

Environmental Protection Agency. Estimating exposure to 2,3,7,8 TCDD. External Review Draft. Washington DC: US EPA, Office of Research and Development (EPA/600-6-88/005a), 1988.

7. Tatsukawa R, Tanabe S. Fate and bioaccumulation of persistent organochlorine compounds in the marine environment. In: Baumgartner DJ, Dudall IM (eds). *Oceanic Processes in Marine Pollution, Volume 6*. Malabar, FL USA: Kreiger; 1990: pp 39-55.

8. Roe D, Pease W, Florini K, et al. *Toxic Ignorance: The Continuing Absence of Basic Health Testing for Top-Selling Chemicals in the United States.*. Environmental Defence Fund, New York, USA; 1997.

9. Brown V. World-Wide Fund for Nature Report: Causes for Concern: Chemicals and wildlife; Dec 2003.

10. Schettler T, Stein J, Reich F, Valenti M, Wallinga D. *In Harm's Way: Toxic Threats to Child Development*. Report from Greater Boston Physicians for Social Responsibility; 2000.

11. Henschler D. Science, occupational exposure limits and regulations: A case study on organochlorine solvents. *American Industrial Hygiene Association Journal* 1990; 51: 523-530.

12. Hays SP. The role of values in science and policy: The case of lead. In: Needleman H (ed). *Human Lead Exposure*Boca Raton, FL, USA: CRC Press; 1992: pp 277-299.

13. Rice DC, Evangelista de Duffard AM, Duffard R, et al. Lessons for neurotoxicology from selected model compounds SGOMSEC joint report. *Env Health Perspect* 1996; 104 (Supp 2): 205-215.

14. USDHHS Seventh Annual Report on Carcinogens, Research Triangle Park, NC:US. Department of Health and Human Services; 1990.

15. IARC Monographs on Evaluation of Carcinogenic Risks to Humans Suppl 7 (Lyon, France: IARC 1987).

A day in the 21st century

16. Brown SK, Cheng M. Volatile organic compounds (VOCs) in new car interiors. In: *Proceedings of the 15th International Clean Air and Environment Conference*. Sydney, Australia, 26-30th November 2000; 1: 464-468.

17. Cioroiu BI , Tarcau D, Cucu-Man S, et al. Polycyclic Aromatic Hydrocarbons in Lung Tissue of Patients With Pulmonary Cancer From Romania. Influence According as Demographic Status and ABO Phenotypes. *Chemosphere* 2013; 92(5): 504-511.

18. Pope CA, Burnett RT, Thun MJ, et al. Lung cancer, cardiopulmonary mortality, and long-term exposure to fine particulate air pollution. *JAMA* 2002; 287(9): 1132-1141.

19. Maheswaran R, Haining RP, Brindley P, et al. Outdoor air pollution and Stroke in Sheffield, United Kingdom. Small-Area Geographical Study. *Stroke* 2005; 36(2): 239-243.

20. Kukall WA. Bowen JD. Dementia epidemiology. *Med Clin North America* 2002; 86(3): 573-590.

21. Wallace L, Pellizarri E, Hartwell T, et al. Concentrations of 220 volatile organic compounds in air and drinking water of 350 residents of New Jersey compared with concentrations in their exhaled breath. *J Occup Med* 1986; 28: 603-608.

22. APHA (American Public Health Association). Resolution 9304: recognizing and addressing the environmental and occupational health problems posed by chlorinated organic chemicals. *American Journal of Public Health* 1994; 84: 514-515.

23. Bethwaite PB, Pearce N, Fraser J, et al. Cancer risks in painters: study based on the New Zealand Cancer Registry. *Br J Ind Med* 1990; 47: 742-746.

24. Steenland K, Kugathasan S, Barr DB. PFOA and Ulcerative Colitis. *Environ Res* 2018; 165: 317-321.

Chemicals and cancer

25. Houlihan J, Wiles R, Thayer K, Gray S. *Body Burden: the pollution in people.* Environmental Working Group. January 2003. https://healthy-materials-lab.s3.amazonaws.com/resources/BodyBurden_The_Pollution_in_People.pdf

26. Cantor KP, et al. Water pollution. In: Schottenfeld D, Fraumeni JF Jr (eds) *Cancer Epidemiology and Prevention.* 2nd edition. Oxford, UK: Oxford University Press; 1996.

27. Lagakos SW, et al. An analysis of contaminated well water and health effects in Woburn, Massachusetts. *J Amer Stat Assoc* 1986: 395: 583-596.

28. Lampi P, Hakulinen T, Luostarinen T, et al. Cancer incidence following chlorophenol exposure in a community in Southern Finland. *Arch Environ Health* 1992; 47(3): 167-175.

29. Fagliano J, Berry M, Boye F, et al. Drinking water contamination and the incidence of leukaemia: an ecologic study. *Am J Public Health* 1990; 80(10): 1209-1212.

30. Osborne JS, Shy CM, Kaplan BH. Epidemiologic analysis of a reported cancer case cluster in a small rural population. *Am J Epidemiol* 1990; 132(Supp 1): S87-S95.

31. Hoover R, Fraumeni JF, Jr. Cancer mortality in US counties with chemical industries. *Environ Res* 1975; 9(2): 196-207.

32. Pickle LW, Mason TJ, Fraumeni JF Jr. The new United States Cancer Atlas. *Recent Results Cancer Res* 1989; 114: 196-207.

33. Najem GR, Louria DB, Lavenhar MA, et al. Clusters of cancer mortality in New Jersey municipalities, with special reference to chemical toxic waste disposal sites and per capita income. *Int J Epidemiol* 1985; 14(4): 528-537.

34. Schneider AP, Zainer CM, Kubat CK, et al. The breast cancer epidemic: 10 facts. *Linacre Q* 2014; 81(3): 244-277.

35. Smith MA, FreidlinB, Lynn A, et al. Trends in Reported Incidence of Primary Malignant Brain Tumours in Children in the United States. *J Nat Cancer Inst* 1998; 90(17): 1269-1277.

Fat-loving chemicals target the nervous system

36. Pritchard C, Mayers A, Baldwin D. Changing pattern of neurological mortality in the 10 major developed countries 1979-2010. *Public Health* 2013; 127(4): 357-368. (See also Chapter 2)

37. Ingalls T. Endemic clustering of multiple sclerosis in time and place, 1934-84. Confirmation of a hypothesis. *Am J Forensic Med Path* 1986; 7(1): 3-8.

38. Kukall WA. Dementia epidemiology. *Med Clin North Am* 2002; 86(3): 573-590.

39. Trapp GA, Miner GH, Zimmerman RL, et al. Aluminium levels in the brain in Alzheimer's disease. *Biol Psychiatry* 1978; 13(6): 709-718.

40. Ehmann WD, Markesbery WR, Alauddin M, et al. Brain trace elements in Alzheimer's disease. *Neurotoxicology* 1986; 7(1): 195-206.

41. Su FC, Goutman SA, Chernyak S, et al. The role of Environmental Toxins on ALS: A Case-Control Study of Occupational Risk Factors. *JAMA Neurol* 2016; 73(7): 803-811.

Endocrine disruption

42. Colborn T, Dumanosta D, Myers JP. *Our Stolen Future*. London, UK: Abacus; 1996.

43. Chandra A, Stephen EH. Impaired Fecundity in the United States: 1982-1995. *Fam Plann Perspect* 1998; 30(1): 34-42.

44. Carlsen E, Giwercman A, Keiding N, Skakkebaek N. Evidence for the decreasing quality of Semen during Past 50 Years. *Br Med J* 1992; 305: 609-613.

45. Merzenich H, Zeeb H, Blettner M. Decreasing sperm quality: a global problem? *BMC Public Health* 2010; 10(1): 24.

46. Irvine S, Cawood E, Richardson D. Evidence of deteriorating semen quality in the Uniited Kingdom: birth cohort study in 577 men in Scotland over 11 years. *Br Med J* 1996; 312: 467-471.

47. Swan SH, Brazil C, Brobnis EZ, et al. Geographical differences in semen quality of fertile US males. *Env Health Perspect* 2003; 111: 414-420.

48. Dougherty RC, Whitaker MJ, Tang SY, Bottcher R, et al. Sperm density and toxic substances: A potential key to environmental health hazards. In: McKinney JD (Ed). *Environmental health chemistry: The chemistry of environmental agents of potential human hazards.* Ann Arbor, MI, USA: Ann Arbor Science Publishers; 1981: pp 263-278.

49. March WA, Moore VM, Wilson KJ, et al. The Prevalence of Polycystic Ovary Syndrome in a Community Sample Assessed Under Contrasting Diagnostic Criteria. *Human Reprod* 2010; 25(2): 544-551.

50. Soto A, Sonnenschein C. The Role of Estrogens on the Proliferation of Human Breast tumour Cells (MCF-7). *J Steroid Biochem* 1985; 23: 87-94.

51. Gao H, Yang B, Li N, et al. Bisphenol A and Hormone-Associated Cancers. *Medicine* 2015; 94(1): e211.

52. Gross-Sorokin MY, Roast SD, Brighty GC. Assessment of feminization of male fish in English rivers by the Environmental Agency of England and Wales. *Environ Health Perspect* 2006; 114(suppl): 147-151.

53. vom Saal FS. Variation in phenotype due to random positioning of male and female foetuses in rodents. *J Reprod Fertil* 1981; 62(2): 633-650.

54. Vreugdenhil HJI, Slijper FME, Mulder PGH, et al. Effects of Perinatal Exposure to PCBs and Dioxins on Play Behaviour in Dutch Children at School Age. *Environ Health Perspect* 2002; 110: A593-A598.

55. Damstra T, Barlow S, Bergman A, Kavlock R, Van der Kraak G. International Programme on Chemical Safety: Global Assessment of the State-of-Science of Endocrine Disruption. World Health Organization 2002; WHO/PCS/EDC/02.2 www.who.int/pics/publications/en/toc.pdf?ua=1" (accessed 23 April 2020)

Chapter 7: Reducing exposure to toxicity

The toxic mouth

1. Levenson J. *Menace in the Mouth*. WDDTY Publications, London. 2000.
2. Hanson M. *Bibliography compiled by Swedish researcher Mats Hanson* The Swedish Mats Hanson Mercury Bibliography 2009: http://hestories.info/the-swedish-mats-hanson-mercury-bibliography-2009.html
3. Vimy MJ, Lorscheider FL. Intra-oral Air Mercury released from Dental Amalgam. *J Dental Res* 1985; 64(8): 1069-1071.
4. Vimy MJ, Lorscheider FL. Serial Measures of Intra-oral Air Mercury: Estimation of Daily dose from Dental Amalgam. *J Dent Res* 1985; 64(8): 1072-1075.
5. Vimy MJ, Takahashi Y, Lorscheider FL. Maternal-fetal distribution of mercury (203 HG) released from dental amalgam fillings. *Am J Physiology* 1990; 258: R 939-945.
6. Danscher G, Horsted-Bindsley P, Rungby J. Traces of mercury in organs of primates with amalgam fillings. *Experimental and Molecular Pathology* 1990; 52: 291-299.
7. Drasch G, Schupp I, Hofl H, et al. Mercury burden of Human Foetal and Infant Tissues. *Eur J Pediatr* 1994; 153: 607-610.
8. Nylander M, Friberg L, Lind B. Mercury Concentration in the Human Brain and Kidney in Relation to Exposure from Dental Amalgam Fillings. *Swedish Dental J* 1987; 11(5): 179-187.
9. Eggleston DW, Nylander M. Correlation of dental amalgam with mercury in brain tissue. *J Prost Dent* 1987; 58(6): 704-707.
10. Westrup D, Ehmann WD, Markesbury WR. Trace Element Imbalances in Isolated Subcellular Fractions of Alzheimer's Disease Brains. *Brain Research* 1990; 553: 125-131.
11. Lorscheider FL. Toxicity of ionic mercury and elemental mercury vapour on brain neuronal protein metabolism. *Neurotoxicity*

15(4): Twelfth International Neurotoxicity Conference. Hot Springs, Arkansas, 30th Oct – 2nd Nov 1994.

Electro-pollution

12. Wertheimer N, Leeper E. Electrical Wiring Configurations and Childhood Cancer. *American Journal of Epidemiology* 1979; 109: 273-284.
13. Tornqvist S, Knave B, Ahlbom A. Incidence of leukaemia and brain tumours in some electrical occupations. *Br J Indust Med* 1991; 48: 597-603.
14. California Report. An Evaluation of the Possible Risks from Electrical and Magnetic Fields (EMFs) from Power Lines, Internal Wiring, Electrical Occupation and Appliances. 2002. www.dhs.ca.gov/ehib/emf/RiskEvaluaion/riskeval.html
15. Savitz DA. Liao D, Sastre A et al. Magnetic field exposure and cardiovascular disease mortality amongst electrical utility workers. *Am J Epidemiol* 1999; 149(2): 136-142.
16. Havas M. Radiation from wireless technology affects the blood, the heart, and the autonomic nervous system. *Rev Environ Health* 2013; 28(2-3): 75-84.
17. BioInitiative Report: A Rationale for Biologically-based Exposure Standards for Low Intensity Electromagnetic Radiation. 7 June 2013
18. ECOLOG Report: A Review of Current Scientific Research in view of precautionary health protection. ECOLOG Institute, Hanover. April 2000.
19. van Wijngaarden E, Savitz DA, Kleckner RC, et al. Exposure to electromagnetic fields and suicide amongst electric utility workers. *West J Med* 2000; 173(2): 94-100.
20. Gorpinchenko I, Nikitin O, Banyra O, et al. The influence of direct mobile phone radiation on sperm quality. *Cent European J Urol* 2014; 67(1): 65-71.
21. Hardell L, Carlberg M, Soderqvist F, et al. Meta-analysis of long-term mobile phone use and the association with brain tumours. *Int J Oncol* 2008; 32(5): 1097-1103.
22. Sadetzki S, Chehrit A, Jarus-Hakak A, et al. Cellular phone use and the risk of benign and malignant parotid gland tumours – A nationwide case-control study. *Am J Epidemiol* 2008; 167(4): 457-467.

23. Wolf R, Wolf D. Increased Incidence of Cancer near a Cellphone Transmission station. *International Journal of Cancer Prevention* 2004; 1(2): 123-128.
24. Naila Study. The Influence of Being Physically Near to a Cell Phone Transmission Mast on the Incidence of Cancer. *Umwelt-Medizin-Gesellschft* 2004; 17: 4. www.powerwatch.org.uk/news/20041118_naila.pdf
25. Szmigielski S. Cancer morbidity in subjects occupationally exposed to high frequency (RF and microwave) electromagnetic radiation. *Science of the Total Environment* 1996; 180: 9-18.
26. Edwards T. *Brain Waves: the autism link. What Doctors Don't Tell You*: Special Report 2007; 19 6-9.
27. Santini R, Santini P, Danze JM et al. Study of the Health of people living in the vicinity of mobile phone mast base stations. *Pathologie Biologie* 2002; 50: 369-373.
28. Tamara JM, Carlo GL. Wireless Radiation in the Etiology and treatment of Autism: Clinical Observations and Mechanisms. *J Aust Coll Nutr Environ Med* 2007; 26: 3-7.

Nanoparticles

29. World Health Organization – Regional Office for Europe. Chapter 3: Formaldehyde. In: *WHO Air Quality Guidelines – Guidelines for Indoor Air Quality: Selected Pollutants* Copenhagen, Denmark: WHO; 1999. www.euro.who.int/__data/assets/pdf_file/0009/128169/e94535.pdf (accessed 27 April 2020)
30. Chen Z, Meng H, Xing G, et al. Acute toxicological effects of copper nanoparticles in vivo. *Toxicology Letters* 2006; 163: 109-120.
31. Kemp A. Food additives and hyperactivity. *Br Med J* 2008; 336(7654): 1144.

Pesticides

32. www.euractiv.com/section/agriculture-food/news/pesticide-residues-detected-in-almost-all-european-foods/1138367/
33. Committee on Toxicity (COT): Pesticides Residue Committee. 2001. https://cot.food.gov.uk/cotwg/wigramp (accessed 27 April 2020)
34. Hites RA, Foran JA, Carpenter DO, et al. Global assessment of organic contaminants in farmed salmon. *Science* 2004; 303(5655): 226-229.

35. Perrotta C, Stainess A, Cocco P. Multiple myeloma and farming: A Systemic review of 30 years of research. Where next? *J Occup Med Toxicol* 2008; 3: 27.

36. Karunanayaka CP, Dosmman JA, Pahwa P. Non-Hodgkin's lymphoma and work in agriculture: Results of a two case-control studies in Saskatchewan, Canada. *Indian J Occup Environ Med* 2013; 17(3): 114-121.

37. Sinner PJ, Cerhan JR, Folsom AR, et al. Positive association of farm and rural residence with acute myeloid leukaemia incidence in a cohort of older women. *Cancer Epidemiol Biomarkers Prev* 2005; 14(10): 2446-2448.

38. Rask-Andersen A. Asthma increase among farmers: a 12-year follow-up. *Ups J Med Sci* 2011; 116(1): 60-71.

39. Garry FV, Schreinemachers D, Harkins ME, et al. Pesticide appliers, biocides, and birth defects in rural Minnesota. *Environ Health Perspect* 1996; 104(4): 394-399.

40. Priyadarshi a, Khuder SA, Schaub EA, et al. A meta-analysis of Parkinsons disease and exposure to pesticides. *Neurotoxiciology* 2000; 21(4): 435-440.

41. van der Mark M, Brouwer M, Kromhout H, et al. Is Pesticide Use Related to Parkinson's Disease? Some Clues to Heterogenicity in Study Results. *Environ Health Perspect* 2012; 120(3): 340-347.

42. Ascherio A, Chen H, Weisskopf MG, et al. Pesticide exposure and risk of Parkinson's disease. *Ann Neurol* 2006; 60(2): 197-203.

43. Parron T, Requena M, Hernandez AF, et al. Association between environmental exposure to pesticides and neurodegenerative diseases. *Toxicology and Applied Pharmacology* 2011; 256: 379-385.

44. Dunstan RH, Donohoe M, Taylor W, et al. A preliminary investigation of chlorinated hydrocarbons and chronic fatigue syndrome. *Med J Aust* 1995; 163: 294-297.

45. Bassil KL, Vakil C, Sanborn M. Cancer health effects of Pesticides. *Can Fam Physician* 2007; 53(10): 1704-1711.

46. Turner MC, Wigle DT, Krewski D. Residential pesticides and childhood leukaemia. *Cien Saude Colet* 2011; 16(3): 1915-1931.

47. Buckley JD, Meadows AT, Kadin ME, et al. Pesticide exposures in children with non-Hodgkin's lymphoma. *Cancer* 2000; 89(11): 2315-2321.

48. Zahm SH, Blair A. pesticides and non-Hodgkin's lymphoma. *Cancer Res* 1992; 52(19 Suppl): 5485s-5488s.

49. McDuffie HH, Pahwa P, McLaughlin JR, et al. Non-Hodgkin's lymphoma and specific pesticide exposures in men: cross-Canada study of pesticides and health. *Cancer Epidemiol Biomarkers Prev* 2001; 10(11): 1155-1163.
50. Woolf MS, Toniolo PG, Lee EW, et al Blood levels of organochlorines Residues and Risk of Breast Cancer. *J Natl Cancer Instit* 1993; 85: 648-652.
51. Hunter DJ, Kelsey KT. Pesticide residues and Breast cancer: The Harvest of a Silent Spring? *Natl J Cancer Instit* 1993; 85: 598-599.
52. Pretty JN. *Regenerating Agriculture: Policies and Practice for Sustainability and Self-Reliance.* London, UK: Earthscan; 1995.
53. Pimentel D, Levitan L. Pesticide Amounts Applied and Amounts Reaching Pests. *BioScience* 1986; 36: 86-91.

Safe as houses

54. Bethwaite PB, Pearce N, Fraser J, et al. Cancer risks in painters: study based on the New Zealand Cancer Registry. *Br J Ind Med* 1990; 47: 742-746.
55. IEH. Indoor Air Quality in the Home: Nitrogen Dioxide, Formaldehyde, Volatile Organic Compounds, House Dust Mites, Fungi and Bacteria (assessment A2). Leicester, UK: Institute for Environment and Health; 1996.
56. Mitro SD, Dodson RE, Singla V. Consumer Product Chemicals in Indoor Dust: A Quantitative Meta-analysis of US Studies. *Env Sci Technol* 2016; 50(19): 10661-10672.

Outdoor pollution

57. Pope CA, Burnett RT, Thun MJ, et al. Lung cancer, cardiopulmonary mortality, and long-term exposure to fine particulate air pollution. *JAMA* 2002; 287(9): 1132-1141.
58. World Health Organization. *Ambient air pollution: A global assessment of exposure and burden of disease.* Geneva, Switzerland: WHO; 2016
59. Yuan T, Shen Y, Shie R, et al. Increased cancers among residents living in the neighbourhood of a petrochemical complex: A 12-year cohort study. *Int J Hygiene and Env Health* 2018; 221(2): 308-314.
60. Knox EG, Gilman EA. Migration patterns of children with cancer in Britain. *J Epidemiology & Community Health* 1998; 52(11): 716-726.

Hair dyes, cosmetics, aerosols

61. Zhang Y, Sanjose SD, Bracci PM, et al. Personal use of hair dye and the risk of certain subtypes of non-Hodgkin's lymphoma. *Am J Epidemiol* 2008; 167(11): 1321-1331.
62. Rauscher GH, Shore D, Dale P et al. Hair Dye Use and Risk of Adult Acute Leukemia. *Am J Epidemiol* 2004; 160(1): 19-25.
63. Wilkenfeld IR. Scents Make No Sense. *The Environmental Physician* Fall, 1991.

Chemicals in water

64. Cantor KP, Hoover R, Hartge P, et al. Bladder cancer, drinking water source, and tap water consumption: a case-control study. *J Natl Cancer Inst* 1987; 79(6): 1269-1279.
65. Hildesheim M, Cantor KP, Lynch CF, et al. Drinking water source and chlorination by-products. Risk of colon and rectal cancer. *Epidemiology* 1998; 9: 29-35.
66. Weisel CP, Wan-Kuen J. Ingestion, Inhalation and Dermal Exposure to Chloroform and Trichloroethylene from Tap Water. *Environ Health Perspect* 1996; 104: 48-51.
67. Calafat AM, Wong L, Kuklenyik Z, et al. Perflouoalkyl Chemicals in US Population: Data from the National Health and Nutrition Examination Survey (NHANES) 2003-2004 and Comparison with NHANES 1999-2000. *Environ Health Perspect* 2007; 115(11): 1596-1602.

Chapter 8: Releasing toxicity

Other associations

1. Kerkvliet NI. Immunotoxicology of dioxins and related compounds. In: Schecter A (ed). *Dioxins and Health*. Chichester, UK: Wiley; 1994: pp 199-225.
2. Gottscalk LA, Rebello T, Buchsbaum MS, et al. Abnormalities in hair trace elements as indicators of aberrant behaviour. *CompPsychiatry* 1991; 32(3): 229-237.
3. Whyatt RM, Santella RM, Jedrychowski W, et al. Relationship between ambient air pollution and DNA damage in Polish mothers and newborns. *Environ Health Perspect* 1998; 106(Suppl 3): 821-826.
4. Tong S, Baghurst P, McMichael A, et al. Lifetime exposure to

Curing the Incurable

environmental lead and children's intelligence at 11–13 years: the Port Pirie Cohort Study. *Br Med J* 1996; 312(7046): 1569-1575.

5. Mayes MD. Epidemiological studies of environmental agents and systemic auto-immune diseases. *Environ Health Perspect* 1999; 107(Suppl 5): 743-748.

The boomerang effect

6. Body Burden: Executive Summary, 2003, Environmental Working Group, Mount Sinai School of Medicine and Commonweal. www.ewg.org/reports/bodyburden/

7. Zieger M. Biomarkers: The clues to genetic susceptibility. *Environ Health Perspectives* 1994; 102(1): 50-57.

8. Onstot J, Ayling R, Stanley J. Characterization of HRGC/MS Unidentified Peaks from the Analysis of Human Adipose Tissue. Volume 1: Technical Approach, Washington DC: US Environmental Protection Agency Office of Toxic Substances (560/6-87-002a).

The polluted foetus

9. Rogan WJ, Gladen BC, McKinney JD, et al. Polychlorinated biphenyls (PCBs) and dichlorodiphenyldichloroethene (DDE) in human milk: effects of maternal factor and previous lactation. *Am J Public Health* 1986; 76(2): 172-177.

10. Body Burden: The Pollution in Newborns: Executive Summary, July 2005, Environmental Working Group, Mount Sinai School of Medicine and Commonweal. www.ewg.org/reports/bodyburden2/execsumm.php

11. Koopman-Esseboom C, Huisman M, Weisglas-Kuperus N, et al. Dioxin and PCB levels in blood and human milk in relation to living in the Netherlands. *Chemosphere* 1994; 29(9-11): 2327-2338.

12. Jensen AA, Slorach SA. Assessment of infant intake of chemicals via breast milk. In: *Chemical Contaminants in Human Milk*. Boca Raton, USA: CRC Press; 1991: pp 215-222.

13. Tilson HA, Jacobson JL, Rogan WJ. Polychlorinated biphenyls and the developing nervous system: cross species comparisons. *Neurotoxicol Teratol* 1990; 12(3): 239-248.

Trans-generational toxicity

14. Anway MD, Cupp AS, Uzumcu M, et al. Epigenetic

transgenerational actions of endocrine disruptors and male fertility. *Science* 2005; 308(5727): 1466-1469.

Early exposure primes later disease

15. Thiruchelvam M, Richfield EK, Goodman BM, et al. Developmental exposure to pesticides paraquat and maneb and the Parkinson's disease phenotype. *Neurotoxicology* 2002; 23(4-5): 621-633.
16. Whyatt RM, Perera FP. Application of biological markers to studies of environmental risks in children and the developing foetus. *Environ Health Perspect* 1995; 103(suppl 6): 105-110.
17. National Research Council, National Academy of Sciences. *Pesticides in the diet of infants and children*. Washington DC, USA: Natl Acad Press; 1993.

The cocktail effect

18. Wade MG, Parent S, Finnson KW, et al. Thyroid toxicity due to a subchronic exposure to a complex mixture of 16 organochlorines, lead, and cadmium. *Toxicol Sci* 2002; 67(2): 207-218.
19. Mehendale HM. Amplified interactive toxicity of chemicals at nontoxic levels: Mechanistic considerations and implications to public health: Mechanistic-based predictions of interactions. *Environ Health Perspect* 1994; 102(Suppl 9): 139-149.
20. Arnold SF, Klotz DM, Collins BM, et al. Synergistic activation of estrogen receptors with combinations of environmental chemicals. *Science* 1996; 272(5267): 1489-1492.
21. Soil Association & Pesticide Action Network, UK. The Cocktail Effect: How pesticide mixtures may be harming human health and the environment. Soil Association and Pesticide Action Network; October 2019. www.soilassociation.org/media/19535/the-pesticide-cocktail-effect.pdf

Dealing with the toxicity

22. Pelkonenn O. Comparison of activities of drug-metabolizing enzymes in human fetal and adult livers. *Clinic Pharmacol Ther* 1973; 14(5): 840-846.
23. Hattis D, Russ A, Goble R, et al. Human interindividual variability in susceptibility to airborne particles. *Risk Anal* 2001; 21(4): 585-599.
24. Hattis D, Erdreich L, DiMauro T. Human variability in parameters

that are potentially related to susceptibility to carcinogenesis. I. *Preliminary Observations*. Cambridge, MA, USA: Center for Technology, Policy & Industrial Development, MIT; 1986.

Reducing the toxic load

25. Mansfield J. *Arthritis, Allergy, Nutrition and the Environment.* Northampton, UK: Thorsons; 1995.
26. Rea W, Pan Y, Fenyves EJ, et al. Reduction of chemical sensitivity by means of heat depuration, physical therapy and nutritional supplementation in a controlled environment. *J Nutr Environ Med* 1996; 7(2): 141-148.
27. Myhill S. *Sustainable Medicine.* London, UK: Hammersmith Books Limited; 2015.

Fasting

28. Ehret A. *Mucusless Diet Healing System.* New York, US: Ehret Literature Publishing Company; 1953.
29. Bennett P, Barrie S. *7-Day Detox Miracle.* Roseville, CA, USA: Prima Health; 2001.
30. Lettieri-Barbata D, Cannata SM, Casagrande V, et al. Time-controlled Fasting Prevents Aging-like Mitochondrial Changes induced by Persistent Dietary Fat Overload in Skeletal Muscle. *PLoS One* 2018; 13(5): e0195912.
31. Cheng C, Adams GB, Perin L, et al. Prolonged Fasting reduces IGF-1/PKA to Promote Hematopoietic Stem Cell-based Regeneration and Reverse Immunosuppression. *Cell Stem Cell* 2014; 14(6): 810-823.
32. Brima EI, Jenkins RO, Lythgoe PR, et al. Effect of Fasting on the Pattern of Urinary Arsenic Excretion. *J Environ Monit* 2007; 9(1): 98-103.
33. Lavin DN, Joesting JJ, Chiu GS, et al. Fasting induces an Anti-Inflammatory Effect on the Neuroimmune System which a High Fat Diet prevents. *Obesity* 2011; 19(8): 1586-1594.
34. Marinac CR, Nelson SH, Breen CI, et al. Prolonged Nightly Fasting and Breast Cancer Prognosis. *JAMA Oncology* 2016; 2(8): 1049-1055.
35. Lee J, Duan W, Mattson P. Evidence that Brain-Derived Neurotrophic Factor is required for Basal Neurogenesis and mediated, in part, the Enhancement of Neurogenesis, by Dietary Restriction in the Hippocampus of Adult Mice. *J Neurochem* 2007; 8(6): 1367-1375.

Chapter 9: How energy can heal

1. McGee CT. *Miracle Qigong: Healing from China*. Couer d'Alene, Idaho, USA: MediPress; 1994.
2. Church D. *The Genie in Your Genes*, 2nd ed. Santa Rosa, US: Energy Psychology Press; 2008.
3. Edwards G. *Conscious Medicine*. London, UK: Piatkus; 2010.

Sunlight

4. Hobday R. *The Healing Sun*. Findhorn, Forres, UK: Findhorn Press; 1999: pp 102-103.
5. Christopher JR. *Curing the Incurables*. 2nd ed. Springville, USA: Christopher Publications Inc; 1977.
6. Smith P. Michael Holick PhD, MD. The pioneer of Vitamin D research. *Life Extension Magazine* Sep 2010.
7. Domene AC. *Multiple Sclerosis and (lots of) Vitamin D*. Odyssey Books; 2016.
8. Vitamin D and cancer – are you getting enough? Cancer Active 23 August 2018. www.canceractive.com/article/Vitamin-D-and-cancer-Are-you-getting-enough
9. Ott JN. *Health and Light*, Columbus, US: Ariel Press; 1973.
10. dos Santos AF, de Almeida DRQ, Terra LF et al. Photodynamic Therapy in Cancer Treatment- an update review. *J Cancer Metastasis Treat* 2019; 5: 25.
11. Dougherty TJ. Photoradiation Therapy – New Approaches. *Seminars in Surgical Oncology* 1989; 5: 6-16.

Exercise

12. Morris JN, Heady JA, Raffle PAB et al. Coronary heart disease and physical activity of work. *Lancet* 1953; 265(6795): 1053-1057.
13. Paffenbarger RS, Laughlin ME, Gima AS, et al. Work activity of longshoremen as related to death from coronary heart disease and stroke. *N Eng J Med* 1970; 282: 1109-1114.
14. Morris JN, Everett MG, Pollard R, et al. Vigorous exercise in leisure time: Protection against coronary heart disease. *Lancet* 1980; 2: 1207-1210.
15. Abramson J. *Overdosed America*. London, UK: Harper Perennial; 2005: pp 225.
16. Paffenbarger RS, Olsen E. *Lifefit: An Effective Exercise Program*

for Optimal Health and a Longer Life. Champaign, Illinois, USA: Human Kinetics; 1992.

17. Holick CN, Newcomb PA, Trentham-Dietz A, et al. Physical activity and survival after invasive breast cancer. *Cancer Epidemiol Biomarkers Prev* 2008; 17: 379-386.

18. Holmes MD, Chen WY, Feskanich D, et al. Physical activity and survival after breast cancer diagnosis. *JAMA* 2005; 293(20): 2479-2486.

19. Graf C, Wessely N. Physical Activity in the Prevention and Therapy of Breast Cancer. *Breast Care* 2010; 5(6): 389-394.

20. Meyerhardt JA, Giovannucci EL, Holmes MD, et al. Physical activity and survival after colorectal cancer diagnosis. *J Clinic Oncol* 2006; 24: 3527-3534.

21. Meyerhardt JA, Heseltine D, Niedzwiecki D, et al. Impact of Physical activity on cancer recurrence and survival in patients with stage III colon cancer; finding from CALGB 89803. *Journal of Clinical Oncology* 24; 2006: 3535-3541.

22. Wolin KY, Yan Y Colditz GA et al. Physical activity and colon cancer: A meta-analysis. *Br J Cancer* 2009, 100: 611-616.

23. Kenfield SA, Stamffer MJ, Giovannucci E, et al. Physical activity and survival after prostate cancer diagnosis in the health professional follow-up study. *J Clinic Oncol* 2011; 29: 726-732.

24. Robbins J. *Healthy at 100*. New York, US: Ballantine Books; 2007.

25. Reeves P. *A Living Miracle*. London, UK: Pathfinder; 2008.

26. Simonton O, Matthews-Simonton S, Creighton J. *Getting Well Again* 2nd ed. New York: Bantam books; 1992: pp 226. (See also Chapters 3 and 5.)

27. Bartion A (ed). *Recovery from CFS: 50 Personal stories*. Milton Keynes, UK: Authorhouse; 2008.

Chapter 10: Healing, vital force and electricity

Healing energy

1. 'Adam'. *Dream Healer: A true Story of Miracle Healing*. London: Time Warner Books; 2006.

2. Bengston WF, Krinsley D. The Effect of the 'Laying on of Hands' on Transplanted Breast Cancer in Mice. *Journal of Scientific Exploration* 2000; 14(3): 353-364.

3. Abbott, NC. Healing as a therapy for human disease: a systemic review. *Journal of Alternative and Complementary Medicine* 2000; 6(2): 159.

4. Benor D. Survey of spiritual healing research. *Complementary Medical Research* 1990; 4(1): 9.

5. Edwards H. *The Healing Intelligence*. London: MPG Books Group; 1975.

6. Achterberg J, Cooke K, Richards T. Evidence for correlation between Distant Intentionality and brain function in recipients: A functional magnetic resonance imaging analysis. *J Alt Complement Med* 2005; 11(6): 965-971.

7. Shealy N, Church D. *Soul Medicine: Awakening your Inner Blueprint for Abundant Health and Energy*. Santa Rosa, California, US: Energy Psychology Press; 2006.

8. Cerutti E. *Olga Worrell: Mystic with Healing Hands*. New York, US: Harper; 1975.

9. Steven L, Fahrion SL, Wirkus M, et al. EEG amplitude, brain mapping and synchronicity in and between bioenergy practitioner and client during healing. *Bridges* 1992; 3: 1.

10. Shealy N, Church D. *Soul Medicine: Awakening your Inner Blueprint for Abundant Health and Energy*. Santa Rosa, California, US: Energy Psychology Press; 2006.

11. Edwards H. *The Power of Spiritual Healing*, 3rd edition. Guildford, UK: Biddles Ltd; 1978.

12. Edwards H. *The Evidence for Spirit Healing*. London, UK: Spiritualist; 1953.

Life force energy

13. Soh K. Bonghan ducts and acupuncture meridian as optical channel of biophoton. *Journal of Korean Physical Society* 2004; 45(5): 1196.

14. Kirlian SD, Kirlian V. Photography and visual observation by means of high-frequency currents. *J Sci Appl Photog* 1961; 6(6).

15. Oldfield H, Coghill R. *The Dark Side of the Brain*. Shaftesbury, Dorset, UK: Element Books; 1988. (See also Chapter 2.)

16. Vries J de. *Cancer and Leukaemia*. Edinburgh, UK: Mainstream Publishing; 1987: 150-151.

17. Eden D, Feinstein D. *The Energy Medicine Kit*. Boulder, Colorado, US: Sounds True Inc; 2004.

18. Sancier KM, Homan D. Multifaceted benefits of medical Qigong. *Healing Tao USA*. https://healingtaousa.com/articles/multifaceted-health-benefits-of-medical-qigong (accessed 12 April 2020).

19. McGee C. *Qigong, Miracle Healing from China*. Couer d'Alene, Idaho, USA: Medipress; 1994. (See also Chapter 9.)

20. Eden D, Feinstein D. *The Energy Medicine Kit*. Boulder, US: Sounds True Inc; 2004.

21. Edwards G. *Conscious Medicine*. London, UK: Piatkus; 2010. (See also Chapter 9.)

22. Callaghan R. *Tapping the Healer Within*. New York, USA: Contemporary Books; 2001.

23. Feinstein D. Energy psychology: A review of the preliminary evidence. *Psychotherapy Theory, Research, Practice, Training* 2008; 45(2): 199-213.

24. Feinstein D, Eden D, Craig G. *The Promise of Energy Psychology*. New York, US: Penguin Group; 2005.

Electromagnetic energy

25. Cornelissen G, Halberg F, Breut T, et al. Non-phototic solar associations of heart rate variability and myocardial infarction. *Journal of Atmospheric and Solar-terrestrial Physics* 2002; 64: 707-720.

26. Ober C, Sinatra S, Zucker M. *Earthing*. Laguna Beach, US: Basic Health; 2010.

27. Applewhite R. The effectiveness of a conductive patch and a conductive bed pad in reducing induced human voltage via the application of a ground rod. *European Biology and Biomagnetics* 2005; 1: 23-40.

28. Li Q, Kobayashi M, Wakayama Y, et al. Effect of phytoncide from trees on human natural killer cells function. *Int J Immunopathol Pharmacol* 2009; 22(4): 951-959.

29. Park BJ, Tsunetsugu Y, Kasetani T, et al. The physiological effects of Shinrin-yoku (taking in the forest atmosphere or forest bathing): evidence from field experiments in 24 forests across Japan. *Environ Health Prev Med* 2010; 15(1): 18-26.

30. von Pohl GF. *Earth Currents: Causative Factor of Cancer and other Diseases*. Frech-Verlag; 1987.

31. www.positivehealth.com/article/environmental/biosensing-to-counter-geopathic-stress

32. Bachler K. *Earth Radiation*, 2nd ed. Galiano Island, British Columbia, Canada: Holistic Intuition Society; 2007.

33. Gordon R. *Are you Sleeping in a Safe Place?* Dulwich, UK: Dulwich Health; 1989.

34. Bearden TE. Vacuum engines and Priore's methodology, the science of energy medicine. Parts I and II. *Explore!* 1995; 6(1): 66-90.

Chapter 11: Energy within and around

Thought energy

1. Linn D. *The Soul Loves the Truth*. Carlsbad, California, USA: Hay House; 2006. (See also Chapter 3.)
2. Ehrsson HH, Geyer S, Naito E. Imagery of voluntary movements of fingers, toes and tongue activates corresponding body-part specific motor representations. *Journal of Neurophysiology* 2003; 90(5): 3304-3316.
3. Keysers C, Wicker B, Gazzola V, et al. A touching sight: S11/PV activation during the observation and experience of touch. *Neuron* 2004; 42: 335-346.
4. Rankin L. The Nocebo Effect: Negative Thoughts can Harm Your Health. *Psychology Today* 6 August 2013. www.psychologytoday.com/gb/blog/owning-pink/201308/the-nocebo-effect-negative-thoughts-can-harm-your-health
5. Roulson J, Benbow EW, Hasleton PS. Discrepancies between clinical and autopsy diagnosis and the value of post mortem histology: a meta-analysis and review. *Histopathology* 2005; 47(6): 551-559.
6. Christakis N, Lamont E. Extent and determinants of error in doctors' prognosis of terminally ill patients: prospective cohort study. *Br Med J* 2000; 320: 469.
7. Rein G, Atkinson M, McCraty R. The physiological and psychological effects of compassion and anger. *Journal of Advancement in Medicine* 1995; 8(2): 87-105.
8. Edwards G. *Conscious Medicine* London, UK: Piatkus; 2010. (See also Chapter 9.)

Organising fields

9. Oschman J.*Energy Medicine in Therapeutics and Human Performance*. Philadelphia, US: Butterworth-Heinmann; 2003.
10. Aissa J, Guillonnet D, Beneviste J. A simple and fast method for in vivo demonstration of electromagnetic molecular signalling (EMS) via high dilution or computer recording. *FASEB Journal* 1999; 13: A163.
11. Aissa J, Guillonnet D, Beneviste J. The molecular signal is not functional in the absence of 'informed' water. *FASEB Journal* 1999; 13: A163.
12. Frohlich H. Long range coherence and energy storage in biological

systems. International Journal of Quantum Chemistry 1968; 2: 641-649.

13. Cohen S, Popp F. Biophoton emission of the human body. *Journal of Photochemistry and Photobiology B: Biology* 1997; 40: 187-189.

14. Sheldrake R. *A New Science of Life*. UK: Ikon Books; 1981.

15. Redfern N, Roberts A. *Strange Secrets: Real Government Files of the Unknown*. New York, USA: Paraview Pocket Books; 2003.

16. Braden G. *The Divine Matrix: Bridging Time, Space, Miracles and Belief.* Carlsbad, California, USA: Hay House, 2007.

17. Agar WE, Drummond FH, Tiegs OW. Second report on a test of McDougall's Lamarckian experiment on training of rats. *J Exper Biol* 1942: 19: 158-167.

Quantum healing

18. Bartlett R. *The Physics of Miracles*. New York, USA: Atria Paperback, 2009: pp 16-18.

19. Bartlett R. *Matrix Energetics*. New York, USA: Atria Paperback; 2007.

The more the better

20. Canfield J, Hansen JV. *Chicken Soup for the Soul*. Florida, US: Health Communications Inc; 1983. (See also Chapter 3.)

21. Church D. Heart of Healing. *Santa Rosa, USA: Elite Books; 2004.*

22. McTaggart L. *The Power of Eight*. London. UK: Hay House; 2017.

Chapter 12: Putting it all together

1. van Baalen DC, de Vries MJ, Gondrie MT. Psychosocial correlates of "spontaneous" regression in cancer. Monograph: Department of General Pathology, Medical Faculty, Erasmus University (Rotterdam); 1987.

2. Zahl PH, Maehlen J, Welch HG. The natural history of invasive breast cancers detected by screening mammography. *Arch Int Med* 2008; 168(21): 2311-2316.

3. Welch HG, Black WC. Using autopsy series to estimate the disease "reservoir" for ductal carcinoma in situ of the breast: how much more breast cancer can we find? *Ann Intern Med* 1997; 127(11): 1023-1028.

4. Nielsen M, Thomsen JL, Primdahl S, et al. Breast cancer and atypia among young and middle-aged women: a study of 110

medicolegal autopsies. *Br J Cancer* 1987; 56(6): 814-819.

5. Nielsen M, Jensen J, Andersen J. Precancerous and cancerous breast lesions during lifetime and at autopsy. A study of 83 women. *Cancer* 1983; 54: 612-615.

6. Nielsen M. Autopsy studies of the occurrence of cancerous, atypical and benign epithelial lesions in the female breast. *APMIS Suppl* 1989; 10: 1-56.

7. Chopra D. *Quantum Healing*. New York, USA: Bantam Books; 1989. (See also Chapter 4.)

8. Ornish D, Weidner G, Fair WD, et al. Intensive lifestyle changes may affect the progression of prostate cancer. *Journal of Urology* 2005; 174(3): 1065-1069.

9. Ornish D, Magbanua MJ, Weidner G, et al. Changes in prostate gene expression in men undergoing intensive nutrition and lifestyle intervention. 2008. *Proceedings of the National Academy of Sciences* 2008; 105(24): 8369-8374.

10. Ornish D, Lin J, Chan JM, et al. Effect of comprehensive lifestyle changes on telomerase activity and telomere length in men with biopsy-proven low risk prostate cancer: 5-year follow-up of a descriptive pilot study. *Lancet Oncol* 2013; 14(11): 1112-1120.

11. Rankin L. *Mind over Medicine*. Carlsbad, CA, US: Hay House; 2013.

12. Carter JP, Sace GP, Newbold V, et al. Hypothesis: Dietary management may improve survival from nutritionally linked cancers based on analysis of representative cases. *J Amer Coll Nutr* 1993; 12(3): 209-226.

13. Faulkner H. *Against all Odds*. London, UK: Community Health Foundation; 1992.

14. Gearin-Tosh MJ. *Living Proof, A Medical Mutiny*. London, UK: Scribner; 2002.

15. Lipton BH. *The Biology of Belief*. Santa Rosa, CA, USA: Mountain of Love/Elite Books; 2005.

16. Robey IF, Baggett BK, Kirkpatrick ND, et al. Bicarbonate increases tumour pH and inhibits spontaneous metastases. *Cancer Res* 2009; 69(6): 2260-2268.

17. Volk-Draper L, Hall K, Griggs C et al. Paclitaxel Therapy Promotes Breast Cancer Metastasis in a TRL4-dependent Manner. *Cancer Res* 2014; 74(19): 5421-5434.

18. Daenen LGM, Roodhart JML, van Amersfoot M, et al. Chemotherapy Enhances Metastasis Formation via VEGFR-1-

expressing Endothelial Cells. *Cancer Res* 2011; 71(22): 6976-6985.

19. Gingis-Velitski S, Loven D, Benayoun L et al. Host-Response to Short-Term, Single-Agent Chemotherapy Induces Matrix metalloproteinase-9 Expression and Accelerates Metastasis in Mice. *Cancer Res* 2011; 77(22): 6796-6796.

20. Park SI, Liao J, Berry JE, et al. Cyclophosphamide Creates a Receptive Microenvironment for Prostate Skeletal Metastasis. *Cancer Res* 2012; 72(10): 2522-2532.

21. Alishekevitz D, Gingis-Velitski S, Kaidar-Person O, et al. Macrophage-induced Lymphangiogenesis and Metastasis Following Paclitaxel Chemotherapy is Regulated by VEGFR3. *Cell Rep* 2016; 17(5): 1344-1356.

22. Chang YS, Jalgaonkar SP, Middleton JD, et al. Stress-Inducible Gene Atf3 in the Noncancer Host Cells Contributes to Chemotherapy-Exacerbated Breast Cancer Metastasis. *Proc Natl Acad Sci USA* 2017; 114(34): E7159-E7168.

23. Karagiannis GS, Pastoriza JM, Wang Y, et al. Neoadjuvant Chemotherapy Induces Breast Cancer Metastasis Through a TMEM-mediated Mechanism. *Sci Transl Med* 2017; 9(397).

24. Morgan G, Ward R, Barton M. The contribution of cytotoxic chemotherapy to 5 year survival in adult malignancies. *Clinic Oncol* 2004; 16(8); 549-560.

25. Day P. *Cancer: why we are still dying to know the truth*. UK: Credence Publications; 2000.

26. Weeks JC, Catalona PJ, Cronon A, et al. Patients' expectation about Effects of Chemotherapy for advanced cancer. *N Engl J Med* 2012; 367: 1616-1625.

27. Frahm AE, Frahm DJ. *A Cancer Battle Plan*. New York, USA: Tarcher Putnam; 1997.

28. Goodman S. *9 Steps for Reversing and Preventing Cancer* Franklin Lakes, New Jersey, USA: New Page Books; 2012. (See also Chapter 3.)

29. Servan-Screiber D. *Anti-Cancer: A New Way of Life*. London, UK: Michael Joseph (Penguin Group); 2006.

30. Servan Screiber D. *Not the last Goodbye*. London, UK: MacMillan; 2011.

Appendix II: More on food and health

1. Woolams C. *Heal Your Gut, Heal Your Body*. Croydon, UK: Health Issues; 2017.

References

2. Tilg H, Kaser A. Gut Microbiome, Obesity and Metabolic Dysfunction. *J Clin Invest* 2011; 121(6): 212-232.

3. Kootte RS, Vrieze A, Holleman F, et al. The Therapeutic Potential of Manipulating Gut Microbiota in Obesity and Type 2 Diabetes. *Diabetes Obes Metab* 2012; 14(2): 112-120.

4. Monda V, Villano I, Messina A, et al. Exercise Modifies the Gut Microbiota with Positive Effects. *Oxid Med Cell Longev* 2017; 2017: 3831972.

5. Perlmutter D. *Brain Maker*. London, UK: Yellow Kite; 2015.

6. Wyburn-Mason R. The Naeglerial Causation of Rheumatoid Arthritis and Many Human Cancers. A New Concept in Medicine. *Med Hypotheses* 1979; 5(11): 1237-1249.

7. Ebringer A, Rashid T. Rheumatoid Arthritis is Caused by a Proteus Urinary Tract Infection. *APMIS* 2014; 122(5): 363-368.

8. Braun J, Kingsley G, van der Heijde D, Sieper J. On the difficulties of establishing a consensus on the definition of and diagnostic investigations for reactive arthritis. Results and discussion of a questionnaire prepared for the 4th International Workshop on Reactive Arthritis, Berlin, Germany, July 3-6, 1999. *J Rheumatol* 2000; 27: 2185.

9. van Kuijk AWR, Kerstens PJSM, Perenboom BA, et al. Early-onset polyarthritis as presenting feature of intestinal infection with Strongyloides stercalis. *Rheumatology* 2003; 42(11): 1419-1420.

10. Sanctuary MR, Kain JN, Angkustsiri K, et al. Dietary Considerations in Autism Spectrum Disorders: The Potential Role of Protein Digestion and Microbial Putrefaction in the Gut-Brain Axis. *Front Nutr* 2018; 5: 40. doi:10.3389/fnut.2018.00040

11. Campbell-McBride N. *Gut and Psychology Syndrome*. Cambridge, UK: Medinform Publishing; 2010.

12. Sandgren AM, Brunmer RJM. ADHD originating in the gut? The emergence of a new explanatory model. Med Hypotheses 2018; 120: 135-145.

13. Akhondzadeh S. Microbiome and Schizophrenia. *Avicenna J Med Biotechnol* 2019; 11(4): 269.

14. Darlington LG, Ramsey NW, Mansfield JR. A Placebo-controlled Blind Study of Dietary Manipulation Therapy in Rheumatoid Arthritis. *Lancet* 1986; 1(8475): 236-238. DOI: 10.1016/s0140-6736(86)90774-9

15. Kroker GFR, Stroud R, Marshall T et al. Fasting and Rheumatoid

Arthritis: a Multicenter Trial. *J Clin Ecology* 1984; 2(3): 137-144.

16. Marshall RRM, Stroud GF, Kroker T, et al. Food Challenge Effects on fasted Rheumatoid Arthritis Patients: a multicenter trial. *J Clinic Ecology* 1984; 2(4): 181-190.

17. Panush RS, Carter R L, Katz P, et al. Diet therapy for rheumatoid arthritis. *Arthr Rheum* 1983; 26(4): 462-471.

18. Kjeldsen-Kragh J, Haugen M, Borchgrevink CF, et al. Controlled trial of fasting and one-year vegetarian diet in rheumatoid arthritis. *Lancet* 1991; 338(8722): 899-902.

19. Warren T. *Beating Alzheimer's: A step towards unlocking the mysteries of brain diseases.* New York, USA: Avery Publishing Group; 1991.

20. Brostoff J, Challacombe SJ. *Food Allergy and Intolerance* 2nd Ed. Edinburgh, UK: Elselvier Health Sciences; 2002.

Appendix III: The use of supplements

1. Micronutrient Information Center, Linus Pauling Institute, Oregon State University. Micronutrient Inadequacies of the US population; an Overview. https://lpi.oregonstate.edu/mic/micronutrient-inadequacies/overview

2. British Nutrition Foundation: Summary of Key Findings from the NDNS Report of Years 7 and 8(combined) National Diet and Nutrition SURVEY (NDNS), published by National Health England. www.nutrition.org.uk/nutritioninthenews/new-reports/ndnsyears7and8. html?__cf_chl_jschl_tk__=9f5709cfc34c8c60f42ecbc9b090f3
f73651d657-1588012566-0-AWIr_uKA0HFvjsTfYTzX6DKq cGqhcnAwsartUCRzy3hKqM1kwmoqG-p-deoXXNfcrDb-pjH0-PC3pVhmApKTYEDbTnLbsGagD0eJaiUBEcsXIV40g FsGiLocxOE2cgQzpJpsptaIrUriOees6HnnQWXlJDutEhz_ wUpCVVK3Kcz_vqFNFhpLw-iXbUM6CJe3KvDR5f0ifghCM--OYNYP_g2LHgYLvji8jsZCObGbVROsZ4yEmVoepnouA t9ipS_DxaPZeimOfosiOTARm5MUm4xu6juYoiKvjIdv6FL Er7FsaadAT1QUsd9ofz3-0Db0g2mxHRMWO5a53sZbfX6-SX0fdvpfahF489dL3Cv6DETZHi-HBzo19iiwcda5lfSvlcYfYEv8H A5iLu3sysTC2vM.

3. Bernade L, Howard T, Burk D. Synergistic killing of Ehrlich ascites carcinoma cells by ascorbate and 3-amino-1,2,4- triazole. *Oncology* 1969; 23: 33-43.

4. Chen Q, Esprey MG, Krishna MC, et al. Pharmacological ascorbic

acid concentrations selectively kill cancer cells: action as a pro-
drug to deliver hydrogen peroxide to tissues. *Proc Natl Acad Sci
USA* 2005; 102: 13604-13609.

5. Robinson AR, Hunsberger A, Westall FC. Suppression of squamous
cell carcinoma in hairless mice by dietary nutrient variation.
Mech Aging Devel 1994; 76: 201-214.

6. Cameron E, Pauling L. Supplemental ascorbate in the supportive
treatment of cancer. Prolongation of survival times in terminal
human cancer. *Proc Natl Acad Sci USA* 1976; 73: 3685-3689.

7. Cameron E, Pauling L. Supplemental ascorbate in the supportive
treatment of cancer; re-evaluation of prolongation of survival
times in terminal human cancer. *Proc Natl Acad Sci USA* 1978; 75:
4538-4542.

8. Riordan HD, Riordan NH, Jackson JA, et al. Intravenous vitamin C
as a chemotherapy agent: A report on clinical cases. *Puerto Rico
Health Sciences Journal* 2004; 23(2): 115-118.

9. Hoffer A, Pauling L. Hardin Jones biostatistical data from cohorts
of cancer patients with a large fraction surviving at the
termination of the study and a comparison of survival times
of cancer patients receiving large regular oral doses of vitamin
C and other nutrients with similar patients not receiving those
doses. *Journal of Orthomolecular Med* 1990; 5(3): 143-154.

10. Murata A, Morishige F, Yamaguchi H. Prolongation of survival
times of terminal cancer patients by administration of large doses
of ascorbate. *Int J Vitam Nutr Suppl* 1982; 23: 103-113.

11. Padayatty SJ, Levine M. Reevaluation of ascorbate in cancer
treatment: emerging evidence, open minds and serendipity. *J Am
Coll Nutr* 2000; 19(4): 423-425.

12. Riordan HD, Casciari JJ, Gonzalez MJ, et al. A pilot clinical study of
continuous intravenous ascorbate in terminal cancer patients. *PR
Health Sci J* 2005; 24(4): 269-276.

13. Pleshette J. *Cures that Work*. London, UK: Century Arrow; 1986. (See
also Chapter 1.)

14. Murata A. Viricidal activity of vitamin C for prevention and
treatment of viral diseases. In: Hasagawi T (ed) *Proc First Int
Congr IAMS*. Science Council of Japan, 1975.

15. Baur H Staub H. Treatment of hepatitis with infusions of ascorbic
acid: comparison with other therapies. *JAMA* 1954; 156: 565
(Abstract).

16. Marik PE, Khangoora V, Rivera R. Hydrocortisone, Vitamin C and Thiamine for the Treatment of Severe Sepsis and Septic Shock: A retrospective Before-After Study. *Chest* 2017; 151(6): 1229-1238. DOI: https://doi.org/10.1016/j.chest.2016.11.036

17. Yamamoto T, Kinoshita M, Shinomiya N, et al. Pretreatment with ascorbic acid prevents lethal gastrointestinal syndrome in mice receiving a massive amount of radiation. J *Radiat Res* 2010; 51(2): 145-156.

18. British Society of Ecological Medicine conference: Advances in Nutritional Therapies held at Charles Darwin House, 30 November 2012. Presentations by Japanese doctors.

19. Bartler FC, Berkson B, Gallelli J. Amanita Toxins and Poisoning: Thioctic Acid in the Treatment of Poisoning with Alpha-Amanitin. *International Amanita Symposium* 1978; 1980: 197-202.

20. Sechi G, Deladda MG, Bua G, et al. Reduced Intravenous Glutathione in the Treatment of Early Parkinson's Disease. *Prog Neurophsychopharm Biol Psychiatry* 1996; 20(7): 1159-1170.

21. Wright JV, Gaby AR. *The Patient's Book of Natural Healing*. Rocklin, California, USA: Prima Health; 1999.

Index

Index

Campbell, Professor Colin, 35, 36,
    68, 72
Campbell-McBride, Dr Natasha, 374
cancer, 2
    alternative therapies, 366
    approaches to healing, 336–338
    books on, 363–369
        authors eventually relapsing/
            succumbing, 353–357
    cell death *see* apoptosis
    chemicals causing (carcinogens),
        60–61, 67, 172, 173, 174, 175,
        176, 178, 179, 180, 181, 183,
        183–185, 210, 212, 219, 229,
        233, 235, 311, 322, 349–350
        difference from other
            chemicals, 311
    chemotherapy, 349–351
    deaths/mortalities, 68, 75, 82, 168
    diet/nutrition/food and, 4–5,
        33–51, 340–341
        books on, 363, 364, 365, 367
        eggs, 87
        fruit and vegetable protective
            effects, 42–44, 75, 76, 77
        macrobiotic, 9, 10, 26, 337
        nutrients, 46–50
        promoters of cancer, 35, 36,
        59, 60, 73
        sugar, 55–56
    electromagnetic fields causing,
        202, 222
    electromagnetic fields of, 21,
        295–296, 296–297, 297, 298,
        300, 301, 302
    energy and, 253–254, 276–277,
        286, 289–290
        thought, 307
    epidemiology, 167, 184–185,
        276–277
    exercise and, 268–271
    geopathic stress and, 295, 296, 297
    hopes for the future, 358–359
    hormone-dependent, 218, 220,
        226, 246

    IGF-1 and, 36, 55, 56, 73, 267
    immune suppressants, 348
    inconsistent results of mind-based
        treatments, 154
    Krebiozen story, 101–102, 330
    metastatic *see* metastatic cancer
    mind and, 101–102, 106, 107, 109,
        115–116, 117–118, 118, 119, 120,

        129, 131–132, 133, 135–136,
        137, 138, 144–145, 147–148,
        154, 155, 156, 157, 158, 159
    mobile phones and, 199
    remission *see* remission
    search for cure to, 357
    spontaneous remission, 328–330
    vitamin C and, 46, 380–385, 386,
        387
    vitamin D and, 46, 263
    see also specific sites/organs/tissues
        e.g. breast; prostate; skin *and*
        types e.g. sarcoma
Cancer (The): The Complete Recovery
    Guide, 339, 366
canned foods, 220
carbohydrates
    refined, 58–61
    soluble fibre, 242–243
carbon filters, 219
cardiovascular disease *see* heart
    disease
Carlo, George, 203
carotenoids, 43, 46, 73
carpets, 212
Carter J.P., 337
casein, 35, 36
cattle *see* cows and cattle
causes
    of disease epidemics *see*
        epidemics
    of toxicity, 206–211
cells
    cancer
        death *see* apoptosis
        resistance to chemotherapy,
        350
        vitamin C and, 380–381
    communication, improving, 48
    extracellular environment,
        339–340
    stem, 38, 338–339
cereals *see* grains
cerebral palsy, 13, 104
cervical cancer, 369
CFS (chronic fatigue syndrome), 209,
    271–272, 337
chakras, 284–285, 287
Chamberlain, Jonathon, 339, 366
cheese, plastic wrap, 182
chelation (heavy metals), 203, 206
chemicals
    in food, 65–66
    toxic *see* toxicity

Index

Index

dental fillings, 194–197, 376
  fish, 85, 207
meridians, 283–284, 291
metabolism, drugs affecting, 17
Metallothioneins, 244
metaphysical approaches, books, 368–369
metastatic cancer, 4, 337
  blocking of metastasis, 47
  chemotherapy, 351
  exercise and, 269, 271
  individual cases/stories, 10, 72, 120, 159, 253, 269, 289–290, 332, 353–355
  to bone, 129, 269
Mexico, 32
  Tarahumara Indians, 107
microbiome in gut (bacteria and other microbes), 371–375
microplastics, 85, 204, 206, 214, 219
microwave radiation, 199, 200, 202, 221–223, 224
  ovens, 224–225
  typical daily exposure, 177, 180, 182, 183
milk, 72–74, 95
  products (dairy), 32, 36, 40, 41, 72–74, 364
mind (and mind–body), 19, 20, 99–162, 342–343, 346
  books, 368–369
  healing, 123–141, 306
  power, 20, 102–107, 161–162, 162
  see also brain; thoughts
minerals
  in fruit and vegetables, 77
  in soil, 90–91, 380
  see also heavy metals
miracles/miraculous recovery, 106, 136, 273, 278, 281, 315, 317, 318
mobile (incl. smart) phones, 177, 180, 199, 201–202, 221–222, 224, 247, 248, 343
  base stations and masts, 199, 202, 223
  brain tumours and, 199, 201
modern medicine see medicine
Moertel, Dr, 381
molybdenum, 243, 244, 246
Moraitis, Stamatis, 119
morphic fields and resonance, 160, 312
morphine-like substances, 110

mortal oscillatory rates, 301
  see also deaths
mortalities see deaths
motor neurone disease, 193–194
  electromagnetic fields and, 200
  Evy MacDonalds, 143, 155
  Steven Hawking's, 116–117
  see also amyotrophic lateral sclerosis
Mount Sinai Study, 183, 187, 229
mouth, toxic, 193–199
multiple personality disorder, 102
multiple sclerosis (MS), 25, 26, 70, 81, 186, 209, 263, 344
  books, 365, 366
  epidemic, 186
  individual cases/stories, 14–15, 25, 26, 118, 287, 365
Murata, Dr A, 383
muscle meat, 71
mushrooms, 50, 53, 76, 387–388
music, 133
myalgic encephalomyelitis (CFS; ME), 209, 271–272, 337
myeloma, 45, 79, 285, 338, 367
Myhill, Dr Sarah, 238

nanoparticles, 204–206, 218
National Diet and Nutrition Survey, 56, 380
National Health and Nutrition Examination Survey (NHANES), 379–380
Native Americans, 29, 33, 40, 154, 294, 318
natural (food labelling), 94
natural flavours (food labelling), 94
natural killer (NK) cells, 6, 48, 50, 126, 127
naturopathy, 11, 238, 241
negative emotions, 144, 145, 146, 162, 308, 323, 340
negative expectations, 111, 112
nervous system
  disease see neurological disease
  parasympathetic, 126, 128, 129, 294, 340
  sympathetic, 125, 128
neuro-linguistic programming (NLP), 149, 150
neurological (nervous system incl. brain) disease/damage, 185–187

Index

Index